SOCIAL
CONNECTIONS
AND YOUR
HEALTH

ISBN 978-1-954095-67-0 (Paperback)
Social Connections and Your Health
Copyright © 2021 Alfred L. Anduze, MD

Yorkshire Publishing
4613 E. 91st St,
Tulsa, OK 74137
www.YorkshirePublishing.com
918.394.2665

Printed in the USA

SOCIAL
CONNECTIONS
AND YOUR
HEALTH

Alfred L. Anduze, MD

TULSA

CONTENTS

DEDICATION

To my children, grandchildren, family and friends for your social contribution to my good health.

To the CENTENARIANS of Ikaria from whom we learned so much about longevity, who set the example to follow and who followed their own example as proof that human life can be long and rewarding at the same time.

To my grandparents and all the grandparents of the world for their wisdom and patience and knowledge of the kind of life that allowed us to become grandparents.

And to Theodore (Ted), a British gentleman guest at the Turim Hotel in Lisbon, who apparently lived there and plied his special talent for meeting people and making them and himself, feel good.

PREFACE

The reason I wrote this book:

Why do some people smile, offer and return greetings when getting on an elevator or entering a room occupied by strangers, and some people avert their gaze, stare straight ahead or at their electronic devices and otherwise ignore others?

Why are some people friendly and engaging and others blank or hostile?

Why are some people social and others, antisocial?

In a new world of social distancing, why should anyone ever learn to be social?

Is sharing hugs and laughter with family and friends different anywhere on our planet?

Is socializing the common denominator that keeps societies healthy?

Why this book is different?

Social Connections and your Health is the second in a linked series of basic strategies for good health; the others being stress control, nutrition, exercise, mental stimulation and toxin avoidance. It identifies the processes involved in how social interactions can lead to connections; provides international experiences (survey results) and results of scientific studies on viewpoints of socializing. It offers an introduction to research on young adults and the effects of electronic immersion and the new social distancing on social interactions and our health. It includes practical solutions via protocols for improving social skills and author experiences based on reality, and not conjecture.

Our planet, Earth, is "shared space". With a population of seven (7) billion people and counting, we encounter each other more often than not. With widespread travel and the availability of internet information, exposure to "different" people is a common experience and no longer a viable excuse for antisocial behavior.

Ants greet each other, exchange messages and plans and get things done. Most animals meet and greet and some fight over territorial and reproductive rights, but none get riled up, angry and determined to ostracize, demonize and separate over such trivia as skin color, ethnicity, class standing or education.

Refusing to acknowledge the presence of another human or refusing to congregate or mix because of minor differences in appearance and culture is abnormal behavior. Setting restrictive rules on socializing, being told explicitly to avoid and to hate others, is unnatural and cannot be of any advantage except to set up a false sense of security, upset and/or irritate a fellow human being. Antisocial behavior is a detriment to human health and well-being and its widespread use and promotion by any group is plainly absurd.

As a pre-kindergartener, I noticed that all children laughed and cried in the same manner and for the same reasons, no matter what their differences in appearance. Why was socializing restricted to certain groups as we grew older?

In the early 1960s, I was fortunate to leave my small community in the Caribbean, venture out into the world and experience a European education. At the wide-eyed age of fourteen, I was blessed with parents and siblings who encouraged the now endangered art of reading and learning about distant lands and cultures. Determined to become "*un homme du monde*", whatever that would be, four years later, while firmly matriculated into a pre-med program on the US mainland, I realized that the students, teachers and people that I had met in those formative years had contributed enormously to my becoming "social". My range and quality of friends and acquaintances ran far and wide and still sustain my mental health and overall well-being, some six decades later.

I am neither a sociologist nor a psychologist, and do not profess to know all the problems and solutions of our social connections, and if it is broken or evolving naturally. However, my scientific training and forty- plus years of practical experience in medicine have provided me with some sense of what is required for a human being to be healthy.

A decent functional social life is essential to good health, while antisocial behavior and loneliness are consistent with poor health. As a physician in training, I learned to approach my patients with a complete history and physical, including a "social history". Frequently, this space in the record focuses on drug use, or is noted as "WNL "(within normal limits). The record then goes on to more important features, such as the scar on the head, the last flu shot, the fracture of the tibial bone, the atrial fibrillation, the drug prescriptions, and loss of vision after repeated vitreous hemorrhages. What were the circumstances that led to these events? It is imperative to remember that everyone's social history matters. What kind of alcohol is imbibed? How often and with whom? How many family and close friends where there, and how often encountered? What is the individual's attitude toward strangers? The answers may hint at the level of stress present and its effect on the endocrine system of hormones. The causes and progressions of many medical dysfunctions are closely related to the environment and social structure of the community. By paying attention to social history as a major contributor to the cause of the condition, it can become a significant factor in the approach and recovery of any illness.

Social interaction in my medical practice has always been an important part of the patient's visit. From the initial handshake or hug of an old friend, much can be made of the warmth or coldness, the expression of one's feelings in a positive or negative reception and how the encounter contributes toward to the relief of tension and anxiety... which in turn serve to aid digestion, reduce irritable bowel syndrome (IBS), constipation, increase absorption, reduce inflammation and relieve nerve problems. The barriers of social distancing will significantly alter this relationship. The long-term effects on health remain to be seen.

Prevention is better than cure.

Of the six basic lifestyle strategies listed in **Natural Health and Disease Prevention**, Social Connections have just as important an influence on one's health as do the other five, adequate exercise, good nutrition, stress control, mental stimulation and avoidance of toxins and bad habits. While research studies in Japan in the early 1990s rated exercise as #1 in reducing stress associated with the disease process, social connections increased in importance and are right there alongside as its relationship with loneliness and depression has been exposed and examined. As longevity rates increase, who will be there to help with stress control; who will help with the basic activities of daily living (ADL) once an individual is incapacitated or at the age where and when assistance is required, who will help plan and prepare with the end of life; who will call the doctor when one is sick, or sit with you and provide some degree of comfort? What impact will the reduction in social interactions have on our collective health in the "new normal" world?

Humans need give and receive the attention of another. This is seen in the relief of loneliness by having a pet, as proven with the success of bringing pets to visit patients in confinement. The need to socialize goes along with the need to have a sense of purpose, which is the underlying drive that supports a good quality of life. Being connected provides daily activities, affection, laughter, love, something to look forward to, and satisfaction of accomplished tasks. Every human being has "issues", large or small, internal or external based on events detrimental to or benefitting general health. While **In Search of a Stress-free Life** presents the role of stress and its biochemical reactions in the initiation and persistence of disease conditions, this book focuses on why and how socializing or not socializing, having friends or enemies, productive rivalries, outright hostilities and abject loneliness can affect one's health. This book examines how people interact and how these interactions lead to connections that contribute to good health and why and how the lack of interactions contributes to poor health. We associate socializing with good health while antisocial and asocial behavior are linked to poor health.

How and why tribal status, caste, and class came to determine the characteristics of social interactions, and why these relationships persist is highlighted as a major determinant of who interacts with whom. Some societies have moved on from tribal restraints and expanded their range of social interactions, and others have not.

Though far from being "scientific", I made up my own "survey" and named it the **ECNS test**. The Eye Contact, Nod and Smile test consists of making eye contact with elevator riders, beach walkers, mall shoppers, and anywhere that groups of people pass or congregate leisurely, while trying to avoid those in a hurry or performing a specific task. Over the course of five years, I did this test in 20 different countries, on four continents, recorded the responses and assigned the "rates of friendliness" to various groups based on their responses. Anyone can do this test, anywhere, anytime and with anyone. (*See technique and rationale in Chapter One and results in Chapter Four*). Basic manners (*for your health and everybody else's*) when entering an elevator, a restaurant, a café or anywhere a relatively small group congregates is to say hello or smile. Looking someone in the eyes and bidding basic greetings elicits the release of good hormones in both parties. When someone else enters and says nothing, avoids eye contact and ignores or does not acknowledge an existence of you or anyone else, the release of bad hormones is almost palpable. A smile is infinitely, ultimately, and universally healthier than a frown or a blank stare. In certain societies, people exhibit and respond to basic manners better and more often than in others.

As I write these notes, "social distancing" in response to the Covid-19 pandemic, is the order of the day. In the USA, interactions requiring social skills were on the decline anyway and how we were treating "others" left much to be desired. Social distancing may have provided a solid excuse to be antisocial. Sincere interest and interactions with "others" are much lower than in most developed countries, and now is being promoted and even set as the rule of law. Especially for the youth, attention directed at improving social skills may be all but abandoned completely. It is possible that the sagging health statistics may drop even more. Though social interactions alone are beneficial to both mental and physical health, the creation of connections serves to solidify and maintain one's good health. Note that one may interact but fail to connect. This happens often when effective social skills are lacking or the situation and participants just don't have the right chemistry or temperament. Successful interactions lead to successful connections that lead to providing positive factors for good health.

What does this book offer?

Besides demonstrating the relationship between social connections and good health, it attempts to show exactly how they fit together and depend on one another. By focusing on the causes of problems, solutions emerge. Rather than treating symptoms of a condition, examination of the how and why can lead to a means of prevention.

Here are a few simple relationships, cause/effects, problem/ solution. Keeping and maintaining good relations with family and friends stimulates the mind and provides security and relative freedom from the fear that ageing brings. Conflict is a ubiquitous obstacle to healthy living, coping with change becomes a major challenge and when effective, can overcome such life-changing events as retirement and feelings of uselessness, losing a loved one, changes in living arrangements, loss of control over one's activities of daily living, and ultimately, one's independence.

In the 21st century, socializing or not socializing has become a matter of choice. Cooperation for building, production and preservation is no longer a necessity as machines and technology can accomplish similar physical results. As preferred policies of exclusion replace the principles of inclusion, the human social structure will change or be torn down. The choice is between socializing and respecting each other's space and worth, or competing to destroy the rival, destroy the self and the environment as a secondary casualty.

Modern European populations appear to value quality of life more than material wealth... though the recent rise of the right-wing populism may put this tenet in deep dispute. The prevalence of hatred and antisocial behavior may well plunge Europe into the depths of poor social skills that would affect the general health of the population, as it has in other cultures.

Every human being has value and is worthy of social interaction. By refusing to socialize with certain people or under certain circumstances, one diminishes the value of the other person. Socializing is a lifestyle strategy that could benefit both individual and global health, by reducing the chemical and physical stresses that lead to anxiety and depression, cardiovascular and neurological diseases. Failure to socialize is detrimental to one's health and to the welfare of the inhabitants of the planet.

DISCLAIMER

If anything in this book offends you or you find your personality described to a tee on these pages, it was not intentional.

If you think that my diatribes and opinions were made in anger, I assure that they were not.

Disappointment yes, anger, no. I am disappointed that so many of my fellow human beings have chosen heartlessness and cruelty over kindness and compassion. That the antisocial behavior of so many has surged to the point where hundreds of thousands of people have died from a pandemic that could have been curtailed by more cooperation and caring, is truly disappointing. That many of our leaders and ordinary countrymen openly chose material profits over the lives of our neighbors is a tough pill for me to swallow.

I am disappointed that my elderly life has so little value to the younger generations that they stride "mask-less" in my face and think nothing of it.

By the end of the book, if it still seems angry to you, I apologize. Try to see beyond the presentation and kindly join me in recognizing the problems inherent in modern human behavior, adjust your own lifestyle appropriately and strive to bring a better quality of life to our fellow human beings.

INTRODUCTION

"Man is by nature a social animal; an individual who is unsocial naturally and not accidentally is either beneath our notice or more than human. Society is something that precedes the individual. Anyone who either cannot lead the common life or is so self-sufficient as not to need to and therefore does not partake of society, is either a beast or a god."
Aristotle, Politics.

Sociality, kindness and antisocial behavior are hard-wired into the DNA of humans. The expression of one over the other depends on the tenor of the society. Both the quantity and quality of social connections are essential to good health. Pro-social behavior is preferred over anti-social behavior and prevails in survival issues and efforts to reproduce.

We associate anti-social behavior with chemically directed stress and though it has serious consequences on the health of both the inflictor and the receiver, remains prevalent in the lives of modern *Homo sapiens*.

What determines the extent of our interactions with "others", anyone apart from oneself or immediate family? What if the Good Samaritan had decided not to stop and help the stranger? In a world surrounded and driven by thievery and aggression on the one hand and indifference and scorn on the other, he could have decided to look the other way and walk past the one in need. What factor or factors made him stop and interact? What makes us pass a beggar on the sidewalk and keep our eyes averted lest they make contact? Must we keep our souls clean and safe from his plea and bodies sterile from the infestation of his poverty Upon chance encounters, what makes us decide to engage or disengage, interact or ignore?

The raw guts of this book are how and why some people are social and others are anti- social; how and why some interactions lead to social connections and others do not; how and why encounters, greetings, slights and rejections among human beings elicit physical and emotional reactions; how and why both affect one's health positively or negatively; and how and why one's health affects the ability and motivation to socialize.

The need to interact and share our experiences with others is universally human, yet some do it better than others. Social interactions are linked to good health, and conversely antisocial behavior leads to adverse chemical reactions associated with loneliness, depression and poor health. Human compassion is innate and heartlessness is learned. Social skills can be natural or acquired with minimal effort.

Vignette #1: John Brown is a physician, speaks three languages, lives in a major city in a First World country. He travels often, sees patients from multiple cultures, which highlights his ability to communicate, and has a wide diversity of friends. JB is in excellent health supported by a nutritious diet, exercise, mental stimulation from science and cultural exposure to different people with all of which he is comfortable. He handles the stresses of life with grace and aplomb and responds with high creativity and productivity. Jack Smith is a physician in the same city, speaks three languages, avoids socializing whenever he can, is short-tempered with staff, prefers to diagnose through laboratory results, limits time with patients and defers follow up visits to associates. He eats alone, is frequently depressed and recently developed hypertension and heart arrhythmias.

Social Interactions

The way a person acts toward and within the group defines his/her sociality. Such behavior may be pleasant and is beneficial to one's general health and well-being. It may be hostile especially when directed toward "others" or when received as threatening or undesirable, and may lead to chemical stress, which is a major risk factor in disease formation. Any social interaction that boosts the spirits will often lead to increased health and likewise when linked to stress is likely to impact one's health negatively. Being sociable means being involved, caring, giving, being compassionate towards others, being humane, and interacting with one another as opposed to the "me, me, me, I win-you lose mentality, I have it all and want more…at your expense and that makes me great". According to Sociology 101, there are five (5) types of social interactions: exchange, competition, conflict, cooperation and accommodation.

There are multiple factors in human interactions; pro-social and antisocial, positive and negative, peaceful and warlike, loving and hateful. Whichever is expressed eventually dominates. The mental and physical state of the individual and of the group, and the health of the environment are significant factors. For example, for a social interaction to occur, the status, appearance, speech, and conduct of the participants and the availability of an appropriate environment must meet basic requirements of acceptance.

The highlight of socializing lies in the Greek "philotimo", the welcoming benevolent treatment of strangers by a majority of its population. In Report to Greco, by Nikos Kazantzakis, on encountering an old lady while on a mountain trail, the stranger receives her hospitality in sharing a meal, a drink, a place to sleep and expresses his appreciation. When asked why she was so hospitable, she replied, "You are human, I am human, too." As humans sharing the same space, the least we can do is acknowledge it. Nature does not specify who is better or worse. There are no inherent rules defining appearance or material wealth as determinant factors in dictating human interactions. What gives one the right to deny the existence of another?

"What makes the desert beautiful is that somewhere it hides a well..."
Anonymous

Interacting with your "environment" can and may elicit a similar positive or negative response, as it does when one interacts with people.

Social interactions have been severely restricted by events such as disasters, pandemics, and wars. Public places of "normal" human interaction, like banks, cafes, and grocery stores are opportunities for people to gather, converse, and perhaps connect. Now we are restricted by Covid-19 distancing, masking and stay-at-home orders. Likewise, using electronic devices for communication has led to reduced opportunities to physically interact with others. A bad ride, a long wait or a tour group that would have led to interactions between strangers, are almost non-existent. Antisocial people who rarely make eye contact, exchange basic greetings or talk to strangers are quite comfortable and satisfied. It remains to be seen what the long-term effects of lack from the lack of touching and adequate social interactions will bring.

Social Connections

Encounter -> Interaction -> Acquaintance -> Connection -> Bond

Social connections are the relationships you have with the people in your life. They may be family and neighbors, close or far away, accessible only with electronic devices or travel, but involve various levels of affection, friendship and trust. Social connections require more emotional energy and sense of permanence than do interactions or acquaintances.

The primary advantage of connections lies in the health benefits, both mental and physical. People who genuinely care about each other live longer and have a better quality of life than those who are resentful and hateful towards each other.

Strong connections usually involve relatives, marriage, close friends, and special individuals within specific groups. Being willing and able to confide private matters is the cornerstone of strong relationships. Group participation or time spent appreciating the environment often leads to quality time spent with friends. In all cases, connections instill a sense of well-being and belonging that enhances one's health. The best relationships are those in which there is no sense of urgency, where money and status are not qualifying factors, and where materials and time are shared equally and sincerely.

Time and emotional energy invested in other humans have value.
Each of us is worth something. "Do not ignore or neglect me."
Author

Having good social connections is the secret to solid mental development, security and a happy life. Meaningful relationships are a prescription for better emotional, mental, and physical health. Identifying and building social connections start with the family unit. One sharpens social skills with relatives, then with school friends and extend to distant acquaintances. The development of inclusive, positive techniques and habits, leads to confidence, which opens doors to meeting and creating more connections.

*The transition from social interaction to connection is natural
and involves mutual need and benefit cemented by "trust".*

Besides good health, social connections are linked to success in endeavors, longevity, better nutrition through association, less depression, less disease susceptibility, and better quality of life. Both providing and finding social support lends to positive relationships, less stress, more reliability, consistency and stability, which in turn contribute to good mental and physical health. With strong social connections in place, the accompanying support ensures a sense of belonging and grounding that reduces chronic stress. In achieving a stress-free environment, there is a natural increase in feel-good hormones and decrease in feel-bad hormones associated with poor health. Support means love, trust, and availability of advice exchanged with others, preferably with trusted family, like-minded friends and people with similar senses of purpose. To maintain the psyche, one needs sustainable and renewable energy to establish belonging, standing in the community, country and world to mean something to oneself and to have purpose. Achieving this state of balance explicitly and implicitly involves other people. External relationships of family and friends provide both mental and physical feelings of success,

*Social connections have an enormous impact on
physical, emotional & mental well-being.*

What do social connections and "socializing" have to do with health? They are directly related. There are many stories and instances of loners existing quite well. Are they "healthy"? Probably not. Biochemically they are deficient and physiologically, they function differently. Social connections are necessary for development of the mind and nourishment of the body by exchanging ideas and events. Internal well-being depends on one's reaction and handling of incidents ranging from minor irritations to major crises. Stress may be acute and repeated as with financial burdens, work-related issues, deadlines, and extended commutes, or chronic, long- term, and perpetual such as racism leveled upon non-white males in schools, streets, home, or job. Not complying with the expected "norm", academic shortfalls because of inadequate facilities or motivation, issues with interpersonal relationships and errant interactions ranging from daily lack of courtesies to repeated lack of concern or attention between one group and another, threats, real and perceived, to one's livelihood, domicile, inner circle and larger group dynamics are not easy hurdles to clear.

Social connections seek to identify and settle the organism into a comfort zone. Multiple positive interactions lead to higher chances of solid connections linked to good health and better chances of survival and reproductive opportunities.

Pro-Social / Antisocial Behavior

Social Connections leading to Friendships are the cornerstones of healthy living. Pro-Social Behavior is natural. Humans need each other and thrive when they are together. Anti-Social behavior along with toxin intake (smoking and drugs) and lack of physical activity, are major causes of inadequate bodily functions and eventual poor health. Socializing is natural and any other doctrine that promotes separation and domination of one group over another, such as Nazism, Fascism, and Institutional Racism are unnatural and detrimental to the health of both the individual and the society. A large inequality gap increases separation along class and ethnic lines, foments resentment, hatreds and lack of interactions and reduces the incidence of social connections. Recently, only 50% of Americans report having meaningful daily face-to-face social interactions (i.e. before the pandemic). The pandemic came along and the already fragmented society appeared to fall apart. While the dominant group has access to safety and material necessities, the vulnerable suffer and experience disproportionate loses. Socializing is reduced for both groups.

Countries with social policies of separation and discrimination will not do as well in containing a pandemic as those with unified societies.

Social behavior in different cultures is often ascribed to tribalism and can go both ways. In excerpts from an interview with Klee Benally, a Navajo activist, as told to Jacqueline Keeler, for NPR, reported 4/20/2019, "Notre Dame and the Fight for Sacred Lands" (Common Dreams.net), he revealed that some built monuments of stone (Meso-America, Egypt, Europe, Asia) as commanded by the privileged few who subjected the many to their needs... and others (North and Caribbean American and central Africa), built tipis and clay huts that housed the communities together and created kinship relationships that merged people, the land and nature. Life value was for the many, not just for the few. Huts were built for the many, not temples for the few.

The Taino people of Puerto Rico and the Dominican Republic, and the Diné of the American Southwest, called themselves "the people", as did several Amerinds in the northern Amazon basin. The Dakota (Lakota) were "allies", "friends". They did not separate into aristocracy and peasantry, haves and have nots, privileged and bereft. They interacted together and forged connections that made them "the people".

A small group of the Penan people of Borneo remain as hunter-gatherers with no sense of time, no salaries, no taxes, very little material possessions and no poverty. Their wealth lies in the strength of their relationships, their group solidarity signals the value of the community. Ties to place and people, the success of high social connections was linked to successful stewardship of the land for tens of thousands of years. When these bonds are broken, the health of all suffers.

"The most beautiful things in the world cannot be seen
or touched, they are felt with the heart."
(recurrent theme.....*Le Petit Prince...)*
and all works on love and wisdom and life

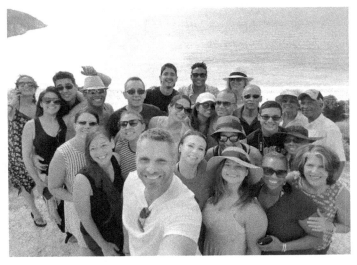

Figure 1. Socially connected at a beach in Kefalonia, Greece.

These friends and relatives took their time and traveled thousands of miles from different localities to meet for this event, as commemorated in this photo. Being and staying connected with a positive attitude, kindness, good intentions and deep friendships serve to build and maintain good mental and physical health.

"It is only with the heart that one can see rightly; what
is essential is invisible to the eye." Le Petit Prince

"Happy right here, right now" as all that matters will be successful. Being genuinely glad to see a friend as well as a stranger, and happy to participate and help out with genuine enthusiasm, contributes to a healthy social life.

"You gotta understand the difference between someone who speaks to you on their free time and someone who frees their time up to speak to you." Awesome Quotes Eva

"Anyone can sympathize with the sufferings of a friend, but it requires a very special nature to sympathize (applaud & support) with a friend's success." Oscar Wilde, poet

Health & Well-Being
as related to and a consequence of social behavior

"Good health is not just the absence of disease. It refers to wellness and well-being." Andrew Weil, MD, pioneer in the discipline of Integrative Medicine

Health is not only the absence of disease, but the condition of being sound in body, mind and spirit. It depends on and is related to genetics and environment (*level of nutrition, activity, toxin avoidance, mental stimulation, stress control, and social connection*) as well as economic status, education level, and access to health care. Unfortunately, the influence of the latter three is often overlooked. All organisms strive for good health to produce a high quality (well-being) and quantity (longevity) of life.

Well-being is the state of being happy, healthy and secure. (*Merriam Webster dictionary*) In all studies on longevity, diet and exercise are assumed factors, then stress reduction, avoidance of toxins is followed by a social life of good friends, good marriage and family support as essential to Good Health. The premise of this book is simple. Being sociable is good and being antisocial is detrimental to your health. Social connections are essential to maintaining one's body and mind in good functioning order. Having the support of friends and family in your life can help you stay healthy. This support usually comes in the form of love, trust and availability of time spent with others deemed essential to human function, i.e. whomever you ascribe the importance of influence and advice, be it real strong friends and trusted family, church associates, clergy, like-minded colleagues, counselors, or support groups. All contribute to initiation and maintenance of human dignity, which is a necessity, like air, water and nutrients for the body and energy in the form of belonging, meaning and purpose, both of which contribute to well-being. Achieving this state, explicitly and implicitly involves other people.

> The achievement and maintenance of Good Health can be reached by using the basic strategies to a viable lifestyle. Perhaps the most important factor is stress control, reducing the chronic release of harmful hormones. Adequate Exercise, avoidance of Toxins and fresh organic Diet will help maintain the body, while effective Mental stimulation and consistent Social Connections are essential factors for the mind and spirit.
> (*Natural Health and Disease Prevention, 2016*)

The key to good health and longevity is a strong functional Immune System for reduced disease susceptibility and DNA repair… strong Social connections contribute to a healthy immune system.

Studies & Statistics

in social connections and your health.

Blue Zones, by Dan Buettner, lists five regions that excel in longevity and are related to basic lifestyle choices for good health: nutrition, physical activity, stress control, safe environment, and social connectivity. Here people live longer and with better quality of life by living "correctly". A major feature of the blue zones is the social circles that support healthy and productive behavior. In Moats, Okinawa, Japan, there are groups of five friends, all committed to each other for life. Loma Linda, California features a faith-based social connectivity. Nicoya peninsula, Costa Rica and Ogliastra region in Sardinia specialize in fresh nutrition and exercise. Ikaria island, Greece, excels in all six basic strategies. The blue zones have these and much more in common. Investing time and love into children as well as quality care and respect for elders and life partners greatly enhance the community lifestyle. Other similarities include a plant-based diet, routine physical activity, high interactive social life, adequate mental stimulation, low toxin exposure, and low stress levels. All share a strong sense of purpose, multiple circles of healthy friends, warm comfortable climate, walkable environment, clean water, high use of herbals, olive oil and red wine resulting in low dementia and high longevity.

The Roseto Effect is a 50-year study of heart disease which concluded that physical activity, plant-based diet (high carbs and low meats), * social solidarity (no loneliness, no stress of exclusion) in an Italian - American community, access to, ability to pay for and attitude towards health care, maintaining healthy habits, weight control, regular checkups and access to medications, S through sharing of worries and concerns, like minded friends, puzzles, meditation workshops, and volunteering, all contribute to good health and well-being.

(Am J Public Health, 1992 August;82(8):1089-92)

Study: In the Social Connections and Immune System, those individuals with six (6) or more relationships were happier, healthier and four times less likely to catch a "cold" than those with three (3) or less. The study concluded that social isolation is a significant health risk factor similar in scope and outcomes as smoking, hypertension, obesity, or sedentary lifestyle.

(Cohen, Doyle, Skoner, Rabin & Gwaltney 1997)

The Framingham Heart Study's healthy effects of socializing showed that both social isolation and perception of social isolation (loneliness) are correlated with a higher risk of mortality and that both are risk factors for cardiovascular disease. Lonely individuals have increased peripheral vascular resistance and high blood pressure. Chronic social stress is associated with activation of the Sympathetic Nervous System and the Hypothalamus Pituitary Axis resulting in selective expansion of proinflammation monocytes and glucocorticoid resistance.

Being connected is good for the heart. (Loneliliness, Social Isolation, and Cardiovascular Health, Antioxidant Redox Signal, 2018 Mar 20:28(9):837-861. Ning Xia and Huige Li.

Statistics linking Socializing to Good Health and Lack of Socializing to bad health: from the National Institute on Aging: National Institutes of Health: US Department of Health and Human Services: Research Suggests a Positive Correlation between Social Interaction and Health. A report on research studies on social interaction and health among older adults suggest that social isolation may have significant adverse effects: That…

- Social relationships are consistently associated with biomarkers of health
- Positive indicators of social well-being may be associated with lower levels of interleukin-6 in otherwise healthy peo-

ple. (IL-6 is an inflammatory factor implicated in age-related disorders such as Alzheimer's disease, osteoporosis, rheumatoid arthritis, cardiovascular disease, and some forms of cancer).

- Some grandparents feel that caring for their grandchildren makes them healthier and more active. (due to strong emotional bonding, active lifestyle, healthier meals, and may even reduce or stop smoking)
- Social isolation constitutes a major risk factor for morbidity and mortality, especially in older adults
- Loneliness may have a physical as well as an emotional impact and is associated with elevated systolic blood pressure, which may lead to hypertension.
- Loneliness is a unique risk factor for symptoms of depression. Both have a synergistic adverse effect on well-being in middle-aged and older adults.

(Am J Public Health, 1992 August; 82(8): 1089-92)

Brigham Young University: Social Interactive people live 50% longer than socially isolated people; social ties delay memory loss; and social isolation is a risk factor for cognitive decline in the elderly.

(Professor J Holt- Lunstad. Study reports from 2004- 2018)

Mass Inst of Tech Study: Socially active people are more productive in the workplace, i.e. that socializing coffee breaks are better than no contact at all.

Univ Chicago Study: Sleep quality in the socially active is better than in the socially isolated. Poor sleep is defined as disrupted, interrupted, insomnia and nightmares)

Journal of Mind, Mood and Memory, July 1, 2014: "Interaction with others helps ward off cognitive decline and depression and promote physical and mental well-being."

*Harvard University Study: Grant: Beginning in 1967, an 80-year prospective, follow up on the lives of people ("relatively privileged") since 1967: suggested that a "successful life" is not about determination to get and have more, but that "the only thing that really matters in life are our relationships with other people". That Rejection of "others" is unnatural, damaging, hurtful, wrong and eventually unhealthy. That a successful life is not about cholesterol levels and BP or intellectual of career achievements, or how much money in your bank account, but about "human connections", parents, siblings, spouses, children, friends, neighbors, mentors, and "others"... is about inclusion, welcoming, openness, ... is about profound moments when you touched others or when they touched you....is about positive behavior in terms of relief of suffering, loss, sickness, death ...is about "healing presence of another". The study concluded that "social connections, i.e. relationships, are best for health and that loneliness is bad for health." Not diet, not exercise, not BP or cholesterol levels but, social relationships (quality and quantity) were the determining factor in longevity.

Vignette #2: The 4-year-old girl upon seeing an older person crying on a bench, snuggles up and stays... when asked what she was doing, replies: "I was just helping him cry".

Study: Socially isolated animals developed more atherosclerosis than those housed in groups. Lack of social support and stimulating environment associates with increased stress reactions and risk of cardiovascular disease.

> *(Effects of social isolation and environmental enrichment on atherosclerosis in ApoE-/- mice. E. Bernberg, et al. Stress 2008 Sp.)*

Study: Low social status has a detrimental effect on the immune system and is associated with heart disease, cancers, diabetes, obesity, and inflammations. Even if bad habits (poor diet, toxins smoking, and risky behavior) are removed, the longevity gap between rich and poor for males remains at 15 years and females at 10 years. The stress of low social status affects the quantity and quality of one's life.

(In Search of a Stress-free Life, 2018)

Study: To highlight the effect of low status in a group of 45 female Rhesus monkeys, the newest member experienced less grooming, less attention, and more harassment, from which she exhibited chronic depression due to the hormonal effects of chronic stress. A blood analysis showed 1600 differences in activity level of immune system genes between those at the top and those at the bottom. The "bottom" immune system runs "too aggressively" (on high due to repeated insults) and gives rise to increased levels of inflammation, which has a collateral damage to tissues and subsequent increased risk of disease. The study concludes that low status (due to factors outside the control of individual) has negative effects on health. The social environment impacts health through unhealthy behavior in the forms of direct and indirect stress.

(J Ting and L Barreiro. Science 354, 1048-1051 (2016)

Study: Early social stress has potent lifelong health effects. Issues with maternal attachment relationships, low maternal social rank and greater frequency and intensity of social conflict, have a negative influence on inflammatory stress response in plasma and CRP (inflammation markers)

(Early social stress promotes inflammation and disease in Rhesus monkeys. E. Kinnally, et al. Scientific Reports 9, article # 7609 (2019)

Study: Grooming in rhesus monkeys was asymmetrically directed toward higher ranking females and in reducing aggression between grooming partners, associates with social tolerance. Social status and connectedness (especially dominance rank) have strong effects on social relationships and is important in health and fitness consequences.

(Social Status drives social relationships in groups of unrelated female rhesus macaques. N. Snyder-Mackler, etal. ncbi.nim.nih.gov (2016)

How the mind handles imperfect or absence of social connections is crucial to health. People in the middle and at the bottom may have "things", materials, but not "status". They "feel" that they are at the bottom (compared to the higher ranks, who have never been at the bottom and do not have a clue as to how it feels). They "feel" oppressed, hated, ignored, detested by those at the top, who set the trends and make the rules. Consequently, they harbor more chronic stress that often leads to poorer health. Study: In Acciareli, Italy (north of Naples), 10% of the population is over the age of 100. In the USA the percentage is 0.002. The reasons researched are as follows:

1. Mediterranean diet of fresh local food, no preservatives, no truck miles, no processing additives), sardines, anchovies, fresh produce high in antioxidants, use tea and culinary herbs, olive oil and low intake of red meat which contributes to low cholesterol levels and low incidence of inflammation. Yet, they smoke, eat fatty food, and drink wine. On the positive side, both rosemary, a favorite herb, and olive oil, the omega 3 staple, aid in circulation health and brain function. Hence the low incidence of dementia with advanced age?

2. The inhabitants lead a happy life relatively free of stress and focused on enjoyment of life. *They enjoy each other. (stress destroys immunity, leads to chronic inflammation, accelerates ageing, by the slow destruction of body, mind & spirit.)*

3. They are physically active with walking, gardening, biking with a purpose and on a daily basis. The environment with hilly steps, natural spaces, long winding roads and active sex into old age contribute to the fulfilling the adequate exercise requirement.
4. The people are "Socially" active, involved, and included well into old age. Spending quality time together with trust, compassion, and group dynamics, slows cellular degeneration.
5. There is little or no use of chemical fertilizers or pesticides in their crops or gardens.
6. The environment is favorable with warmth and sunshine, which facilitates the absorption of vitamin D with its multiple benefits, unpolluted air, and sea breezes, which contribute to a pleasance that enables immortality.

As a result, there are low levels of heart disease, dementia, and obesity. Blood chemistry analysis showed low levels of adrenomedullin (a peptide hormone that widens blood vessels). Centenarians have wide blood vessels and therefore low production of adrenomedullin (much like younger people in their 20's). As a result of their lifestyle, they have healthy blood vessels so there was no need for adrenomedullin production. (i.e. In the normal & accelerated ageing, there is an increase in adrenomedullin needed due to narrowing blood vessels. The Acciarelians have naturally occurring wide blood vessels, enabling good circulation, and have no need for adrenomedullin production.) Study: Loneliness had a direct link to depression and to Cardiovascular disease, which increases the risk of death. Researchers found more evidence for the link between depression and all-causes for Cardiovascular mortality. *JAMA Network Open 2020, Meng R, et al.*

Study: The spread of obesity in a large social network over 32 years is associated with poor health and increases in incidence and prevalence when friends are also obese and decreases when friends lose weight. This is attributed to peer group behavior. Females have superior support systems than males, which contributes to their increased longevity, as they express feelings of grief, anger, and intimacy more than males.

N A Christakis, New England Journal of Medicine (2007)

Eat right, Be happy, Stay fit, Enjoy friends.

While the USA spends more on "health care" per capita than many other countries combined, its life expectancy has decreased for the third year in a row (2015, 2016, 2017). The increase in deaths has been ascribed to an increase in opioid use, gun violence and suicide. Another reason lies in its failure to deliver on health care for all its citizens. Exorbitant expenses are poured into diagnosis and treatment, while prevention through attention to the causes of disease is largely ignored. Millions of dollars are assigned to the production and sales of designer drugs to block internal signals, the technology of triple bypass heart surgery and stem cell organ replacements, while little or nothing is directed toward prevention. Next to nothing is directed to promote safe environments, clean air and water, high quality public education so that everyone has access to a decent job with decent wages. Poor disadvantaged people get sick earlier and more often, and fail to recover completely and/or turn to drugs to alleviate their pain, mental and physical, then are blamed for their poor choices.

Stress control is perhaps the single most widely misunderstood or totally neglected contributor to some 80% of these disease processes. A sedentary lifestyle, poor diet of artificial foods coupled with overeating, a penchant for toxin production and exposure, and low mental stimulation due to low access to good education all contribute to the general picture of a society in poor health.

Good health is associated with strong Social connections and an open cooperative society. It is no surprise that poor health is reflected in a country that favors individualism over community, withholds health care from its most vulnerable citizens and promotes separation and antisocial behavior. The six strategies of good health are ALL interconnected. Avoiding toxins involves environment and what you ingest for nutrition. Lack of exercise affects the brain and the body with accumulation of toxins. Stress releases toxic chemicals and cell damaging hormones. Mental stimulation from the input of others is exercise for the mind. And is affected by lack of exercise and social interactions for adequate brain blood flow carrying oxygen and nutrients. Lack of social connections is associated with depression, cardiovascular disease and adverse responses to chronic stressors. Nutrition for the body is affected by dining together instead of alone. A perfect diet is no good if it cannot be digested properly. Nutrition for the soul comes in the form of art, music, literature, laughter, entertainment, support, and belonging. Exercising together is preferable to exercising alone.

Health and well-being depend on the composite environment of quality of air, water, food, shelter, level of activity, social and economic status, mental stability (the six basic strategies) neither strategy alone is as effective as all six together.

ECNS: Eye Contact, Nod and Smile testing

What happens upon first encounter with a person in a public space? Upon giving a basic greeting consisting of "Eye Contact, a Nod of the head and a Smile", what is the initial reaction?

I recorded the results of this test on the beaches of Puerto Rico, the elevators and cafeterias, hotel breakfast areas, cafes, museums and public squares of world cities (20).

There are those who return a simple greeting and those who do not.

For whatever reason, some are pro-social and some are antisocial. Some people view the greeting as an opening for an interaction that is unwanted and some jump at the opportunity to interact. I should preface this by saying that (1) this is not a scientific study and (2) I am a gray-haired, slim to medium build, older gentleman, with brown skin tones who is of no threat to anyone.

A hint to the results, in general, 9 out of 10 Puerto Ricans returned the greeting as opposed to 2 out of 10 Americans on the same beach or in the same restaurant. It is amazing how few people know how to smile and at least nod hello.

It does not cost anything to be friendly, neither
in energy expended nor in coinage.

When someone looks you in the eye, acknowledges your presence and smiles, and you turn away or look through or past them, for whatever reason, you are antisocial. Refusing a basic greeting in either direction could result from poor parental instructions or example, bad habits, simple laziness, or failure to see another human being as important enough to warrant a simple greeting. This behavior is usually learned. Refusal to be friendly to other people or being averse to the company of others is behavior deviant to the natural norm. The rejection of a basic greeting can sometimes lead to adrenalin bursts and cortisol seepage in the bloodstream, which eventually affects organs and leads to adrenal gland fatigue and chronic stress that wears on the heart, respiration, Central Nervous System, and digestive system. Yet, sometimes it makes one "feel good" to be aloof and cold toward others. But this is only for a short time. Habitual rejection of basic greetings will eventually lead to deprivation of spontaneous interactions, which can become detrimental to one's health.

I am aware of your presence, we share the same space, we have equal access, let us be civil and "humane", let us just say "hello". Ants and other insects pause upon encountering each other. Most primates greet each other, as do most mammals, yet many humans are adept at ignoring each another completely. Does it make them feel superior? Does it make them feel safer?

"Much hostile and aggressive behavior among animals is the expression of social insecurity" Yann Martel

How much inner insecurity at not being good at being social is there. All humans crave love and affection, yet a sizeable number prefer to ignore and eliminate the potential source of their cravings. Unable to give, they will not receive. There is no excuse for refusal to acknowledge the presence of others. There are only two fears that humans are born with… fear of loud noises (due to the acoustic-startle reflex seated in the spinal cord and innate for defense) and fear of falling (due to depth perception development for self-preservation). There is no innate fear of strangers, large animals, fire, water or "others", This fear is taught by self-serving elders and weak adults and learned by follower humans.

A simple greeting should be acknowledged even if never returned.

The why, how, what and what we can do to improve our social skills, create a viable social life and maintain good health, are discussed in the ensuing chapters.

Summary of Contents

Chapter one explores the history and science of the processes of social interactions and connections, with a focus on the biochemical and physiological reactions involved with the release and response to feel-good and feel-bad hormones. Cooperation plays a major role in defense, protection, food distribution, and formation of culture, with its management of forgiveness and revenge. Social and antisocial behavior saw a major shift when *Homo sapiens* changed from egalitarian mobile hunter-gatherer society to a more stationary agrarian one. Though mechanisms of socializing like music, dance, dining, and conversation that began at the campfires in Africa, changed with adaptation to different environments, the effects on health remained the same. Compassion and Heartlessness in which a "kind" or a "cruel" DNA was expressed became the defining bases of a dualism in human personality. Empathy, altruism, and trust are basic foundations of human interactions, but can be overcome by aggression and evil. Communications and touch are essential tools for humanness and play major roles in Tribalism, with its identity markers designating who are included or excluded. In setting the parameters for Us and Them and designating all outsiders as "others", we see the same scenario on display in the 21st century. The question of with whom do we interact is just as poignant today as the lines of separation is deeply etched in historic social behavior.

Chapter two explains the health benefits of social behavior with reference to the biochemical and physiological advantages of positivity. Belonging to the group and fitting in with the environment shape our personalities and sense of purpose. Social skills, kinship, and friendship are major players in promoting good stable health and well-being. Displaying basic kindness and good manners results in dignity and respect from and for all those encountered. The highest test of prosocial behavior is one's interactions with strangers.

Inclusion with unlimited access will present the best opportunities for connections.

Chapter three examines the basis for and consequences of antisocial behavior. It is often characterized by social anxiety and isolation and consists of two arms. *Inflicting*, with rudeness and disrespect may be due to lack of skills, gratification in humiliation or pure hostility, includes snobbery, use of socializing drugs, self-interest and system blaming. The sociopath makes full use of the Us versus Them ideology to gain and maintain satisfaction. On the *Receiving* end of antisocial behavior are the sufferers of loneliness, lack of self-worth, depressives and high incidence of stress diseases of the heart, central nervous and immune systems. The results of the concentrated use of electronic devices and social distancing as the result of the Covid-19 pandemic, are yet to be determined. Asocial (autism) is the purest form of antisocial behavior.

Chapter four presents social experiences in other cultures, including the Blue Zones, Mediterranean, Europe, Middle East, Asia, North and South America, and the Caribbean. Similarities and differences occur along environmental and historical lines. The interplay of all six basic health and five socializing strategies in forming social connections is emphasized as a major factor in human behavior. The results of the social survey conducted in Athens and the Eye Contact, Nod and Smile testing show that some societies are more friendly than others.

Chapter five presents solutions in the form of suggestions for the management of social interactions and connections, by forming and honing social skills. A social skills protocol that focuses on self-confidence, eye contact, body language, basic manners, communication, flexibility and cooperation, seeking interactions, positive intent, and basic humanity is provided.

CHAPTER ONE

ORIGIN AND HISTORY OF SOCIAL INTERACTIONS

"Man is by nature a social animal; an individual who is unsocial naturally and not accidentally is either beneath our notice or more than human." Aristotle

"Lions, wolves, and vultures don't live together in herds, droves or flocks. Of all the animals of prey, man is the only sociable one. Every one of us preys upon his neighbor and yet we herd together." John Gay

"All children laugh and cry in the same way and for the same reasons. We are all the same and will get along just fine." (observation by the author at age four on first day of attendance at a multilingual kindergarten)

Pre-History

Australopithecus afarensis, 3.8-million years ago, **a** hominid, climbed down from the trees and *walked upright* on two legs into the savannas of the Afar region of the East African Rift Valley. Nicknamed "Lucy" by modern archaeologist/anthropologists, her brain was 20% larger and her spine was more vertical than that of a chimpanzee or an ape. She still had a plant-based diet and she retreated to the trees for protection and food. Occasionally she used sharp tools (probably found, not made) and she cared for her children, while developing rudimentary cognitive and social skills that helped her form and maintain a small group of similar individuals. "Socializing" rewarded her with a comforting response within the group and an effective defense response to predators and those outside the group. Her identification with the group defined the competition for space, food and reproductive rights, all parts of basic survival.

Homo habilis roamed freely in East Africa between 2.3 to 1.4-million years ago. The handy man, made and developed the first tools, displayed distinctive group behavior, had *l*anguage skills, and dietary diversity in consuming some meat and bone marrow. Most importantly, he passed on tool making skills to the next generation or to another group in what became *instructive education.*.

Homo erectus,1.9 to 0.7-million years ago, upright man, with a body more adapted for long distance running, extended his movements in the savannah, formed hunting and foraging groups for division of labor through cooperation and collaboration and organized food distribution. Advancements in his lifestyle led to major increases in brain size to satisfy extended needs. He learned to control fire, which allowed the adoption of larger animals with energy-rich meat as a source of protein (cause and/or result). Enjoying a longer childhood for learning and development of a social brain, he interacted with larger groups of people, and further developed social behavior

2

in order to keep track of the individuals and groups and maximize their efficiency. Whether from climate changes, pursuit of game animals, in search of more abundant forage, or just innate urges, Homo erectus moved. He traveled, took his family, friends and acquaintances, and started the migrations out of Africa into Eurasia.

"If you want to go fast, go alone. If you want to go far, go together." African proverb

With fire in their pouches and time on their hands, they could socialize at night. In providing warmth, light, protection from predators, opportunity for myth, storytelling and teaching, they had good reasons to "gather". In addition, cooked food had a better taste and digested easier, so they ate more. Protein contributed to increased brain size and more connections of white matter; provided safety from bacterial and parasitic infections; allowed signaling, rituals, and discussion that led to planning and group coordination. Cooperation for the hunt, the move or the shelter, wood collection and type of defense to put in place, all required and grew out of social interaction. It created more time and less stress for them to sit together and socialize. They survived by banding together, sharing food, and working to create a comfortable living space.

Greater social behavior led to better survival.

(The "me-first" society of modern times would never have survived; the capitalistic, opposition to sharing, selfish society would have been destroyed in an instant, by both external and internal elements.)

Big game hunting required Cooperation. It provided sufficient and excess meat, which led to sharing through altruism and egalitarianism, with benefits to the entire group. Equal access to all, provided a reduction in alpha power and expulsion of meat thieves and cheaters.

Social selection with its indirect reciprocity for altruists, advantage in directing gene selection, and exclusion of alpha males, favored the cooperative moral male. His social status reputation led to sexual success and reproduction of more like himself. As self-restraint survived there was less risk of rebellion (conflict avoidance), more personal autonomy, and better breeding opportunities. Socializing strengthened the bonds required for success in the hunt. Sharing reinforced morality and strengthened the group with nutrition for all. Success led to internalization of the rules supported by a sense of shame (man is the only animal with a "blushing" autonomic reflex). Using symbolic communication (gossip) as in fireside chatting was an effective control of the group by providing reminders of morality and extra-familial generosity, and the rewards of moral conduct.

Homo sapiens, 160,000 to 40,000 years ago, wise man, moved out of Africa and into Eurasia and surrounding lands. Besides having more brain growth, they developed another tremendous advantage. The capacity to anticipate what a partner was thinking led to huge gains in cooperation, coordination of activities and elaborate planning. The ability to address a situation and interact to get results, thereby creating problem solving networks within the brain and functional groups outside that promoted more social well-being, the most important being that survival depended on becoming and remaining connected. The societies that formed were not all perfect, as group beliefs and values could also lead to trouble rooted in the fear of threats from various sources, environmental and other humans. With larger groups, more complex lifestyles and shifting values, social behavior could convert to aggressive and antisocial behavior.

Homo neanderthalensis, 500,000 years ago, Neanderthal man, (derived from Homo erectus' earlier migrations into Europe) cared for their sick and injured, buried their dead, and displayed the strength of attachment between individuals much closer to the social connections we have today. In possession of social cognition, they could distinguish between subjective and objective, real and unreal, belief and truth, and opinion and fact. Social interaction led to the emergence of joint attention and coordination of perspectives, allowing one to appreciate another's experiences and learn objectives as things that exist other than oneself. The cave dweller encountered the toolmaker, merged, interacted, grew and receded, with the cooperative planner emerging on the survival chart.

Another wave of more modern *Homo sapiens*, 60,000 years ago, left Africa and spread further across the globe. This group had evolved further, was better equipped and had developed a more complex society through natural selection that functioned whether stationary or mobile. Humans raised in groups had better social skills than those living alone. They encouraged selected features like the capacity for learning, teaching and social skills for the benefit of the individual and the group, which were passed on, while personalities that favored selfishness and antisocial behavior, were discouraged.

Successful groups displaced, dominated and pushed to extinction other groups with which they came into contact. This feature persists throughout our existence.

Modern *Homo sapiens* moved from scavenger to gatherer to hunter through social skills that favored cooperation. The rewards were direct and more abundant when work was done in groups. From cooperation came connections, built on trust and cohesion of kinship. Groups that worked well together were more successful at hunting, cooking, and protecting than those who stayed alone. Kin selection, where one would risk all to help or save a relative, and trusted friends, were major factors in groups forming societies.

The society that resulted from the interaction of two or more human beings, grew through communication, cooperation, conscience and trust, the combination of which made humans more social than other primates and previous hominids.

*Social Interactions grew into connections through
the process of natural selection, then into groups and
societies as a principal means of survival.*

Social Selection

Early humans chose their partners and friends based on success and survival of the entire group, through food procurement, shelter, and defense. The preferred features necessary for group success were dependency on a partner or partners for foraging and hunting skills and ability and tendency to treat others with a sense of compassion and fairness. The group ejected aggressive alpha styles, cheaters and hoarders or did not choose them for future endeavors.

Social Interaction was the original group behavior of the human species, based on cooperation and sharing, which led to enhanced survival (better food supply and protection) and ensured progression to the next generation. When humans ceased to be "social", the group would fail. The act of hunting and gathering led to mental growth via social development in the form of personal relationships. Interactions leading to success bred trust and reliability, set up alliances, bonding, sexual contact, and loyalties. They gathered and lived together with and without kinship, developed a wide range of social networks and experienced success.

Groups got larger and split off due mainly to availability of resources and variety of mates, which led to competitive rivalries, dominance, deception and betrayal. Despite the proven advantage of group over individual behavior, there was also a compulsive need to belong to a group. Pro-social behavior outshone antisocial, but the latter maintained a constant presence. Despite being ostracized, enough of these uncooperative individuals survived, perhaps through the kindness of their peers and through their wits, to keep their genes in the general pool.

Cognition

How did *Homo sapiens* become "wise"? Prior to the acquisition of "wisdom", hominids grouped together for protection and acquisition of essential nourishment. Deliberate socializing and thinking are linked. Which came first, is debatable. First order thinking involves being aware of one's own thoughts and the thoughts of others. *Homo sapiens* "knows and knows that he knows". Second order thinking involves what the self thinks another person is thinking of self. An increase in number of individuals in the group led man to use cognition to keep track of individuals through recognition and eventual communications. Group planning of procurement of food, distribution and improved chances of being picked for a choice chore the next time, led to significance of adornment and ornamentation of identification and to social behavior acceptable to the group. How one person thinks that others think about their own thoughts is the core of complex social interactions. The birth of thought, to know that you know that you know (introspection), defined becoming human.

Adam and Eve ate the forbidden fruit of awareness of themselves (nakedness) and were evicted from Eden since they were no longer "innocent". They had gained awareness, had become "social", interacting with others, and "human", thinking about it and no longer needed to be there. *Homo sapiens* could view themselves as objects and see what they looked like to the others, how they were seen, and what they thought about how they were seen. This was the basis of male/female interactions that led to courtships that led to the reproduction that enabled survival and multiplication. The ability to predict another's behavior went a long way to enhance group hunting, warfare, coordinated exploration and acquisition of supplies that enhanced the survival rate when compared to others without this ability. By outsmarting large animals, bringing some under control, ensuring their safety and enhancing their food supply, they increased their intelligence through feedback, learning and reciprocity.

Third order thinking advanced to complex planning and cooperation for who, what, how and where, followed by the why of art, religion, and society construct. Efficiency provided time to contemplate oneself thinking of others and others contemplating us.

The defining moments in human cognitive development played out over thousands of years. The social interactions that resulted in and from cooperation, organization, and eventual success prompted hominids to repeat the process over and over until it became part of essential existence.

How they presented to others including self-adornment, appearance and behavior, were the social skills required to move forward in organizing a successful society. These interactions that grew into social connections had as its basis, awareness of self and awareness of others. This "autobiographical memory", being able to link past and future, using interactions for survival, came about some 60,000 years ago and presents as "intelligence". Awareness of self, of others, and thinking about themselves thinking about themselves, formed "cognition" and enabled deliberate social interaction. The more "social" the individual, the higher the chance for survival.

The wave of *Homo sapiens* that migrated from Africa to populate the world were intelligent, self-aware, introspective and empathetic, all the features needed for effective social interaction. They developed personalities suited to group travel, with extroversion, openness, agreeability and tolerance at the forefront. Positive interaction and fair treatment of others were absolute requirements for group behavior on such journeys. They interacted with stable, positive, courageous others, rather than unstable, fearful, threatened and threatening individuals from inside and outside their group.

Man, the social animal

"Society is something that precedes the individual. Anyone who either cannot lead the common life or is so self-sufficient as not to need to, and therefore does not partake of society, is either a beast or a god." Aristotle, Politics

Man's inherent instinct is to live in a society with other human beings. The 50,000 year-old man was well on the way to becoming a social animal using language as a tool to promote cooperation to manage making and building things that enhanced his physical and mental safety, his health and his mobility. For the hunter-gatherers, everything in nature was "connected" and this especially applied to his own groups. That life and survival depended on connections was the root of their belief system. Social interactions in the form of ceremonies, were used to explain and share the meaning of things, and in understanding what someone else was thinking (intentions) and reacting accordingly. Social connections have their origins in innate genetics consistent with human evolution through natural selection that favored release of "feel good "hormones that accompanied human development from infancy to adulthood, where cooperation enhanced chances of survival and disconnections were often fatal. Where did the interactive characteristic of human life come from and how did it develop into the social interactions we have today?

We are hard-wired for social interaction as a necessity for survival, good health and well-being.

The origin and evolution of social behavior, like most things, is multifaceted. That society was a natural product of human beings (Jean Jacques Rousseau, French philosopher) and that man's drive for survival used social interactions for peace and harmony instead of conflict (John Locke, English philosopher), were two of the many theories in contention in the 17th century. That society arose as a natural order and evolved through social selection to reward survivors and punish violators is the most accepted norm.

Social behavior is 50% genetic and 50% environmental

Since nothing in nature is 100% one and not the other, human nature evolved as a dichotomy, a mixture of feelings, chemistries, reactions, behaviors based in part on genetics and part on environment. The origin of social life is from innate moral senses, that go on further to be shaped by experience and learning. An innate sense of fairness and reciprocity lead to cooperation. There is an innate sense of morality (right vs wrong) in the principles required for survival, which is the foundation of social behavior. Every society values kindness and cooperation as positive and cruelty and conflict as negative features.

Science of Social Connections

All creatures use the same 3 letter DNA coding combination to make the same amino acids and the same proteins essential to life. We owe our existence to a single origin of life and that only through "sharing" did we all proceed through survival and development. Contrary to the mindset of some modern humans, we need each other. We survived and thrived only through communication and sharing, not isolation, not exclusion, not protectionism, not selfishness. We survived with a mixture of basic instincts, altruism, empathy, trust, genetics and lots of luck in having all the essential elements come and stay together.

All humans have shared inheritance, the capacity to live with one another, to socialize, to find meaning and love in families and friends, to respect value and to cooperate in groups. This is common humanity. The science behind the development of social beings grew through natural selection of hormones that shaped our behavior toward cooperation, learning, love, friendship and building of a functional society.

Vignette #3: Imagine a small town in the middle of somewhere. It is a place where everybody knows everybody else and helps each other to overcome obstacles and maintain a quality existence. Town meetings are held to resolve the large problems and home life more than resolves the small ones. It is a place where each leading citizen, of which there are fifty, gives to Popi, the town beggar an ample share of food, basic shelter and a dollar a day, for twenty years. Though he is not too bright, Popi has a good feeling each time he stashes the money into a hole in a wall and never spends it. When the mayor declares bankruptcy as the result of poor decisions, ill-advised deals and bad luck, and after a flash flood destroyed half the town's infrastructure, Popi retrieves his $365,000 and saves the town. He does it out of the goodness of his nature.

Is Popi's behavior innate or learned? What anatomical arrangement and chemicals are so prominent in his brain to produce this behavior?

To examine the science behind pro-social behavior, one may look at social connections in the kingdom that has been around a lot longer than ours, plants. Trees and plants care for each other. They share water, warnings, and communications, through a root system, produce phytochemicals for protection and show their "feelings" through physical and chemical reactions. Forest trees live longer than isolated trees partly from protection in the group and partly by community existence. The advantages of working together are evident in protection, keeping each other alive through supporting the "forest" as micro-biosystem, sharing resources equally in a form of social security. (Modern wealthy humans and many not so wealthy, refuse to share). Loners, trees isolated on a windswept hill, are inherently weaker, less healthy, and more susceptible to attack by insects, parasites, and pathogens than those in a forest.

In the animal kingdom, chimpanzees, great apes, elephants, ants, bees and birds, whales and dolphins are naturally "social" and exhibit forms of a society, small but functional. Smaller animals grouped together to defeat larger animals, for offense, defense, and comfort. Big and small contributions benefitted all, regardless of amount.

Organized social behavior originated and developed with us cooperating and in response to the increasing numbers of participants. There was safety, success and progress in numbers. Innate DNA transcribed social connections in response to environmental needs through natural and social selection. Individuals banded and bonded in groups of loose individuals (mixed sexes) instead of just in pairs from the inception of the split of primates from lemurs and other prosimians some 52-million years ago. From the wild, wandering *Homo erectus* to the tamer, more settled *Homo sapiens* groups survived because of collective friendliness and pro-social behavior.

Neuroanatomy of Social Interactions

The key area in the brain active in social interaction is the frontal cortex. Within its confines are the superior temporal sulcus (STS), fusiform face area (FFA), orbitofrontal cortex, medial prefrontal cortex (site of experience and correct social behavior) and the limbic system (site of emotions, affection, and memory). The limbic centers regulate autonomic and endocrine function in response to emotional stimuli. The frontal cortex controls cognitive skills, emotional expression, communications, judgement, sexual behaviors and problem solving. It is the area designated for interactions with others in a natural response to identity "markers" and tribal group behavior. As hominids accessed more proteins their brain and body size increased. But as the small-brained hobbits on the island of Flores in Indonesia (20,000 years ago) can attest, they made tools and had language. Intelligence is not solely dependent on brain size, but more on brain "cytoarchitecture, neural density and development of culture and language specificity. The advent of VEN cells (Von Economo Neurons) deep in the gray matter of large brains, provided faster and more efficient connectivity of signals, and long spindle cells associated with "humane" behavior, gave us empathy, sympathy, cooperation and compassion. These cells signaled the endocrine system to produce classic feel-god and feel-bad hormones responsible for much of human social behavior.

Coincident with the increase in brain size and composition, *Homo erectus* (1.7-million years ago) formed hunting and gathering groups for division of labor, protection, toolmaking and sheltering. The development of language (Broca's and Wernicke's areas in the forebrain) enabled cooperation and planning in securing and preparing a food supply, group protection and ensured reproduction. It also provided social intelligence, awareness, attention and concern for the group. The brain areas that receive and process social information include the visual centers of the occipital cortex seeing other human bodies; the temporal cortex hearing other human voices; the central pSTS region for determination of intentions, feelings, thoughts in anticipation of the proper response; the prefrontal cortex in charge of social skills, judgement, aggression management, emotion regulation, planning and reasoning and the amygdala, seat of powerful emotions. (*The Social Brain, National Institute of Health*)

The area of the brain associated with understanding the minds of others is larger in people who have bigger social networks. Activity in specific brain regions coincide with active social life. The regions that process social signals, facial expressions, names and faces are larger in people with more Facebook friends. Research shows that monkeys that live in larger groups grow bigger brains, in processing space to accommodate more complex social networks. The orbital prefrontal cortex (right behind the eyes) is one area used for directing appropriate social behavior and interactions with others. *(Stephanie Pappas, Live Science. Jan 31, 2012)* Both the prefrontal cortex and paralimbic systems involve emotional reactions that influence social behavior and self-control. The limbic system, seat of emotions like anger, anxiety, fear, and pleasure, contain determinants of social interactions, such as friend or foe. The amygdala, a pair of small almond-size structures in humans, expresses fearful, more aggressive emotions and are much bigger in large wild animals. Human psychopaths with small amygdalae are fearless and show minimal social cooperation. They have high fear recognition, low morality and will kill and feel no remorse. People with antisocial behavior have large amygdalae, readily blame and show hatred for "others", and react with aggression when approached or reproached. Treatments with selective serotonin reuptake inhibitors (SSRI's; drugs to increase levels of serotonin) to make them more social and less aggressive have met with some success.

High serotonin levels, more social interactions (pro-social).
High cortisol levels, less sociability (antisocial)

Feel-Good and Feel-Bad Hormones
The Biochemistry of Social Connections

What causes that good feeling one gets with the anticipation of seeing a friend? What is that sudden rush of happiness when you meet your tennis buddy to hit some balls and catch up on the local gossip. What gives you that energy boost in the middle of a long run or at the beginning of a loving hug? What gives you that butterflies in the stomach feeling when faced with the prospect of a potentially embarrassing encounter? What causes that sinking feeling at a sudden rejection or loss of a loved one? What leads to that sick feeling of depression from loneliness or being far from the security of home? All these feelings result from variations and expressions of hormones released from the endocrine glands and nervous system upon encounter, interaction and connection. Hormones are molecular forms of proteins, made of peptides and amino acids that bind to receptors on target cells and affect behavior. Social behavior is regulated and influenced by the properties and amounts of these chemical reactions produced by these proteins. Oxytocin, dopamine, serotonin, adrenalin, noradrenalin, endorphins, and cortisol are some of the hormones, which in combination or in varying amounts, have a direct effect on mental and physical health and indirect effects on nutrition and stress levels.

Babies are "social" from before they are born. They react and interact with mother in formation of pathways essential to growth and development and eventual survival. Separation of an infant from its mother or source of survival leads immediately to anxiety over loss of warmth, care, love and eventually to extreme distress and even, death. The separation leads to a release of cortisol and concomitant suppression of oxytocin that leads to social and cognitive deficits, behavioral and learning difficulties, and brain alterations in social areas. The pain is like that of drug withdrawal and the painkiller is re-connection. The same neurochemicals that ease the pain of social separation distress in an infant, also ease physical pain. Oxytocin also has a rage component in anticipation of rejection or loss. The infant thrives when both biological (food, water, shelter) and psychological (social connections) needs are met, and fades when either is deficient or absent. Social pain can be influenced by suggestion, hypnosis, i.e. it has a mental component, and by physical pain, neglect and rejection. Memories of social pain linger on, are recurrent and many times are more intense than memories of physical pain. Social pain is real, universal and described in the same terms as physical pain in all languages. Study: In an experiment by Dr. Jack Panksepp, an Estonian neuroscientist in 1978, puppies were given non-sedating (low) doses of morphine and then separated from mother and siblings. On brain scan, social and physical pain were found in the same area, anterior cingulate cortex (ACC) of the brain. (It is absent in reptiles.) The ACC has the highest density of opioid receptors, which respond to both social and physical pain and links to the mother/infant attachment behavior in mammals. Females are more "social", more intuitive and better at assessing the character of the "other" than males. The female hormonal structure developed more innate abilities for "socializing" with assurances of safety and acceptability in addition to her natural infant bonding skills.

Oxytocin (OT), the "cuddle" hormone, is a neuropeptide released through closeness with another person, or a pet or cherished object (stuffed animal), physical touch like a hug, intimacy, and in women during childbirth (parturition) and breastfeeding (lactation). Triggered from the hypothalamus (reward center of the brain) into the bloodstream during social bonding, attention and falling in love, in response to pro-social excitement and in the female during orgasm while the male releases vasopressin, it rises to high amounts during long term relationships. The amount decreases with increasing time (ageing). In addition to being the natural support for the infant's well-being, oxytocin motivates and changes the process that promotes "approach" behavior. Do it and you will receive pleasure from the love and trust hormone. Pro-social caregivers have high levels of oxytocin. Antisocial loners have lower oxytocin levels. In cases of learned antagonistic behavior toward others, oxytocin production and release will be lowered. Oxytocin release from the hypothalamus is often accompanied by concomitant dopamine release to enhance the motivation to gain the reward. The antisocial behavior of neglect with low levels of both hormones and low drive to social interaction is evident in the blank faces of victims of Parkinson's disease. In the lower primates, the release of oxytocin signals avoidance in situations of distress, sending the message, "get help". In non-primates, it stimulates aggression toward strangers in protection from threat to offspring. High oxytocin in groups is associated with generosity and protection.

Oxytocin is associated with enhanced feelings of trust and positive response to others, like reaction to social signals of eye contact, fairness, cooperation, proximity to and understanding of the intentions of others. Discernible levels are severely reduced in autism, hence the asocial behavior. In multiple studies on rats, oxytocin release and sensitivity are higher in females during social interactions than in males. High levels are associated with maintaining a sharp memory, less drug use, lower stress levels, and better mental health and indication of some "reversal" of Alzheimer's plaque buildup. Reduced levels are associated with increased rates of ageing. Oxytocin promotes favoritism and caring to the "ingroup" and hostility to "the ou group". While its levels help to discern the dividing line between friend and foe, for strangers, the response could go either way.

Dopamine is the "happiness" hormone, associated with anticipation of reward, a good event, a tasty food like chocolate or oysters, and meeting someone you like for some quality time together. It is the "fall-in-love" hormone, along with norepinephrine and epinephrine, that makes your knees shaky and your heart rate increase, which also occurs when faced with the horrors of possible rejection. Large amounts release in periods of stress, at the sense of danger. Getting on an elevator with "other" imparting a sense that one's purse is in danger, seeing an "other" in the park, bird-watching, triggers the increased production and release of dopamine, adrenaline, and cortisol to increase alertness, spout anxiety and prompt calls to 911. When chronic, in excess and repeated, dopamine co-opts cortisol, leading to stress on the body and mind. When the effects wear down, the subject is apathetic, mean, unconcerned, and "burned out. Both in excess and in depletion, there are harmful effects, usually of anxiety, fear, bad feeling, and dread. Sustained levels of dopamine and cortisol are detrimental to good health. Dopamine, well-known as a natural high, is used to relieve symptoms of Parkinson's disease. Released from the substantia nigra and ventral tegmental area of the brain, dopamine expresses its social interaction features in relation to the number, concentration and activity levels of receptors in the particular individual depending on the history of stress levels and reactions of his/her forbearers. The release and reaction are genetic and subject to mutations in either direction. That one entire group may be aggressive and another group more passive, suggests that the variable nature of the dopamine reaction may be learned. Being "social" is associated with" normal" amounts and antisocial behavior, more than normal or less than normal. The actual response depends on the ratio of dopamine to serotonin receptors and their activity, the amount released and the response of the individual to excess or depleted dopamine.

(This supports the presence of "cruel vs kind" DNA in social behavior; feel-good dopamine at normal levels, vs feel-bad dopamine at high or low levels)

Serotonin, the "mood" hormone, contributes to happiness and feeling of well-being and responds to social factors and behavior in a better or worse manner. Acceptable social behavior coincides with just the right amount of serotonin, while high levels correlate with social anxiety and low levels link to depression. Hunger, over-eating, over-exposure to sunlight and too much exercise triggers the release of excess serotonin. The gut produces 80% with the rest coming from the brain and blood platelets.

An event or trigger mechanism releases feel-good or feel-bad hormones into the bloodstream. A positive feedback releases more a negative feedback shuts it down. More release may lead to repeated triggers which may become addictive. The same brain areas light up with feel-good activity as they do with cocaine. There are also the same withdrawal symptoms of reduced sleep and induced depression. Other social hormones include endorphins, which are released mainly upon exercise and lead to increased stamina and performance, lowered anxiety, calming and reduced pain and physical discomfort. Melatonin, a sleep regulator which also contributes to a calming mood; phenylethylamine, which acts like a "love molecule" of chocolate and sugar; ghrelin, a stress reduction hormone that leads to relaxation and regulator of hunger and satiety; and testosterone, released in both male and females when holding hands, caressing, eyes meeting, an arouser of sexual desire, especially high in females when ovulating, can all be classified as other social hormones. Tryptophan, a precursor of serotonin, and gamma-aminobutyric acid (GABA), an anxiety calming neurotransmitter, are also in the mix.

The main stress hormone is **cortisol,** which is released along with adrenalin in the presence of threat to elicit a fight-or-flight response. When the threat passes, cortisol turns off and full recovery occurs. However, when released in a constant drip as a chronic stressor, the receptors become overwhelmed, tolerance decreases and a slow deterioration of tissues and organ systems occur. Like dopamine, cortisol releases both feel-good and feel-bad hormones, the most prominent expressed depending on the situation and the individual. In addition, it influences the release of other hormones of aggression, like epinephrine, norepinephrine, plus hydrogen ions and reactive oxidative species (ROS), which may cause tissue damage by themselves. The response depends on the amounts, the trigger, and the individual involved in the response. Other social hormones include ghrelin, melatonin, and acetylcholine. Study: In research that began in 1958, the Siberian fox to dog experiments, Dmitri Belyaev, a Russian biologist researcher proposed that domesticated foxes had genes for social behavior as opposed to antisocial genes in wild foxes. The social foxes produce more serotonin (happy) and oxytocin (cuddly) than testosterone (aggressive). He and his team bred generations for friendliness and suggested that nature selected humans in the same way. The friendliest survived, thrived and reproduced, thus passing on the "social" genes. Though the study has flaws now under evaluation, the results suggest that we can breed foxes and other animals for friendliness. Running over 60 years and now being carried on by 85 year-old Lyudmila Trut, a biologist at the Russian Academy of Sciences, the experiment selects the tamest foxes and breeds each generation for increasing friendliness. We can also note that both the appearances and cognition of the foxes changed. The domesticated ones featured floppy ears, curved tail, and rounded snout; and were better at problem solving than their wild forebearers. The increase in cognition in foxes was associated with change in social behavior. Some 150 genes in the frontal cortex showed changes between aggression and tameness. "Behavioral temperament" appeared to be linked to the amount and type of protein produced, and by the genetic code for oxytocin, dopamine, serotonin and other social hormones.

The Genetics of Social Selection
(Kind and Cruel DNA)

Genetic instructions make proteins that affect social behavior.
Evolution selects those attributes that contribute most to survival.

Animals do not behave for the good of the species, but for the good of the individual to reproduce. The survival of the group enables reproduction, which is the primary drive behind social behavior. Male birds prancing and posturing to attract mates put themselves in danger by the showy display. Social behavior maximizes the chances of passing on copies of genes to the next generation.

The most cooperative early *Homo sapiens* enjoyed the best access to food and shelter, the best opportunities and chances for reproduction and the highest chances of survival within the group. They had the most kids and pass on their "social" genes. More oxytocin release had a positive effect with reward feedback for acceptable behavior. The oxytocin-dopamine reactions would have promoted a good feeling, heightened mood and a learned regulation of dopamine for the additive reaction instead of the blocking action. These actions and reactions had a positive effect on the early *Homo sapiens* in strengthening the bonds of their groups, bands and tribes.

As the population grew and groups ranged further into more threatening environments, interactions varied between hostility and pacifism. As man settled into villages and towns relying on agriculture and stored food surplus and material possession, threats and fears arose that triggered the expression of cruel DNA.

What sort of human deliberately kills his brother and family to secure his place as leader or for any other reason? What kind of people sweep in and slaughter an entire village and take its possessions? What DNA coding instructions produce the proteins that urge the brain to abduct and sell human beings into a life of abuse and destruction? What temperament produces a plan to gift small-pox infected blankets to Native Americans for their extermination? What sort of mind orders the wholesale murder of rubber workers in the Congo or an entire group of Europeans to be starved, gassed and shot? What people stand around and cheer as their compatriots burn another human being at the stake or lynch a neighbor from the limb of a tree? And what kind of heart sits by as the authorities take children from their parents at an imaginary border as punishment for the sin of being poor and desperate? These events occur when cruel DNA- produced hormones overwhelm the system to promote bad behavior.

Homo sapiens are programmed to be both social and antisocial. Whichever behavior dominated, depended on the type and amount of chemical reaction initiated by the genetic make-up, the environment and the prevailing situation.

Vignette #4. The Strange Case of Dr. Jekyll and Mr. Hyde by Robert Louis Stevenson, (1886) illustrates the duality of human behavior. The good, kind doctor experiments with his dark side and returns to "normal" by a self-concocted potion. When the transformation becomes automatic during sleep and waking, and then uncontrollable, all ends in disaster for those around him and for himself.

What makes some people friendly and others so unfriendly?

The answer is many factors: social selection granting access to reproduction, social mobility, rank on the social hierarchy, access to food and shelter, and health benefits. Primates have 98% the same DNA as humans and studies of gorillas, chimps and bonobos are helpful in illustrating this behavior. They live in groups; are willing and able to attack members of the same group, and adopt a hierarchy with a distinct alpha male in charge. Humans (hunter-gatherers) were more egalitarian, with shared power and materials, and the realization that cooperation worked better than domination and bullying. Basic sociality is genetic, but the gene expression as sociable or unsociable, is phenotypic and depends on environmental triggers.

The social life of the chimpanzee (*Pan troglodytes*), relies heavily on touch, communication sounds and responsive behavior, as does that of humans. There is intimacy and dependency often with an older sibling sharing in the infant's care. Group contact includes all individuals and socializing is free among all. When the group grows too large, it splinters off into subgroups that are more manageable (fission-fusion). Unlike early hominids, there is a ladder of importance with the alpha male and dominant females on the top in all activities, hunting-gathering, food sharing and grooming. Life is in the company of "others", where interaction equals success, reproduction and survival. Cooperation leads to food, comfort and defense, and conflicts are resolved by war. Murders and massacres are common.

Bonobos (*Pan paniscus*) have a female leader, are more social, and conflicts are resolved by grooming, as a greeting or to strengthen ties. Interactions lead more readily to connections and peace. With a brain wired to "connect" with others through social interactions, instructed predominantly by kind DNA, the new reactions used the previously unused cruel side of humans, also for survival. The good interactions and social relationships that were mutually beneficial to the group, were now showing how avoidance and shunning could benefit the individual and their closest relationships. In the body and mind, the oxytocin-dopamine effect shared chemical space with the cortisol-epinephrine effect. Good interactions store up positive hormone releases and bad interactions result in bad hormone releases. Chronicity leads to increased susceptibility to disease as the immune system becomes imbalanced. Natural social behavior, is when you hear a scream and get a chilling effect. When you see someone hurt, you feel the pain and rush to help. Endorphins, oxytocin, tryptophan and serotonin levels increase and cortisol decreases. Cooperation, group well-being, compassion, empathy, altruism, trust and bonding is all in effect. Antisocial behavior sees the craning neck at the site of an accident with no intention of assisting, desire to see someone in pain, to see a murder, individualism comes first, self-interest, I won't get involved with "others", is at the forefront. The chronic dripping of cortisol is prominent, while serotonin and endorphin levels are low, and oxytocin is almost non-existent.

In the natural world, the primary purpose of life is survival as a means toward reproduction and passing on of genes. Social interactions work toward this goal by ensuring good health and affording ample opportunities. As the brain developed it evolved social patterns of actions based on the degrees of threat present that would maintain safety and survival. While physical and emotional pain are received and acted upon in the same manner, the building of well-organized groups, with cooperation and effective social behavior, enhanced survival. Social connections enabled *Homo sapiens* to dominate and secure success.

Cooperation

In his social development, *Homo sapiens* 45,000 years ago established an egalitarian order based on sharing, which directly improved the health of the group through more variable and higher quality food, less conflict, more safety and more comfort. Survival behavior developed through active cooperation, the purpose of human interactions and trust, the basis. Together they enabled safety and survival through behaviors that benefitted the group over the individual. Hunting larger animals required teamwork, planning, and group participation based on social behavior. Cooperation reduced the stress of daily living since now he had someone else to depend on, to rely on, and to deliver. Cooperation lights up the brain's reward system, like chocolate and sugar. The society with a strong social structure has cooperation as its foundation. The society with a natural tendency to social interaction has more cooperation, which then fosters further cooperation. As the group enlarged, despite defectors and loners, its survival depended on the cooperators and their responses. Increased social activity led to stronger identity, friendships and more cooperation. Social interactions through teaching and learning promoted culture, which rewards the participants. It enabled the transmission of knowledge, attracted new ideas, diversity and advanced the society. With progress came a rapid evolution of intelligence and further complexity of the social structure.

Vignette #5. The Phoenicians worshipped a peaceful goddess instead of warlike male gods as in Judaism, Christianity and Islam. Excelling in "reading people", they chose social interactions instead of conflict to boost their trade. As they understood and respected each other and "others", the focus was on society building instead of on destruction. Without pre-occupation with a military, they made full use of cooperation skills to ensure success in preparing their boats for successful journeys and trade throughout the Mediterranean. With a singular purpose in trade, shared profits and expansion of trade routes, they managed to get along well with others, learned their ways and offered respect in exchange for group success. In 970 BCE, King David of Israel, died and was succeeded by his son, Solomon. Upon encountering King Hiram of Tyre (Lebanon), with mutual admiration and appreciation the two cooperated instead of going to war. Hiram gave Solomon cedar and fir timber to build the Temple in Jerusalem, and to make boats and Solomon gave Hiram 20 thousand measures of wheat for food for his household and 20 measures of pure oil. (Bible: 1 Kings 5:1-12).

When status competition and self-interest replace group cooperation, there is a decrease in social interactions. When greed and antisocial behavior emerge as "good" principles beneficial to the individual over the group, there is a decline in cooperation.

The mantra becomes, "Every man for himself."

Vignette #6: The Göbelki Tepe temple in Southeast Turkey is the oldest human constructed temple in world circa 11,000 BCE. Appearing before agriculture, it is a work event that required the cooperation of large group without domesticated animals or plants nearby for food. Without evidence of a "leader" or hierarchy, they did it with egalitarian means and purpose, to bring the people together. They accomplished this during times of high pro-social behavior. After 9000 BCE, large groups settled down, grew crops, owned land, set up enclosures and chose leaders. Eventually, as they gathered possessions and material became more important than relationships, some lived better than others and aggression dominated. Individual wealth outshone group success.

Cooperation to benefit the entire group continued, but it became more forced and less social. (Group-oriented behavior eventually gave way to self-interest, individualism and the profit over people we see today.) The history of the success of human settlement still relies on social harmony, morality, basic trust, alliances, defenses and community concerns. Hunter-gatherer groups became part settler/part nomadic so movement/migration had to be well- Coordinated with safety as a priority. Group success depended on the morality which was established through conscience. Sharing and punishment contributed to the social selection of participants whose activities benefitted the entire group. They suppressed alpha males by ostracizing, exiling or killing them. To attain a state of morality that worked for all, there was an internalization of rules, with any deviation punished by the group through shame, gossip and embarrassment and reward for participants, all effective factors in social selection.

Man is the only animal that blushes. This is because of a release of adrenaline as part of the fight or flight reaction, which dilates sub-epidermal blood vessels as evident by a reddening in light skin tones and a more subtle flush in darker skin tones. This reaction occurs in all humans in response to threat, being overwhelmed, or being caught breaking a social code. Suppression of the blush reflex may occur when one is so accustomed to breaking the rules or is unaware that anything is wrong that remaining calm controls the hormonal release. Lying as a way of life is devoid of embarrassment or anxiety. Blushing shows that one cares what other humans think of them. It is an innate physiological mechanism.

Gossip shapes public opinion in socializing, in shaping morality, in discouraging "big shot" mentality by shaming, incites collective action, and is very effective among friends who trust each other. Usually designed to bring the deviant into line and induce fear of a bad reputation, it is an early normal agent of social control. Abnormal gossip designed to hurt and repel, is dangerous and negative for the group.

Social selection preferred those with a "**conscience**", who had internalized the rules and stood by a solid morality, to ensure a fairer food distribution, punish alpha males, reward participants with better choices in quality nutrition for energy to further benefit to the group. Gene selection (usually by females) that allowed "cooperation and conscience" to evolve and flourish led to sexual success which favored more social genes. She chose the provider over the bully. Social selection evolved in favor of gossip to reduce poor reputations and enhance communications (language skills), genes for self-protection, self-control and reduced aggression. Social life required elements of conscience, adherence to group rules, punishment through shame and gossip, to make its contribution to the health of the group.

Cooperation played a significant role in survival and determination of balance between social and selfish genes. Genes were selected to benefit the carrier. Though early selection favored the "social", later genes moved toward the "selfish". A social carrier of selfish genes survived over a selfish carrier of selfish genes. With human development, migration, and settlements, the duality of behavior became more evident, with natural drivers being evolution, selection based on selfish principles, and social behavior, selection based on survival principles.

While still in small numbers, hunter-gatherers formed band societies, kept track of each other through identity markers and trusted each other through cooperative efforts. With survival success came time for social interactions and more reliable connections with each other and with the land. (Still not with materials). Wandering, collecting, toolmaking, they did all for the good of the band. Improved skills and weapons provided larger animals, more food, more protein, larger brain size and more time to "socialize". Morality and social control proved to be more efficient for group success than greed and hoarding. Social contacts with related and unrelated individuals slid easily into binding connections that enhanced the group. The dictum, "Do unto others" appears as standard behavior in ALL human groups since the Paleolithic era and was the groundwork of belonging and stress-free living.

Chimpanzees care for injured mates and later take part in an all-out vicious war. Elephants reassure youngsters in distress and visit graveyards to show remorse. Dolphins support sick companions, raise and support them near the surface of the water to breathe (prevent drowning). Humans show compassion, empathy, and meticulous care for one another, especially in times of catastrophic disaster, yet decline to wear face masks in a respiratory pandemic, as a clear slap in the face to elderly, disabled and most vulnerable, and reject social distancing, in refusing to sacrifice for the "common good". Social vs Antisocial behavior.

Early natural and social selection favored feel-good hormones over feel-bad hormones. Kind DNA dominated in the times of hunter-gatherers and cruel DNA emerged in the agricultural through Industrial Revolution and into modern times. Stress reactions were acute in the form of immediate physical threat rather than chronic in response to time constraint, responsibility, debt, intolerance, fear of loss of status, rank and war. Later humans with more complex lives tended experienced the reverse. The "Greed is Good" Gordon Gekko speech from the 1987 film, Wall Street, laid bare the modern societal mantra that led to the obscene wealth of CEO's and abject poverty of the unfortunate masses in the 21st century. Health-wise, the poor die early from disease, while the wealthy, having better access to prevention and treatment, are "immune". This level of inequality has a pronounced effect on social interactions and connections in the modern world.

Mechanisms of Socializing

Exhibiting open behavior and talking to people in a friendly way, acting in a manner that is acceptable to society, adapting to social needs or uses and actively taking part in a social group are all manners of socializing. The term came into use around 1765 and is synonymous with fraternizing, mingling, mixing, rubbing elbows with, going out with… (*Merriam-Webster Dictionary on line, Springfield, Mass, 2017*) Ancient man developed social skills from natural sources that were successful in procuring friends and partners in any setting and based on tribal loyalty, group safety and innate honor. Evolutionary requirements shaped social behavior. Successful social behavior was rewarded, and unsuccessful behavior was not. To be social, one needed both mental and physical capabilities. Self-confidence, an understanding of the habits and norms of the group, impulse control, recognition of identities, and acceptance of the value of others were the main factors required for success. On the encounter, the ability to communicate and imply emotional openness to enable the interaction, followed by the capacity to make the connection and keep it all but ensured further success.

The intention of social interactions was to achieve social connections that would benefit the group initially, and the individual eventually. Social connections grew out of quality interactions and desire to avoid loneliness. The solitary individual was vulnerable to the elements, predators and the inner decay of loneliness. Relationships cemented the societal groups and strengthened them. From these connections came the development of conscience, meaning and value, ascribed to self and other human beings.

The herd instinct, a concept of the group mind, afforded social behavior determined by survival instincts and the social environment. When in danger, the individual has a better chance when herded together than in isolation. Likewise, the individual does better emotionally and physically, when in a friendly environment, as opposed to a hostile one.

"People may forget what you said, but they will never forget how you made them feel." Carl W. Buechner

Hominids split from chimpanzees some 6-million years ago, ventured out into the savanna about 300,000 years ago, grouped together for defense, shelter and essential nutrition, improved physical size, locomotion and brain size and composition, pooled innovations and raised social connections to another level with cooperation and language. Shared labor, meals and planning for the future led to increased social bonding and solid group formation, with old and young, leaders and followers, thinkers and doers, all working together to increase creativity, production and enhance success. Socializing developed furthest around the African campfires. There was a natural desire to gather and interact. Storytelling, myth building, identity formation, planning, ritual, music, art, dance, dining and religion all laid foundations, grew and flourished.

Division of labor and character also took seed and grew. Some were better than others at the hunt, at the campsite, and on the trail. Food distribution and competition for reproductive rights were stimuli for social development. Some were better at planning, some were physically stronger and more dexterous, and others had better social skills. Homo sapiens are born with genes for social and anti-social behavior whose dominant expression is influenced by parental investment, kinship experience, and group culture.

Social interaction around the campfire revealed that those good at public speaking were accepted and those who were not, were rejected. Pro-social genes maximized and antisocial genes minimized.

Vignette #7: The social life of Marie Antoinette, archduchess of Austria, dauphine of France, Queen of Versailles was a disaster as she never "connected" with her court or her subjects. She hated etiquette, avoided the pomp and circumstance, avoided "people", yet wanted their affection, though "attractive and elegant", she was only nice to those she favored, did not handle hostility well, felt pity at the distress of the poor, but never knew how to express it effectively. Not good at choosing her "friends", she had social interactions, but failed miserably at "connections". She had a few friends (Madame Polignac) but no meaningful relationships. The King, Louis XVI, was her "puppet", lived apart most of the time and had little meaning in her life.

Vignette #8. Some people are better than others at social skills. My daughter, Sharilyn, is the classic "social butterfly", a term given to her by her kindergarten teacher. Friendly, kind, funny and positive, she became the legendary friend, the one any and everybody turns to when confronted by impending depression; the one to suggest and organize the party; and the one who can turn a nerdy recluse into a happy gallant. These traits are innate in everybody, but the art of socializing in any setting is truly a gift and expression of natural talent.

Communication: Successful socializing involves two aspects, non-verbal and verbal communications. The basics involve four phases, encounter, interaction, connection, and bonding. One does not always lead to the other. The encounter entails body language, reduced threat, attraction, and welcome. The salute, wave and extension of the hand showed no weapon no threat. The interaction entailed use of communication, first through touch (infant and mother, siblings, extended family) then by language development to show intentions more precisely. Connections arose through repetitive group hunting, food sharing, entertainment, and conversation. As carnivores around campfires, they shared mythology, imagination, biological needs, and discussion, all toward a unity of purpose, ensuring survival and perpetuation of the genes. The satisfaction centers in the brain were rewarded with a positive sense of belonging and establishment of security.

"Entertainment is the greatest socializing
force in the world." Daniel Beaty

Man has an innate desire to gather, entertain and be entertained. Homo erectus, the upright man, 400,000 years ago, gained control of fire, set up protective shelters and cooked food. Fire extended the day into night, providing time for leisure and socializing. Storytelling, art, music, and theater all enhanced the feel-good hormones as well as delivery of instructions. The power of being able to feed information into a group of people on which to act, constructively or destructively provided a powerful impetus to gather.

In northwest Amazonia, the urge to gather brings the people of distant tribes together for festivals, myth recitals and ceremonies, on a regular basis. Providing a time and place for young men and women to meet, interact and marry, it also serves to avoid incest. In more than one group, the mate should speak a different language and it is incumbent for each to learn that of the other.

Storytelling around the fire, in the caves, was a social interaction in a safe environment and a chance to practice "communications" and provide entertainment. The better communicators were heroes, second ones fed (after hunters and warriors) and had the second-best chance at reproduction. With better nutrition, relaxation time and intellectual stimulation, brain size increased and stories became more complex. The hunt, origins, fantasies, dream telling, past and future, tales of "others", gossip as behavior control, things that work, trust, and understanding, all designed to release feel good hormones. The campfire provided the venue to keep track of everyone in the group, their morality, unity, and keeping children close (fear tactic myths).

Vignette #9. In Denmark, home comfort (hygge) is the art of creating a warm atmosphere and enjoying the good things in life with good people. It uses the warm glow of candlelight and the warmth and pleasure of the fireplace for entertainment and to reinforce social connections.

Stories connect people, help to define who we are, where we came from and where we are going. They instill and maintain the morality essential to effective functioning of the group. Successful leaders use pertinent stories to connect with their subjects and build trust. Ineffective ones tell lies or impart nothing at all. The ability to communicate, to make the listener feel the story, is very effective unifying force in a group. Stories can put distance between something good and something bad; can help you relax, sleep, and regenerate; and can suppress fear and threat. There are born storytellers and attentive listeners; the talent is both innate and learned. Every culture has its tradition of stories derived from the campfires of Africa and the migration trails to all six inhabitable continents and surrounds.

Vignette #10. A pre-school boy all of three years old used to bring the same pile of books for his father to read aloud before they took their afternoon siestas. The little boy knew all the stories by heart and would continue reading long after his father fell asleep, in order to put himself to sleep. It worked. That little boy was me.

Vignette #11. President Xi Jinping starts every major speech with a story depicting some aspect of China's history. It works to engage and hold the audience for what follows.

Just like the innate biological reaction of "blushing" reinforces conscience and morality, shared **laughter** is a social reaction to internal or external stimulation and associated with the expression of emotions. Laughter enhances inhalation, stimulates the heart, lungs and muscles, increases endorphins (feel-good hormones) release from the brain. Besides being good for health, it enhances social interactions and connections. Like yawning and aping, laughing can be "catching".

Music as communication, cooperation, campfire entertainment, messaging, and imparting of ideas derives from and influences social connections within the group. Bird bone flutes from 14,000 years ago provide some archaeological evidence of music as a human instinct. Brain wiring to receive and deliver music (like in animals) is in the pleasure centers and areas of heightened emotions. Music joined stories in giving pleasure and serving to enhance social bonding, along with athletics, body decoration, art, etiquette, folklore, joking and family dining. Around age 12, the individual "notices" music, at 14, one identifies with it and at 20 becomes dexterous and perfect in mastering the delivery. Music crosses group lines. The South Americans enjoy African Benga music and the Chinese gravitate to European classical. When friends appreciate the same sounds, it becomes a social event. Music brings different groups together and can be a vehicle for social bonding. It can be a mark of group identity and a link to personality formation.

Vignette #12: In the 1870's, chamber music at the home of Louis and Pauline Viardot on the rue de Douai, in Paris, on Thursday nights in the 1870s, drew in friends, artists, composers, and conversationalists for the enjoyment and appreciation of the arts and of each other. Similar parties on other nights of the week at friends' homes started the development of a stable network of personal connections, which continued to thrive in the salons and now the cafés and restaurants.

Music is an adaptation trait useful for sex selection as in mating rituals, social bonding and cohesion (collective music-making and appreciation encourages social cohesion), campfire songs, promotion of feelings of togetherness, and cooperation (marching songs). Certain individuals with demonstrable brain damage and mental impairment, like Williams Syndrome, are good at playing and listening to music and are social. While Autism Spectrum Disorders (ASD) are asocial, incapable of empathizing and do not comprehend or feel music (may play but not "feel it"). Prior to the nineteenth century, music was primarily a background to social interactions, in parties, at dinners, and balls. With compositions and symphonies, it was transformed into an art form to be heard and appreciated in the silence of concert halls, chambers, and opera houses.

Ancient humans likely **danced** to attract mates some 1.5-million years ago. The ability to came with the same muscles, body shape, flexibility and balance required for walking and running. Dance was a natural form of expression of pleasure and desire for courtship.

The good dancers displayed their fitness and coordination as positive attributes for selection. It is not much different today. Dance moves could communicate, bond and entertain around the campfire and were a powerful social factor. According to research by Dr. Steven Mithen, archaeologist at the University of Reading, England, good dancers had genes for higher levels of serotonin and vasopressin, two behavior hormones that made them more social. Besides releasing happiness chemicals from the brain, dancing afforded exercise with increased blood flow in healthy small blood vessels, increased cognition if following a dance sequence, movement that connected the physical body to nature (imitation of animal and plant motion), and the release of additional happiness chemicals, oxytocin, and dopamine.

Study: *Frontiers in Aging, NeuroScience, April 2018.* In subjects in their 60s and 70s, researchers tested the white matter specialized cells of the brain for wiring efficiency in messaging between neurons. Young cells showed rapid transmission and older cells were considerably slower. Testing by MRI in three groups (a brisk walk, gentle stretch and balance training, and dance with country choreography), by aerobic fitness and mental capacities revealed that: the first two groups showed "degeneration "of white matter, slight thinning of size and number of connections between neurons which was evident in the oldest and most sedentary subjects. The dance group showed improvement in white matter in the fornix in terms of speed processing and memory. All did better on cognitive tests even if the white matter was skimpier, however, activities that involved both moving AND socializing led to an increase in mental abilities of ageing brains.

Music and Dance have positive influences on
socializing, as well as on health.

Dining emerged around the campfire where and when food was shared, the correct amounts, intentions read and cognitions developed, reciprocity exhibited, new ideas exchanged and trust established within and between groups. *Companero*, a combination word from the Latin "copain", with bread, in Spanish indicates a friend with whom one shares a meal. Besides providing nutrition, food offers a social environment second to none. Sharing food is an evolutionary activity in which social bonds are expressed. Friendship over hoarding. The stranger is always welcomed with food. Gifts of food were made as symbols of friendship and recognition of need. Social structure was developed over food; ideas and planning of the hunt; best food gathering sites; division and assignments of labor; who would lead and who would submit; news and gossip; and food preparation itself. The brain grew further from a change in food source from plants to meat, new tools to cut and retrieve the meat, fire to cook it, the development of enzymes to digest it and better wiring from the addition of seafood. More complex nutritional options afforded better ways and opportunities to interact while eating. In-cave or cave-side dining became not only for nourishment, but a time for social bonding.

Dining today is a sign of a settled society, a ritual offering of gratitude and appreciation, a triumph of society over the untamed world through the taming of food. The transformation of wild animals and plants by humans into food is a social act requiring cooperation, skills and "socializing" in "breaking bread", sharing and interaction. The setting itself with pottery, cooking fires, ovens, utensils and accompanying conversation is "social". Dining is a natural phenomenon.

The forest and savannas and oases gave way to the agora, the site of trade of goods and information and goodwill, became the marketplace present is almost all cultures and societies. Markets would have originated at territorial borders, to swap goods and stories, do business face-to-face and interact. Success of the participants would carry over to the next generation. As interactions lead to connections subsequent encounters may have led to marriages between members of different societies, to contribute to the health of the society. Spouses visiting "home" would have entailed different languages spoken. Being bilingual because of intergroup connections was always desired and valued. Even today, the ability to talk one's way out of a compromising situation un another language is a valuable tool for survival.

The tradition of *"Buen provecho"*, when someone wishes you in Spanish to "enjoy your meal", whether they are passing by your table or said by the server after delivering your meal, is especially evident in Puerto Rico, Mexico and several other Latino countries. Literally it means "good profit", it is a greeting for and by anyone having a meal and indicates the wish for the diner to have good digestion. More than anything, it is a courtesy acknowledging the presence of others. The feel-good hormone reaction elicited by this greeting, relaxes and aids in digestion. Remember that 80% of serotonin is made in the gut. And just as important, it is a courtesy acknowledging the presence of others at the dining site.

Dessert, like fine wine, is an experience that brings everyone together. It helps to close the appetite, add carbohydrates for balance, and is meant to be shared, as cake is sliced, cookies divided up and pudding is dished out. Note the Greek restaurant tradition of giving a free small dessert at the end of the meal, especially to strangers. Besides being a perfect way to end the meal, it endears the server to the recipient in a "connection", often, forever. Dessert prolongs the visit, adds to the comradery, conviviality (eat, drink and enjoy). There is a difference in the meal's value, between solitary eating and communal dining, as measured in social bonding, the results of cooperation. Dining moved from the prehistoric campsites to the taverns of the new settlers. Babylonian homes had built-in counters from which the women served homemade beer, bread, sweets, soups, and leftovers to neighbors and travelers It became an extension of the home, as one of first places for "socializing", discovering relationships about each other and about themselves.

Fast forward to the 18th century when dining together became a French art form. The taverns grew into bistros, brasseries, cafes, and restaurants. The Paris "bistro" became a social institution where people would lunch together at the same spot for years on end. After the Revolution (1789) when the chefs of the aristocracy were suddenly out of work, they opened eateries to serve all three meals at moderate prices developing into art forms of degustation and conversation. By the 1860s, people of all trades met and connected over shared ideas, politics, trade, art and gossip. The diners became the offices of the actively involved. Les Deux Magots, a brasserie opened in 1885, at 6 Place Saint Germain des Pres, in Paris, (my favorite) opened as a "coal café" selling coffee, wine and beer then home-cooked meals to visitors, workers and locals. This site saw many a social introduction that led to interactions and connections that influenced the twists and turns of Parisian history.

Several Spanish tapas bars, like Madrid's Restaurant Botin, originated as a waystation for travelers by horse into and out of the city and quickly became meeting centers for the movers and shakers as well as the professional gossips. The German brauhaus, English pub, Italian trattoria and Greek cafes all started with the provision of food, space for congregation and impetus for conversation, where everyone had a right to an opinion and strangers could become friends. (*Contrast this way of life with the American saloon, which excluded others (Native Americans, Blacks, Mexicans) where guns and gambling were the units of conversation, which gave way to fast-food establishments hardly the place for friendly congregation, TV dinners, desk lunches and home delivery, quite the contrary to social interaction and connections.*)

Cell phones and social distancing provide further disconnect from each other).

Dining with someone else in a relaxed setting provided the atmosphere for good digestion and absorption, and release of feel-good hormones from both internal and external stimuli. Communal dining improves eating habits and healthy choices providing your companions are aware of the advantages of diverse cuisines in offering a good chance to explore the world, and a better chance that the interactions will become connections.

"Do not tell me what you had for dinner, tell me with whom you dined." Greek saying

"Knowing how to behave at a fine restaurant is a telltale measure of social maturity."
Marilyn vos Savant, columnist and writer

"Excellent food and good company are two of life's simplest yet greatest pleasures."
Pinterest.com

Travel can be both uplifting and an educational contribution to being "cultured". Learning new things, communicating, and interacting with foreigners, "travel is fatal to prejudices, bigotry and narrow-mindedness." (Mark Twain, Innocents Abroad, 1869. Fear and hatred become dispelled as the unknown becomes known. Acceptance leads to socializing. Which expands the range and increases your choices of encounters and connections. Or travel can promote snobbery. "I have been there and you have not." Or it can become a way of life.

"I feel like a nomadic Tatar. The sense of settlement is not in me. Any house I have is like a tent." (Ivan Turgenev, Russian writer)

Social interactions across cultures show other ways of interacting with each other. Gift giving, an offer of interaction and invitation to reciprocate, to unite and establish bonds of connection, was an ancient form of social engagement. Man, the social species adopted ten commandment rules for community survival in practically all cultures, as the basis of a society. In many Polynesian cultures, empathy and kindness were valuable social skills which displayed courage and strength. And then, there were the Spaniards, whose obsession with gold led them to commit atrocities against and alienate so many native cultures. Human nature contains the capacity for interaction and friendship through cooperation and empathy, which builds toward social connections that are productive and last throughout life. Biology and sociology are interrelated and natural selection favors both. The duality of man, the social animal, manifests itself as calmness and kindness, Jesus, Buddha, Gandhi or as aggression and violence, Hitler, Stalin, PolPot. *Homo sapiens* can be innately good or innately bad, and most are a bit of both. There appears to be two systems, *Social Kindness and Antisocial Cruelty*, each involving a chemical hormonal release mechanism. We seem to love those like us and hate those unlike us (others). (*Recently heard at US rallies "lock her up," "send them back," "build that wall."*)

Study done at the University of Amsterdam concluded that kindness is limited to one's own group. There is affection for friends with expressions of unity and aversion to strangers seen as threatening enemies. We are hard-wired for kindness and also for cruelty. Hence the niceness of Scandinavians towards each other and animosity towards "others". The kind Danish hygge and the vicious Viking cruelty to "others" in repeated raids and institution of slavery. We saw the dual personalities classic, Jekyll and Hyde, play out in the gleeful anticipation of revenge in the first Gulf War in 1990 (GHW Bush) "to destroy and kill as many Iraqis as possible to punish Saddam Hussein for being Saddam Hussein." For the Iraqi War of 2003, (GW Bush) there was a total commitment and happiness with the invasion, to destroy as much of the country and kill as many Iraqis as possible, although they did nothing. Social or Antisocial? The massacre of Tutsi's and Twa and moderate Hutus, by radical Hutus (1994 Rwanda), wholesale genocides of Jews by the Nazis, Africans & Native Americans by "settlers in America, were all fueled by fear and threat dressed up as hatred. This cruelty is DNA ingrained, the same as kindness. The capacity to show reactive aggression, such as killing for passion, justified defense, and loss of self-control may be explained in terms of self-preservation as a part of survival. Planning and carrying out an execution is both antisocial and natural.

The Greater Good Science Center at UC Berkeley examines the scientific roots of human kindness with a focus on the science of happy and compassionate people with strong social bonding ability and altruistic behavior. Their publication, the Greater Good magazine, issues articles on peace-making vs war mongering, selfishness vs sharing, and meanness vs caring, as both features are in our DNA. Which one gets expressed over the other, depends on environmental circumstances and specific situations warranting a response. The origin of each expression lies in motherhood and infancy, with oxytocin promotion of love, trust and generosity and cortisol taking the lead in cruelty and aggression. The development of the socializing mechanisms takes another hit when confronted with the social caste system of India. Over millennia, priests outranked kings, over warriors, merchants, artisans, serfs, and untouchables, Dalits, on the bottom. They held these positions from cradle to grave with each life being a punishment for past heritage. Social humiliation was okay and expected. The rape of women was and still is the only time the upper classes can touch a Dalit. This is not very social and not good for collective health.

Health Benefits of Socializing

Social factors are a huge determinant of good physical and mental health and well-being (life quality). Health is "the ability of a biological system to acquire, convert, allocate, distribute, and use energy sustainably." (*World Health Organization*). Good health is the positive status of the body, mind and spirit, and not only the absence of disease. The combination of happiness (joy and contentment) and good health contributes to wellbeing.

There is a direct association of social interactions and connections with good health through relaxation (feel-good hormone release) that reduces the chronic immune response intensity and frequency, reduces inflammation, and boosting health. The endogenous brain releases neurotransmitters, serotonin, oxytocin, dopamine, endorphins and epinephrine in just the right amounts to control happiness and cortisol and adrenalin with ample recovery to ensure protection and feelings of security. The genes for mood and behavior make just the right proteins for kindness, compassion, and happiness. Low social activity, antisocial behavior, fear of threat, anxiety, and social isolation release high levels of stress hormones. The constant assault on and erosion of the immune system makes the body weaker and more susceptible to disease and addicted to whatever brings relief. The constant release of cortisol and adrenalin without recovery leads to depression, misery, inner loneliness, and nerve, muscle and organ dysfunction.

Friendliness releases feel-good hormones, pro-social positivity enhances the immune system. Fear and anxiety raised upon encounters with strangers, promote antisocial negativity, releasing stress hormones that enhance inflammation that leads to tissue and organ dysfunction. Study: The social behavior of mice and humans and of ants and humans:

#1 meets #2: they are strangers: -> both increase stress hormones, decrease empathy/ close, and both show health issues

#1 meets #2: they are strangers: -> #2 blocks stress hormones, shows compassion /opens up and beams or becomes vulnerable and develops anxiety, both show health issues

#1 meets #2: they are familiar: ->both reduce stress hormones, both increases empathy/ both open and connect, both remain healthy

Martin LJ, et al. Curr Biol. 2015. Reducing social stress elicits emotional contagion of pain in mouse and human strangers. They show that empathy for pain in others in both humans and mice is stronger between familiars. It is less evident among strangers because of higher stress levels between strangers. The pain from the stress of a social encounter with an unfamiliar can be blocked by blocking the endocrine stress response. *Martin LJ, Tuttle AH, Mogil JS. The Interaction between pain and social behavior in humans and rodents. –NCBI Curr Top Behav Neurosci. 2014* How social interaction, empathy, learning and social stress can modulate pain sensitivity and behavior. There is biochemical evidence that energizing effects result directly from powerful connections to family and friends, community support and belonging. Mental sharpness and physical energy can overcome adversity by activating the stress response system (SRS) to conserve energy via the HTP (hypothalamus-thalamic-pituitary pathway) oxytocin and the 5- HTP (tryptophan/serotonin) activity to maintain contentment and well-being.

Social vs Antisocial… which prevails? What makes one social and the other, selfish? In early man, social behavior that arose and evolved within and between groups had definite health benefits. Cooperation in hunting, building and defense against a common predator led to physical safety and mental security. Socializing reduced the likelihood of disease transmissions by development of group resistance as opposed to the loner being more susceptible to predators and at risk of disease upon encountering pathogen. Socializing increased the reproductive chances and effects. Compassion, empathy, and friendliness were more appealing in a small group than the solitary me-first, too-bad-for-you, always anxious outsider.

Socializing promotes good health in several ways. It creates new neural connections between brain cells, helps build a protective reserve of functional neurons to minimize memory loss later in life and reduces toxic levels of oxidative products in the neurons of the hippocampus (memory and learning center) by reducing stress hormone levels (cortisol). Low levels of cortisol are linked to better cognition. Connecting with others increases a state of relaxation that reduces levels of interleukin-6, a substance usually associated with chronic inflammation. High levels are associated with dementias, heart disease, cancer and neurological disorders. Neural mechanisms drive social behavior and can be identified by functional magnetic resonance imaging (fMRI) which shows which areas of the brain are activated by social positive and negative factors. Some areas correspond to other mammals and some are unique to humans. "*The 'I' in illness is Isolation and the crucial letters in wellness are 'we'* ", a quote from The Heart Speaks: A Cardiologist reveals the secret language of healing, by Mimi Guarneri. From Medical News Today (1/5/19) A study in the Journal of Brain, Behavior and Immunity, by Jennifer Graham-Engeland of Penn State University… showed that negative moods have a direct effect on the immune system. Frequent experiences of or exposure to negative emotions (antisocial behavior) from both sides led to immune system dysfunction, inflammation (increase in proinflammatory cytokines) and stress and anxiety with discernible effects on physical health. Chronic stress has a direct effect on memory and acute or chronic distress affects heart health with increased risk of stroke.

Study: *Hostility and Pain are related to inflammation in older adults. JE Graham et al.* Repeated hostility and pain perception lead to anti-social behavior, which associates with chronically elevated inflammation factors in the immune system, that may maintain negative emotions and more pain. 2006

Study: In *The Healthy Ageing Brain:* Psychotherapy in Australia, Louis Cozolino draws from brain research that good health is linked directly to the human relationships we form and maintain as we age. In a California study, Preventing dementia, women over age 78, with large social networks and daily social contact had 26% less risk of developing dementia than those without such relationships. (Contact via email and telephone also were relevant.) Many other factors come into play, but the basic establishment of social connections is clear.

Study: Researchers at Johns Hopkins University, tracked 147 pairs of male twins for 28 years. They found that men also benefit from social connections in that cognitive and social activity during midlife significantly reduced the risk of dementia in later years. The activities consisted of visiting friends and relatives, participation in club functions, and home hobbies shared with others. Study: Harvard researchers compiling data on over 50-year-olds found that those who were most active socially had a lower rate of memory decline than those who were more isolated. Study: The MacArthur Foundation Research Study on Successful Aging (1985-1996) found that strong social networks were associated with lower cortisol levels in people aged 70 to 79 years old, who had better cognitive performance and overall health.

Interacting with other people exercises the brain and keeps it healthy. The anatomy and biochemistry of social interactions is the same for physical and mental stresses. Love and hate, physical and mental pain occupy the same brain areas. The mode of actions and reactions are similar.

Avoiding pain (threats) and deriving pleasure (rewards) are the driving forces in the motivation to socialize. The first great need is the infant- mother care relationship. Any threat to this connection is painful. It shapes social behavior and feelings well into adulthood. It can be harmful both if unsatisfied and when supplied in excess. It is the basis of the social network and foundation for basic physical and emotional health. There is a direct association of socializing to relaxation (feel-good hormone release) which leads to a "normal" immune response intensity and frequency, a low inflammation index, good health and slower ageing. Study: In Getting Social: The impact of social networking usage on grades amongst college students, Matthew Stollak, et al, exposed the positive consequences of high social connections as GPA increases in intellectual performance, better cognitive functions, and increase in dopamine receptors in the lateral prefrontal cortex. Socializing in a school setting (K through college) is essential for good health. Lack of social interactions with low connections often lead to low social development and low age-appropriate social behavior. Social Pain is evident in not belonging, being bullied, a decrease in cognitive resources, leading to physical and mental pain, and decreased health.

The benefits to health from social interactions include avoidance of isolation, anxiety, depression, loneliness and the reduction of risk of cardiovascular disease and dementia. The release of feel-good hormones and expression of kind DNA gives a significant boost to the immune system, mental sharpness, and central nervous system function. Especially for seniors, when social interactions take the form of volunteering, charity work, taking a class, learning new, group physical activity, cuisine, and combine with stress control and toxic avoidance, it fulfills the six basic strategies for good health. (*Natural Health and Disease Prevention (2016): balanced diet, exercise,*

stress control, mental stimulation, avoidance of toxins and social connec-
tions.) A L.Anduze, MD

Doing Good provides health benefits and goes both ways.

The main health benefits of successful social interactions are the prevention of feelings of loneliness, sharpening of the memory and cognitive skills, the establishment and increase in sense of well-being that prevents metabolic disease from negligence, better quality of life and the overall increase in longevity.

The adverse effects of antisocial behavior from self-interest, egoism, aggression, posturing, and survival of the fittest mentality giving rise to hierarchal inequality manifests as anxiety, hypertension, cardiovascular disease, neurological and gastrointestinal disorders, depression, paranoia and mistrust and rises to prominence in times of scarcity in which constraints like conscience and morality seem to disappear. "They are coming to take our jobs, our guns, our women. They are coming to take America," is a recent example of the mantra designed to instill fear and anger, for the purpose of arousing violent behavior.

A paradox arises. The initial biochemical reaction associated with antisocial aggression is the release of "feel-good hormones", delight in hurting others, from the expression of cruel DNA. In those with a slight "conscience and tinge of morality" this rapidly transfers to the release of "feel-bad" hormones, that take a toll on the body and mind. In those humans with a total lack of guilt and shame, the feel-good hormones dominate, "normally" associate with aggressive behavior and continue to benefit the mind and body as long as nothing interferes with the process. Most times, the absence of conscience continues unchecked. Other times, the mind becomes diseased with aberrations and the body too eventually fails. The Roman emperors, Nero and Caligula, went quite "mad" during and after their maltreatments of fellow humans. It can also be argued that the genes (cruel DNA), in place long before the acts took place, directed the atrocities committed.

It is not the materials you own or how long you live, but the quality of your life that really counts. And good health is a powerful factor in determining that quality. Unfortunately, many treatments for antisocial behavior involve taking antipsychotic drugs and complicated psychoneurological procedures, with little or no attention given to the root causes of the problems. With antisocial behavior, try using with nourishment with foods rich in L-tyrosine, a dopamine precursor, that boost serotonin levels in the blood, (duck, turkey, dark chocolate, oatmeal, cheese). The best treatment is not to get sick in the first place. Avoid the "what can I take for this and that?" and, use instead, "what can I do to achieve good health". One of the most enjoyable and natural strategies for good health is engagement in social interactions that lead to stable connections.

A good friend and a neighborly chat, volunteering in the community and group activities contribute to the personal and the well-being of the entire society.

Heuristic Thinking

The Survival brain evolved to escape from predators, endure climate changes, find food, resist disease, and socialize for reproduction, comfort, and the innate drive to belong. Brain growth concentrated in the neocortex (outer layer), which became the seat of social activity. As the groups enlarged *Homo sapiens* needed to keep track of all the participants. Recognition of friend or foe, needs and intentions, and development of trust drove further increases in size and intelligence. Selection then provided the means of developing the Heuristic brain enabling someone to learn something new for themselves; such as multiple uses for a simple tool or a new concept; cooked food being easier to digest than raw. Thinking outside the box; a "gut feeling" for use of something for other than traditional use; away from automatic thinking. When successful, feel-good hormones would release in abundance. Social skills became favored as being open to "others"; open to diversity; open to change. Interacting with those of different cultures, they widely accepted as original what they had to offer as new and effective. Ancient humans freely and readily went outside his comfort zone and found social interactions and connections that provided opportunities for stress relief and a higher level of comfort and security. Heuristic thinking provided innovations that challenged the neocortex to put aside automatic thoughts for a while and use new ones to develop further. The ultimate result was better health.

Study: at Durham University, UK, Drs Julie Van de Vyver, asst professor of psychology and Professor Richard Crisp, Head of Department of Psychology examines the health benefits of heuristic thinking. To raise creativity levels in thinking, they asked participants to imagine someone outside the stereotype, for example, a male nurse, female neurosurgeon, female truckdriver, male nanny, i.e. performing a different function than expected. Or the experience of living abroad or outside the neighborhood. These thoughts enhanced creativity and performance across the board. Engagement and inclusion are beneficial to brain health. A southern USA backyard barbecue gathering that includes all ethnicities in the vicinity, watching foreign films, reading books about different people and cultures, and making new friends by volunteering or otherwise seeking interactions, is far better for your health than shouting abusive slogans and brandishing guns at "those people". When one "crosses over" and engages all groups of all ages, cultures and ethnicities, whether in the arts, literature, theatre, and music, (jazz musicians attending an opera, reggae and rappers attending a Broadway musical), one enhances connectedness and general kindness, nurtures new and inclusive friendships, and increases personal growth and knowledge. These extraordinary interactions, promote good health for both the individual and the society.

The ageing brain shrinks (atrophy) and exhibits cognitive decline after the 40s at a rate of about 5% each 10 years, then declines at a higher rate in the 70s, because of less blood supply, oxygen and nutrients available and the natural apoptosis (self-destruction) of the frontal cortex. Thinking exercises, along with a balanced diet, adequate physical activity and quality sleep increase blood circulation in the brain to maintain some semblance of good health. With natural ageing, there is less word usage and storage space. This shows that more communication, making new friends and learning new things as we age are good for brain health.

Social Connections In Nature

On the study of trees in a forest, the strong need the weak to act as a unit to protect against excessive heat and winds and hold the soil fast. Paradoxically, sturdy trees get sick or injured and depend on the weaker ones for support through sharing water, essential chemical and physical protection, efficient signaling and extensive root networks. A tree can only be as strong as the forest that surrounds it when acting like an intact community. People who hate and fight each other are weaker than if they stand together. This fact of nature is universal.

"A smile will gain you ten more years of life."

Practical Benefits of Socializing

Conserving energy, bonding and sense of belonging, loving and being loved, being useful and needed, all calmed the Central Nervous System. Positive social interactions had a direct soothing and energizing effect on the entire organism. The appreciation of and for others, the love and support of family, friends, and community are all energy-boosting, while unbalanced and unhealthy relationships are energy-draining. The act of socializing, having much to do with a society's perception of its members and its response to those in need by those with plenty, is a purely humanitarian response. Drawing people in can build a society positively. A country that excludes others and walls itself off based on negative perceptions of others, loses both physically and mentally. Socializing confers dignity upon the donor and value upon the receiver.

*"Voici mon secret: Il est très simple: on ne voit bien qu'avec le Coeur; L'essentiel est invisible pour les yeux." Le Petit Prince....*It is only with the heart that we see well; what is essential is invisible to the eye… the little prince, in a lesson from his friend, the fox.

Every human has both inner and outer worth, dignity, which others must recognize and acknowledge in order to fulfill a successful life. Socializing is a means of recognizing one's existence and conferring this basic dignity. (*When you pass me on the beach or in a hallway or in a restaurant) and avert your gaze, you deny my existence, you deny me the right to dignity.) Francis Fukuyama in "Identity"*…

The human drive for recognition is an engine that propels the need for socializing.

Compassion and Heartlessness

Social Selection: we pass genes on for compassion, altruism, empathy, conscience, extra-familial generosity, shame, heartlessness, punishment and direct cruelty.

How and why were some people kind and others cruel? How and why were some communicative and creative and others averse and destructive? Why are some people peaceful and others warlike? Why do some lives matter and others do not?

The compassion instinct is a sympathetic awareness of the distress of others and a desire to alleviate it that arose and evolved from hominids needing each other for survival. This disappeared for some 500 years of heartless mistreatment of native peoples, with exploitation and racism, which has continued into modern times with group brutality, hate crimes, withholding of healthcare for the vulnerable, and basic human rights, meanness, humiliation, dehumanization and taking children away from their parents. The refusal of some groups to live in a society of social equals is not a natural behavior of early *Homo sapiens*. A society where some citizens cheer at the misfortunes of the poor is not a healthy one.

What kind of person will you be? Which brain will win out? The intelligent frontal cortex side provides access to better food and sex through compassion and morality. The primitive reptilian limbic side supplies heartlessness and cruelty, that takes what it wants without concern or consideration of the group. In ancient man, there was a natural dislike of injustice as seen in an instinct for fair food distribution that benefitted the entire group. Cooperation and sharing was preferred over hoarding and fighting over food and sex. Since numbers enhanced survival, the elimination of an offending individual was a less viable option than inclusion with forced modification of the offensive behavior. The response was innate and DNA-oriented.

Compassion was an essential tool for survival, a sympathetic consciousness of other's distress and an instinctive desire to ease it. Babies cry in reaction to sensing or seeing hurt in others but are as yet incapable of doing much.

The group-oriented human under threat learns compassion contributes to building confidence. A determined, confident group with reliable members for support would contribute more to survival than a group with neglectful members lacking in feeling and loaded with meanness.

What are the consequences of lack of compassion? Feel-good hormones released from both responses, are eventually transformed into feel-bad hormones in the presence of heartlessness. It requires more energy to produce and sustain meanness than kindness. Cruel abusive humans are constantly distrustful and on guard. True relaxation and stress-free development is in short supply.

It takes more energy to be cruel than to be good

We make choices to perceive some as friends and designate others as enemies. Putting others first, interacting and connecting reduces anxiety and provides inner peace. Putting others as enemies ensures constant conflict requiring protection against a real or perceived force, and keeps one in a perpetual state of defense. This turmoil sickens both the mind and the body.

Humans developed a brain built to feel others' pain (kind DNA) as well as to inflict pain on others without remorse cruel DNA. Whichever was expressed the most depended on the quality and quantity of that present, the environment, character of the threat or the fear, and the society's traditions. The humane in humanity may only be good if and when a disaster threatened all. Though both were innate, compassion with the release of feel-good hormones resulting in good health all around competed with heartlessness based on fear with the chronic release of stress-related hormones leading to ill health over time. Hunter-gatherers were nomadic and handled their survival with more compassion than the later settlers did with fear, adherence to possessions and associated heartlessness. Protection of the tribe and its possessions was ascribed to the strongest and the best by virtue of holding others at bay using tactics of heartlessness. Though early hominids were wired for togetherness, sharing, cooperation and fairness, the perception of threat has allowed the actions of cruelty, avoidance and heartlessness to dominate more modern *Homo sapiens.*

The unkind person has no comprehension or concern of the suffering of others. The kind of person that tortures and kills without guilt, exterminates large groups of people perceived as a threat, developed from wild nomads into civilized monsters. Compassion did not die off with the advent of agriculture and importance of possessions. It just shared space with the development and expression of heartlessness. All humans are born with compassion and kindness hard wired in our DNA, which is expressed early in the mother-infant relationship. Whatever innate meanness and cruelty are suppressed until evoked by circumstances that bear forth its existence and growth. Social comes early and antisocial develops later.

Study: From the classic, Dr. Jekyll and Mr. Hyde, to Rutger Bregman's recent masterpiece, Humankind; William Golding's Lord of the Flies; Richard Dawkins' The Selfish Gene; Jared Diamond's Easter Island massacre (which didn't happen) and Stanley Milgran's Shock Machine, which urged ordinary people to deliver painful or deadly voltage to fellow human beings, shows that everyone has the capacity for evil. That people would follow instructions to inflict pain on "others", with half thinking it was fake so kept doing it, and half thought it was real. Some refused to pull the lever to execute, but many did it anyway, bowing to authority, or did it because they felt it was right thing to do. Some were cruel because they liked it. To kill someone especially if they were "other", ordinary human beings are capable of extraordinary cruelty. *Homo sapiens* are easily led from good to evil, and grew to accept and like it, especially when in groups. (lynching, burning at the stake and war).

In the 21st century, we are seeing the progressive loss of compassion by an entire society. Does kindness really matter or do only power and material gain have meaning? Does collective conscience and group morality still exist? Is cruelty gaining a foothold that is becoming the "normal"? Does the absence of punishment for immorality have anything to do with the apparent prevalence of cruelty? How will "getting away with it" affect the kindness/cruelty balance inherent in humanity? Taking children away from their parents as a means of punishment for seeking asylum; tear gassing them at the border; cheering wildly at the mention of the building of a wall to keep "them" out; electing a leader based on the promise of "exclusion" and on the fear of "inclusion" while the entire society does nothing about it. There is no group kindness in an America based on stolen land, genocide of "them" and separation and discrimination against "them".

Empathy

How and why are some people kind and others cruel?

Empathy is when one feels the suffering of another and joins them in the suffering. Baby #1 cries when it sees baby #2 is hurt and in distress. Empathy is what makes us human. Mother #1 feels the hurt of other mothers, through a social bond. As long as the cost of caring is not too high, they join in and feel the pain collectively.

Vignette #13: Upon witnessing the deadly motorcycle accident of my friend, with all the senses alert and on edge, I still experience the deep feelings of pain and agony that accompany those images of some six decades ago.

Examination of the scientific roots of human kindness elicited more questions than answers. At the Greater Good Science Center at UC Berkeley in California, the focus is on happy, compassionate people. All have strong social bonding ability and altruistic behavior. On peace-making vs war mongering, both are in our DNA. They have determined that expression of one over the other depends on environmental circumstances. With selfish vs sharing and meanness vs caring, the origin lies in motherhood and infancy. Oxytocin promotes love, trust and generosity, while lack of it gives way to the opposite, fear, distrust, hate and violent behavior. Which comes first, oxytocin to elicit kindness or kindness to stimulate oxytocin? What factors determine the lack of oxytocin? Parents' behavior? DNA availability of the hormone? Child's reaction to the hormone? Are emotions controllable? And if so, by what means? What determines the difference between true compassion and what's- in- it- for- me selfishness? Are meanness and aggression simply instruments of self-preservation? Or are they as inextricably ingrained as compassion. Compassion, the concern for the welfare of another is visibly absent in some societies, where benevolence is seen as unwanted weakness and heartlessness is seen as valuable toughness. Both exist as part of biology. How each develops depends on genetics and environmental experiences.

Empathy derives from the German "einfühling" or "feeling into", as a connection with the experience of another. "I feel your pain" is natural and DNA-based. Newborns cry at the sound of another baby crying. By 1-year-old the infant attempts to comfort those in distress, and by 14 months old, shows helping behavior. Understanding and sympathizing with the feelings of others are the cornerstones of social relationships and lead heavily into connections, determining well-being. The genes for social selection depend on the female's choice of a preferable male, a provider, not a bully. Compassion is the most important human characteristic that leads to success of the group. With it comes cooperation and collaboration. When inequality arises, social behavior adopts envy and scorn, and rationalization by the less fortunate that the rich deserve and are entitled to have more (at their expense), the society dissolves. With human nature transforming from kindness to cruelty. Social cohesion breaks down, leading to segregation, reduced trust, increased stress hormones and poor health.

The Good Samaritan parable, as told by Jesus in the Gospel of Luke, is about a traveler, stripped and beaten by robbers, who is left near death at the side of the road. Passed and ignored by a Jewish priest and a Levite, another traveler, a Samaritan, finally helps him. The value of human kindness was displayed. Historically, the Jews and Samaritans did not like one another. In this case, the presence of feel-good hormones suppressed the release of self-interest feel-bad hormones? Empathy appeared and evolved from animal precursors to preserve the integrity of the group. We flinch when someone sustains an injury or when we see them standing on a dangerous ledge. This is reactive empathy. We imitate their pain with a squinched up face as a nervous reaction. This is mimicry. The apes do it also. Happy or sad, we mirror the actions of others, yawns and laughs, as a vestige of our innate empathy.

With prenatal care 200-million years ago, the female most sensitive to her offspring produced more and more survived because of the responsive attention. The most sensitive genes were propagated and this emotional reaction, one infant crying and another joining in, developed well before and was the precursor of socializing.

Empathy appeared with the development of the limbic system, the feeling, emotional, pleasure brain, that would determine family life, social friendships and social bonding. The advantages lay in security for the individual and social companionship for the group. This feeling coincides with that of food satisfaction. With empathy one gathers information on someone else and copes the emotions. Louis Armstrong: "When you're smiling, the whole world smiles with you" is pure positive reactive empathy. Facial and body postures and movements can empathize" and display social connectivity. The blank faces of Parkinson's disease does not. The prefrontal cortex and para limbic system house the emotions and sense of morality, that influence social behavior and promote self-control. Destruction or removal of these areas results in the psychopath, one without feelings or remorse, absent empathy. The sociopath is without care for or understanding of the feelings of others and continually breaks rules without shame or guilt, impaired empathy. In modern times, there are many sociopaths with purely selfish interests and severely lacking in social and moral values.

Empathy comes from having an interest in others, deriving pleasure of seeing the happiness of others, and putting it together with cooperation for group survival. In France the celebration of "Fraternite" arose from the 1789 revolution. In the USA, after Hurricane Katrina, those with cars sped away, as "the misery of others is none of our business. People were left behind to die, like animals." (Most animals don't leave their injured behind) The Covid-19 economy was repeatedly touted ahead of the misery and deaths of the afflicted. The lack of empathy displayed by a large portion of humanity was on display. Self-interest bad hormones suppressed the release of feel-good hormones of fellowship.

Empathy vs pitilessness, what makes one individual social and the other, selfish? The advent and emphasis on materials and possessions has reduced sociality to levels seen before man developed common sense. Are we our brothers' keepers? No, we look out only for ourselves. Do we have a sense of compassion? Or are cutthroat realism, eye for an eye, and Me First the laws of the day. The collective Common Good has given way to the rule of Individual Freedom (refusal to wear a mask to reduce the risk of infection both ways) Empathy is innate, comes from reliance on each other as a means of survival, from food and safety first, and from obligatory maternal love and care without which the child becomes a non-reactive zombie and dies. We listen to a sad story and our heads sag, bodies slump and we groan. For humans meant to have a social life, solitary confinement is a punishment worse than death. The value of human contact, time spent with family and friends to fulfill emotional needs, has been replaced with the value of high levels of money, success, and fame.

> *"Nothing is more important than empathy for another human being's suffering. Nothing. Not career, not wealth, not intelligence, certainly not status. We have to feel for one another if we are going to survive with dignity." Audrey Hepburn*

Study: Testing by Cambridge University in 2018, on men and women to determine their levels of empathy, revealed that women score higher than men. Based solely on "social" factors, no genetic basis was found. As power was vested in men, from male perspectives there is a decrease in empathy in the society. They concluded that as testosterone increases, empathy decreases. As oxytocin increases, empathy increases. Aggression and cruelty are perceived as manly strengths, while compassion and empathy are perceived as feminine weaknesses. Sympathy is proactive when you do something about someone's situation, i.e. having concern about another and the desire to do something about it.

Morality is the natural sense of right and wrong, and acting upon it accordingly. "I feel the need to help" determines the morality of the individual and the group. Actions had consequences in the developing world, and when it ceases to play out, the society breaks down. Taking children away from parents, mistreating them is immoral, mean and totally devoid of empathy. Those who perpetrate it are immoral and those who allowed it are equally at fault. Turning away from sufferers yet proclaiming to be "Christian" is immoral, heartless, wrong and devoid of empathy.

The link between giving and receiving is **gratitude**, the foundation of social life in many cultures. The pleasant feeling is from feel good hormones. Society depends on gratitude to stick together and move forward. When appreciation for and of each other breaks down, so does the society. When winner take all, rape victims are portrayed as perpetrators, and the poor are demonized as weak and unworthy of compassion, the foundation of the society weakens. Gratitude is humility, the recognition of the importance of the contribution of others. We link it to health, happiness and solid social connections. In the absence of gratitude, heartlessness, meanness, cruelty, and self-interest dominate as anti- social behavior. Those "friends" exist for whom a favor is not appreciated and may actually be resented.

The kinder, more pleasant to be around, welcoming, more inclusive the person, the higher the quality of the social interaction. In repaying the kindness of others, there is an increase in the feeling of well-being.

Do empathy and morality come from inner human senses, or are they mere products of rules for maintaining society?

Study: At the Greater Good Science Center at UC Berkeley found that those with gratitude and forgiveness had higher health and well-being values, with fewer complaints and physical illness than those with feelings of disappointment, anxiety and envy. Gratitude motivates people to socialize because of more stable emotions, self-confidence, and experiences with positive interaction results. Those with appreciation had more social ties, a better sense of interconnectivity, and a better sense of personal worth than those with more self-centered and antisocial grounding.

Altruism

The unselfish regard for and devotion to the welfare of others also promotes cooperation and sharing and enables group success. Although altruism may be harmful to the individual herself, we do it for the benefit of the others in the group. "It is more blessed to give than to receive: Acts 20:35 (Jesus of Nazareth) Young children help others solve problems with utter delight at success, even when the other is a stranger, and when they receive no benefit at all.

When a society opposes sharing shelter, health care and nutrition, it is against open socializing and is usually lacking in meaningful connections within and outside the group.

Study: University of Buffalo (NY) researchers found a link between selfishness and untimely death. Altruism reduced stress and risk of premature death, and increased life expectancy. High blood pressure and cortisol levels were associated with less money given away. Volunteering to work at a soup kitchen provided a natural high associated with endorphins release. Altruistic individuals at the workplace were more committed, happier, and had more stable mental health associated with well-being and overall life satisfaction. The study also found that most charity is selfish as it gives satisfaction and monetary reward (mainly in tax deductions) to the donor. Only agape, giving expecting nothing in return, is true.

Borrowed from the Greek for "brotherly love", agape has become associated with a Christian love feast. The warm welcome, regarding with affection, and offering protection, it embodies the purity of love for all human beings and that "others" are worthy of respect, sympathy, acceptance and future access to interaction. "Therefore all things whatsoever ye would that men should do to you: do ye even so to them." Matthew 7:12… (Do unto others: Jesus of Nazareth, Sermon on the Mount) Whole-hearted love with pure objectivity is difficult to attain and maintain unless one is of pure heart.

Over five hundred years before the ministry of Jesus, the concept of "ren", composed of compassion, altruism, goodness, virtue and love, was taught by the Chinese philosopher, Confucius. His "Golden Rule "of kindness to others was so effective within the entire society, that it spread outwards to other cultures..

Study: American Journal of Psychiatry, 1964. Rhesus monkeys refused to pull a chain that delivered food to self if a companion received a concomitant shock. Chimpanzees and great apes are protective of sick companions. Elephants rescue a slower or sick companion and mourn their demise with a display of emotional connection and appreciation. Many modern humans do not show this basic empathy.

Empathy and compassion are hard wired in our DNA as inner responses to group threats that assist with survival. Heartlessness, also hard-wired, appears to increase later as a cultural response to threats to survival. Initially, both can release feel good hormones, with the latter lingering on and releasing chronic stress hormones. Schadenfreude, the pleasure at seeing or hearing of the misfortune of another comprises envy and jealousy, especially of a friend. The social mind makes powerful connections in response to need and makes strong alienations and rejections in response to threats. Whichever is manifested depends on the genetics and experiences of the individual and on the societal trends of the time.

The urge to connect is natural, evolutionary, enhanced and reinforced through need and proven success, as a tool of survival. Empathy, sympathy, and altruistic feelings are based on the motivation to help, comfort and care for others are pro social. Since social pain and pleasure use the same neural mechanisms and pathways as physical pain and pleasure, the urge to connect and ability to understand others, especially in small groups, in the making of an effective social being. When the groups enlarged and spread out, the societies changed and though the goals of survival, pleasure and avoidance of pain remained the same, the methods of attainment evolved. Altruism, fairness, and niceness are innate, and are evident early in life. Antisocial, uncooperative behavior is also innate but appears later and at the ends of some prodding, usually from parents, peer groups and a self-interested society.

Study: Happy and Healthy USA Survey by Harris poll in 2017 revealed that a substantial bank account gives physical and emotional pleasure and the perception that high income goes along with well-being. Though having money does not buy happiness, it is better than being broke. In a society that built itself around material wealth and possessions, happiness is decreased as one is always trying to preserve it.

Trust

The evolution of Sociability has its origins in the genetics of empathy and compassion, and cultural development of conscience, morality and trust. From 200,000 years ago, Homo erectus evolved into *Homo sapiens,* through internalization of rules for survival. The active ingredient to success was through social connections which built societies upon family, friends, marriages, organizations, social networks and trust that contributed to well-being—not based on income.

When you put more value on possessions than on human beings, for preservation, you segregate yourself from others you consider unworthy of being a part of your social circle. You lose range and diversity of experience; you lose possibility of pleasures unseen and unrealized; and you use valuable energy in trying to remain aloof and unsociable. You risk compromising your health.

Gifting, the ancient tradition arising from humans recognizing other humans and being grateful for their presence; is a means of socializing; of setting up a relationship; setting up a future interaction; It is "as I do for you and someday you will do for me". Be careful not to set up as a system of debt, as this may lead to resentment.

Trust is the assured reliance of one individual upon the ability, strength and truth of another individual. The key to the science of trust is oxytocin. From its first release to the smooth muscles of the uterus to induce contractions in childbirth and promote lactation after birth, oxytocin reduces social anxiety and promotes bonding and "trust" between mother and infant. High levels help to overcome distrust of other humans and foster social interactions and establish social connections. Trust is both hormonal and cognition interactive to produce a social interaction, add cooperation to get the connection.

The foundation of all social life is trust.

Frequent interaction among diverse sets of people in peaceful setting produces general reciprocity and yields high levels of creativity and production. Trust as a driver of reliability is a key ingredient in cooperation. Distrust, exclusion, fear and separation behavior of its constituents reduce the general health of a community.

Study: Medical students established meaningful connections with one another for social support and reducing the harmful effects of stress. From the initial engagement, through group and individual identification to true connections, there was a high level of trust that reduced fear and increased productivity. A lack of trust in each other led quicker to burnout. *RC Ziegelstein in*

> *"Creating structured opportunities for social engagement to promote well-being and reduce burnout in medical students and residents.* Acad. Med, Dec 26, 2017

> *Fifty years after graduating from medical school, the same group of friends hold tightly to each other through bonds based on caring and cemented by trust. (The author)*

Vignette #14. The Scorpion and the Frog, a Russian fable, in which the scorpion begs the frog for a ride on his back across the river. The frog refuses, citing the high probability that the scorpion would bite him. The scorpion pleads, the frog gives in, agrees and they enter the water. Halfway across the river, the scorpion stings the frog. As the frog was dying, he asked, "Why did you bite me?" As he was drowning, the scorpion replied, "I couldn't help it. It's in my nature". Nature programs a scorpion to destroy its prey. It can never be trusted. There are vicious people who cannot resist hurting others, even when it is not in their best interest.

> *"Trust is the glue of life…it is the foundation principle that holds all relationships".* Stephen Covey

Trust is the key to a healthy, functional society. Distrust leads to breakdown of the same society. The cost in energy spent, wasted, and dispensed, is higher with distrust than with trust. With distrust, there are questions, fear and stress. Survival is possible, but good health is not. Economists found strong correlation between GDP growth and social trust. This is high in Scandinavia and low in Central America.

In principle, all biological systems divide into cooperative groups, specialize and serve the Group. Any benefits enjoyed by the individual come as a courtesy of the group. Trust in someone's word can move an entire tribe or group successfully from place to place and at top efficiency. Mistrust calls for too many checks and balances and uses up valuable energy. Without trust, there is no cooperation and the system breaks down into "every man for himself". Trust is a good friend, a dog, a horse. Flocks of birds, herds of deer, schools of fish, and swarms of insects, all display different types of social behavior based on principles of cooperation that enhance survival. There is safety in numbers for protection, but they also share knowledge of the best feeding sites and best mating opportunities. At this stage, natural selection increases the welfare of the group at the expense of the individual, like in apoptosis, where old cells self-destruct on cue to allow the birth of new cells. Failure to do so results in cancerous growths. With social behavior, altruism is selection at the group level and selfishness is selection at the individual level. When *Homo sapiens* moved from hunter-gatherer to settler, the group moved to individual options to cooperate or compete, lead or follow or separate and form own group within the larger whole. Genes develop for both sociality and antisociality and are expressed with the goal still being that of preservation of the species. Groups with too many selfish individuals inside do not survive. Any threat to the group from outside relies still on altruistic genes where some sacrifice for the good of the many defensive wars.

Homo sapiens are wired for fairness, niceness and for doing good, but possessions and materials stimulated selfishness to the point of domination. We have three strengths and one weakness. That weakness prevails when it gets more results than its competitors. The Golden rule appears in just about every ancient society, and the Christian dictum, "It is more blessed to give than to receive." Acts 20:35 promote social behavior. In the long-term, the benefit that kindness would be reciprocated when needed came up against self-interest. This pushed the psyche of the group into a dual role. They needed trust for the system of indirect reciprocity to work, that help will be there for you when needed (on the rebound). It was an insurance system of sharing and cooperating with someone in need, whether they be kin or non-kin. Helping to build a shelter, weeding a field, or bringing food to the needy in time of disaster, still prevailed as the feel-good system remained intact. The poor, ragged stranger in Paul Theroux's The Pillars of Hercules, who, upon seeing the traveler's frustration at not being able to buy a bus ticket for lack of local currency, gives him his own ticket and expects nothing in return…as he may never see him again. This is pure altruism. A sudden, unsolicited kindness that warms the heart with a gush of endorphins and love hormones is pure *Homo sapiens*, circa 10,000 BCE.

In 2020 AD, we blame the less fortunate for their own misfortunes, cast them aside, and leave them to fend for themselves. The wealthy take more than they need or can use and the meanness genes flourish while pursuing more. In the distant past, those with compassion survived to pass on genes of empathy that helped the group survive. In more recent times, the heartless divided and weakened the group, and only the individual grew stronger.

Trust can give rise to conflicting urges and actions, as both forgiveness and revenge are social instincts. One is a tool of peace and the other an instrument of war. The first is a conscious decision to release feelings of resentment or vengeance to a person or group who has harmed you, regardless of whether they deserve it and is the ultimate expression of being "social".

The epitome of forgiveness is President Nelson Mandela of South Africa. After 27 years in prison and a lifetime of apartheid abuse and humiliation, he forgave his captors, pursued a course of reconciliation that saved his country and rose way above them all. He said no to war and yes to peace, no to racism and yes to democracy. Using reason, compassion and the tribal morality he learned as a child, he governed with responsibility, humanity and moral sense. He learned the language and spoke to the Afrikaners, bringing everyone together to interact in hopes of connecting. The Zulu phrase, "Umuntu ngumuntu ngabantu" means that a person is a person because of other people. Archbishop Tutu (1986) says that " Úbuntu", refers to gentleness, to compassion, to hospitality, to openness to others, to vulnerability and to know that it binds you with them in the bundle of life. It means "I am because you are". *

Revenge is also a natural trait via DNA built-in to satisfy the desire to return the hurt or harm that was or perceived to have been inflicted. Spawned in parts by fear, resentment, and sadism, it serves as warning to deter aggressors, to punish and prevent victims from retaliating. Forgiveness brings peace, satisfies the group, is used to gain more social cooperation and makes the group stronger. Revenge is self-satisfying, promotes war, and makes the group strong in competition.

The choice of one over the other depends, like all other instinctive learning reactions, on the environment and the genes. If one does not share food, they ostracize him. Not cooperating or contributing to the group could risk exile or death. (*Tell that to Jeff Bezos or Elon Musk*). In the chronicles of humanity, half choose forgiveness and half choose revenge. Reconciliation repairs valuable relationships damaged by aggression and regains benefits of cooperation, like food, shelter and security. Revenge motivates the group to act on providing emotional satisfaction at having dominated the assailant, can be used as a deterrent to high crime and disorder, and as a means for the group to appear strong.

Forgiveness promotes mental, physical and spiritual health as it gets rid of negative emotions and feel-bad hormones and increase positive reconciliation. You face down injustice by changing the negative to positive. Increasing the positives results in better health. Increasing the negatives, hostility, fear, and hatred harbor the stress hormones, compromises the immune system and leads to poor health (especially cancers and neurodegenerative diseases).

"Before you embark on a journey of revenge, dig two graves."
Confucius, Chinese philosopher, 520 BC

*Racism will continue as long as there is little or no contact, interaction, connection between the antagonists.

Communications

Cognition, social selection, socializing, compassion, coopera-tion, empathy, altruism and trust appear early in prehistoric man and relate closely to genetic and environmental factors. All living organisms "communicate", but humans went further in using com-munication to plan and organize the future.

From basic greetings, to gestures and sounds that enabled pair-ing, organized cooperation, understood intent, they developed lan-guage primarily as a survival tool. When conversation became an art, *Homo sapiens* went way beyond and above the others. From smoke signals to pathfinding to navigating rivers to road building to tele-graph and telephone, electricity to internet, campfire socializing to global interconnectivity, Homo sapiens was the phenomenal.

Chimpanzees, macaques, and bonobos make eye contact and "smile", some bare their teeth silently in greeting one another to show that it is safe. The same sign with a higher intensity shows that you are a threat, and injecting a little fear indicates a call for help. Facial expressions, gestures, and sounds of varying intensities are features of communication.

In Theroux's travel journal around the Mediterranean, the author encounters a pair of villagers in Aliano, near the ankle of Italy's boot, who very clearly and enthusiastically relate to him that where "Worlds can't meet worlds, people can meet people." Another villager gestures that though I am busy at the moment, "I acknowledge your presence".

My ECNS (Eye Contact, Nod, Smile) ongoing study continuously reaffirms the facts that some people are naturally "social" and others are not. It takes less than a second to acknowledge a simple greeting, yet there are those who feel better with ignoring your presence entirely and others to which a simple nod is too much of a bother.

From the last common ancestor (LCA) around 400,000 years ago (the split from chimpanzee to "human"), early hominids used gestures, facial expressions, body postures, and sounds to communicate their intentions and rudimentary thoughts. The nature of the message called for them to assign specific features to each to facilitate understanding. Communication enabled interaction by getting joint attention to a reference point and became part of the daily routine, getting things done. Cooperation leading to collaboration in acquiring food and ensuring safety required partnerships, which used social skills, of which language was a prominent feature. The way in which the group used words and symbols in the same way to express ideas and intentions, developed from the rudimentary gestures and indicative grunts we associate with prehistoric communications. Animals communicate but do not have language or symbols to convey shared ideas. Social interactions to coordinate foraging, hunting, food distribution, shelter preparation and movements are uniquely human. With two minds and two bodies being better than one, those who were social responded to gestures and invitations to engage, to attend a joint venture or to take part in an event. Someone without interest in communicating or who ignores the gesture or invitation found themselves ignored and eventually ostracized.

True language that conveyed the message and generated stories, concepts, and plans, past, present and future, greatly enhanced social connections. Homo erectus, 200,000 years ago, gathered into larger groups for more successful hunting and defense against predators, pooling and sharing resources and ideas, child raising and care of the sick and elderly, introduced migration, reactive and planed. Social living and coordinated movements of the group entailed keeping track of each person's personalities and whether they could be trusted, were kind and cooperative or heartless and selfish. Group activity required social skills especially communication, to coordinate the activities and cooperate with decisions. For modern Homo sapiens lack of social skills with antisocial behavior may lead to embarrassment and casual shunning. For Homo erectus social behavior was a matter of life and death. Across the savanna, into the valleys, along the rivers and through the mountains, sharing ideas and comprehension of basic creations, new tools, and culture led to increased brain power. The gene mutation FOXP2 enabled the development of speech areas in the brain (Brocas and Wernickes) in the frontal and parietal lobes, plus the laryngeal muscles and tongue. With the brain capable of symbolic thinking (theory of mind, introspection), language developed along with self-awareness and awareness of others' thinking to explain and define one's own thoughts, "hear oneself think", then to convey a thought from one head to another. Once communication became the spoken word conveying meaning and emotion, it brought people together through its powers of expression and ability to grasp the essence of a subject. A phone call is still better than an email in the social world). The spoken word is a better gauge of social sincerity and storytelling still elicits more emotion than the written word, hence appeared first and developed further.

Humans use symbols for abstract reasoning to create and produce. A unified group was needed for this development. Once they internalized instructions, the cognitive resources of the group increased. The goal of human social learning is to conform to the group, gain acceptance, and increase chances of survival. Apes learn by imitation and humans learn by conformity. Both want to show "that I am like you". Using language is one of the most important human markers within and about a society. If they speak the same, with the same word usage and accent, they are more likely to be a unified society. If they speak differently, chances of cooperation and cohesion is less. Two groups separated by markers of skin color and culture, though occupying the same region, do not speak to each other, hence syntax, vocabulary, and accent are different.

From the social interactions of the campfires, increased closeness of winters, need for communication in the hunt, to cooperation and collaboration, construction of settlements and villages, elaborate storytelling, writing, to telegraph and telephone to café culture, email and Skype and snapchat, humans developed language as an essential means of socializing and unification. The same language spawned conflicts, animosities, jealousies, instabilities, surplus members to be distributed elsewhere, exclusions, wall building and wars. How it was conveyed, was of utmost importance to the interpretation.

Vignette #15. A cave dweller around the campfire related the story of his encounter with a wolf. If the delivery was meek and mild, the story fell flat. If exuberant and forceful in his triumph, even if not true, the story became legend. The performance won him fame and more girls, so it was repeated the next time and emulated by the rest of the group.

The art and science of effective communication relies on and encourages the development of social skills. The effect depends on delivery and appropriateness. After a crisis, if you are telling the wrong, inappropriate story to the wrong group, you are more likely to be banned, at least from telling stories in the future. If planning a raid and you give the wrong or incomplete information, like telling of a canary instead of a giant python just outside the cave, you will have a serious problem. Communication skills were very important to the survival of the group. Attention, focus and proper interpretation were just as important as speaking appropriately and used many of the same skills.

Engaging your audience using dialogue skills was required to elicit the desired reactions. Providing appropriate information, a beginning a middle and an end, were essential. In relating the existence of a lion on the other side of the river but omitting to tell of the crocodile on your side, could lead to some serious problems. A good storyteller was essential to the survival of the group.

The environmental differences in separate regions had some influence on social interactions. The northern winters' hibernation patterns and close quarters for warmth drew people together, and enhanced communications. An agrarian society required cooperation for spring and summer sowing and harvest and the celebrations that followed. In the tropical jungle and savanna, the presence of dangerous predators drew people into groups where precise and elaborate storytelling with complete audience connection became a distinct art form. Effective communication built more confidence and the quality and quantity of interactions, connections and relationships grew further.

Human evolution and differences derive their roots from migrations, not from biology. Moving from one location to another, provided the best advantage for survival and "thriving". For this, effective communication was a necessity. Modern humans result from hundreds of thousands of years of mixing of populations during migrations to produce an "interconnected family" created by "social interactions", using communication skills.

Study: The US Dept of Education focus is on STEM fields (science, technology, engineering and math). The goal is to improve the quality of life through inventions and technology. Very little or nothing is allotted for social skills, like geography, history, languages, and cultures. Hence communication skills suffer. Poor communicators have deficient social lives. Social skills during adolescence contributes to brain development and sharpness for facts and analysis. Social skills enhance teamwork, supervision, efficient organization skills, and eventual success.

Social interaction with active positive communication promotes good health. Negative or hurtful communication like bullying, bad manners, and willful neglect promotes a physical and emotional assault. A condescending look from a stranger can be a physical dagger while a kind look and a smile can be reassurance of safety in any environment. Real or potential separation from caregiver or group can trigger serious distress (the dorsal anterior ungulate cortex and anterior insula), while giving and receiving care enables social bonding (the amygdala) and activates the reward system. Almost all social interactions involve the process of communication.

Touch

"Hay palabras que no llegan como abrazos; y hay abrazos que no necesitan palabras." Mexican saying
(there are words that do not arrive like hugs; and there are hugs that do not need words)

Many primate research studies highlight the importance of touch. Grooming, cuddling, caressing and hugging release feel-good hormones. The human infant needs tactile sensation for normal growth and development, good health and security, be it maternal caresses or a blanket, toy or pet.

Historically, touch was always a part of human interactions. The extension of the open hand indicates a removal of or reduction in animosity. Shaking hands is a basic greeting and shows the absence of a weapon or intention of malice. You shake on an agreement. In Ancient Greece, on a Parthenon column, Hera, queen goddess of marriage, birth and jealousy, shakes hands with Athena, goddess of wisdom and war.

Touch is the first indicator of communication of, by and for babies from birth and throughout infancy. The comfort of the release of feel-good hormones (oxytocin), the conveyance of emotion, pain alleviation and as an aid in communication during conversation, caresses for reassurance and closeness are all physiological benefits to the health of the infant.

Study: The importance of touch in development: Evan L Ardiel, MSc and Catherine H Rankin, PhD. The infant brain growth and development heavily depends on social interactions and connections. Developmental delay is common in children deprived of normal sensory stimulation as substantiated by animal models. In rats, maternal pup licking provides the mechanosensory stimulation required for positive growth and development as manifested by their behavior as adults. In the roundworm, *Caenorhabiditis elegans*, physical interaction with other worms promote growth and proper responses to stimuli.

Study: Abraham Maslow's Hierarchy of Needs, a 1943 paper: A Theory of Human Motivation, in Psychological Review, the physiological and anatomical needs of the infant are supplied by love and a sense of belonging through touch and communication. The social connection established with the caregiver develops self-esteem and contributes to self-actualization toward completing one's full potential. Study: The soothing function of touch: affective touch reduces feelings of social exclusion. Mariana von Mohr, et al examined the mammalian need for social proximity and belonging in terms of survival and reproductive success, as opposed to strong negative feelings of social exclusion induced by ostracism. The slow tactile affective touch reduces social pain (of rejection or exclusion) and is modulated by a C tactile neurophysiological system vs a faster neural touch of physical pain. Specific relation between affective touch and social bonding.

(published on line Oct 18, 2017, Research department of Clinical, Educational and Health Psychology, University College London, UK. Hands on Research: The Science of Touch. Dacker Keltner, Sept 29, 2010 UC Berkeley, Greater Good Magazine

Similarly, in the older child and adult, a pat on the back conveys reassurance or congratulations. A light touch on the arm by the speaker during conversation keeps attention and gives emphasis in making and keeping the connection. Touch is an integral part of the basic fundamentals of human communication and bonding.

Vignette #16: Dr. A touches his patients upon arrival and greeting, with a handshake or a hug depending on familiarity. Dr. O does not. When patients feel more "connected", they are more cooperative, take part more fully in their treatment regimen, and the outcomes are better.

For primates, "grooming" is touch, and is a sophisticated medication

Study: Sidney Jourard, Canadian psychologist: Conversations of friends in different parts of the world in a café. The "Coffee House Study" is an observational study focused on dialogue, as a means of human interactions. They observed patrons in cafes in different cultures and noted their intimacy. Though one may dispute the accuracy, the findings indicate the level of touch during conversations. In London, England, there were zero touches between participants during a one- hour conversation. In Gainesville, Florida, there were an average of two touches per hour. In Paris, France, there were 110 touches per hour per conversation, and in San Juan, Puerto Rico there were 180.

(I live here and can vouch for the veracity of this finding.) Dutton J, etal. Journal of Mass Communication & Journalism.

Touch is essential to the normal development of infant health. A simple touch to a neonate, infant or child activates the orbitofrontal cortex in the brain, linked to reward and feelings of compassion, stimulates brain activity for receptiveness to affection (skin-to-skin contact), initiates and improve immune system development and lead to higher resilience to stress and better coping with fear. Touch enhances the development of better cooperative relationships, reinforces reciprocity between people and stimulates the compassion response. ("There, there. It's going to be all right")

According to the McGill Program for the Study of Behavior, in 2021 studies with mice, soothing touch provides physical calming, reminders of affection and support. The cuddled infants showed a reduction in heart rate, whether it be by parents or strangers. Hugs stimulated the release of oxytocin that reduced blood pressure in both the breast-feeding child and mother. It goes both ways. Hugs turn on or off certain genes that influence the DNA of infants in what is now known as epigenetic ageing, changes that can last for generations. Grooming increases acetylation that promotes the glucocorticoid receptor gene, which in conjunction with changes n methylation, can increase affection. Frequent, sincere touching resulted in an increase in loving individuals able to alleviate stress and anxiety.

Social grooming using touch for purposes of cleanliness related to good health, is a prerequisite for mating in most animals. Without touch, the individual could become shabby, unkept and in poor health, which went nowhere with socializing and reduced chances of reproduction. The infant receiving loving touches, cuddling, and hugs showed good neural development in the vagus nerve bundle (*10ᵗʰ cranial nerve, spinal cord to stomach*). Delayed or incomplete development led to an impaired ability to be intimate or compassionate. There are two touch systems with different sensors and nerve fibers involved. The factual system is for finding or identifying items, fast, and concentrated in the hands. The emotional one is for processing mothers' affections, intimate contact, social bonding, and grooming, slowly. It is especially attuned at the back, neck, and intimate areas. Touching and being touched stimulate the systems to release feel-good hormones that enhance health. A sincere hug and a slow back rub can reduce pain and systemic blood pressure as oxytocin blocks the release of cortisol together with the touch to skin, activating the Pacinian corpuscle receptor, which signals the brain to reduce the blood pressure.; reduce stress and anxiety; boost the immune system by the release of other anti-infection hormones; reduced muscle tension from the increase in blood circulation, which promotes additional blood flow into tissues; to increase mood by releasing more oxytocin, serotonin, endorphins, and dopamine combination, all of which bring happiness and joy; improve memory and brain health from the overall stimulation of the parasympathetic nerve system that regulates calmness activity.

Hopefully, everyone has felt those butterflies in the stomach at the first touch of a prospective date and mate, thanks to oxytocin release plus a bit of serotonin and dopamine in the mix, making it into a delightful after-feeling.

There is a cultural component to touch/hug mechanism. Initiation and positive responses are high in Latin America and

Mediterranean countries and low in England, USA, Scandinavia and Asia. Latino traditions are high on touching, hugs, embraces, men to men, men to women, women to women in touch reinforcement. Written letters are closed with "abrazos y besos" (hugs and kisses). The French "bise" the artful kiss on both cheeks for men and women, sometimes with touch and sometimes without. In one raised by huggers, there is likely to be hugging as an integral part of established connections. Linking arms, holding hands provides nurture to a family with physical touch as a custom.

In the absence of connections or contacts, there is a distinct underdevelopment of the vagal system. Not everybody wants a hug. Confusion or misplacement of intent can result in and from unwanted hugs. Some with childhood issues, trauma, or just programmed to avoid touching, experience physical contact as a negative response. Cortisol released instead of oxytocin leads to apprehension, fear, and repulsion.

Study: The Carnegie Mellon University found that some 72% of individuals liked interpersonal touch and 27% did not. Those who were positive tended to be pro social extroverts. Those who were negative tended toward antisocial introversion. Two-thirds of those studied did not like being touched by strangers. The frequency and acceptability of touch decreased with increased age and with increased passage of time (era changes). They concluded that consensual touch is good for one's physiological and psychological health.

"I need a hug."

Tribalism, Identity and Social Markers

The behavior and attitudes that result from a strong loyalty to a particular social group is referred to as tribalism. A fundamental human trait, we use it in defense against a rival group or as offense for gain. The tribe comprises natives, and may include allies, converts, and forced abductees, who identify themselves by markers, names, self-adornments, language, and appearance that indicate belonging. Similar markers can identify other people as a threat or start antagonism against others with different markers, clothing, attitude, or skin color. Local ant colony A invades and destroys foreign ant colony B that has different hydrocarbon markers on their bodies. They designate each other as enemies. Colony A tolerates but recognize as "slightly different", colony C ants with slightly different hydrocarbon markers. Likewise, the body's immune system cells seek out and attack foreign body cells with the "wrong" markers. Hence the making of a vaccine to teach the immune cells whom exactly to attack and whom to leave alone.

Tribe derives from the Greek, "tribus", indicating a social group composed of families, clans, dependents and adopted strangers forming a community, often claiming descent from a common ancestor. Artifacts of self-adornment from 40,000 years ago include beads, needles, bits of clothing, ochre for body painting and figurines indicating identification markers and signs of "relationships" like marriages, friendships (gifts), and interactions between individuals and groups. Evidence of extension of contacts with other tribes shows strong social connections. Clothing was then as is now, a marker of self-identification and attachment to a group. From Otzi, the Austrian ice man, dressed in skins, to the hippies of the 1960s, with long hair and the 1950s crew cut, skin heads, bellbottoms, business suit and kilt, was an indicator of group attachment which provided safety through familiarity. Modern *Homo sapiens* progressed past other primates and insects, in adopting extensive social markers, flags, caps, T-shirts with messages, team recognition, and many identifications as part of the group. Speech patterns, word usage, accents, socially acceptable forms of dress, colors, style, gait, and attitude, all showing the customs and badges of appearance, and signifying conscious intent. Knights raised their visors to reveal their identity, which contributed to the traditional salute. Identity, who you are, and where do you belong? From where did you come? Who are you? Uncontrolled cues of skin color, hair texture, facial features and body shapes were later added.

These identity markers signaled permission to interact or react with aggression to the threat of differences.

Pre-historic innovations were slow. Ancient *Homo sapiens* relied on each other for news, information, security, new ideas and fashion, so that social interaction was more prominent than it is today. Markers identifying the group took precedence over those of individual status. Skin tone, hair texture or appearance features carried no social meaning so mattered very little. They required early society interactions in both daytime routines of food gathering, repairs, shelter and defense, and nighttime storytelling, dramatic acting, and teaching. Proper social behavior grew out of interactions of "us" and "them", which were essential for tribal safety and survival.

As the tribe grew in numbers, 150 being the average for efficient use of resources, access to reproduction and keeping track of each other, smaller groups split off, moved around independently or joined another group for the hunt that brought larger game, better food quality and higher quantity. They gained these advantages through enhanced social interaction skills. Tribalism fulfilled the group capacity and need. The sense of belonging, identity as "us", and sense of purpose provided a healthy reduction in stress through loss of threat, and building of self-esteem.

The egalitarian hunter-gatherer groups survived 200,000 years with these rules of identity by appearance and mode of language, characteristic behavior and more inclusion than exclusion, as in the cases where small groups welcomed and encouraged the inclusion of strangers. Man became the classic social animal by acknowledging others, recognizing their identities, registering the similarities and differences, engaging, responding to markers, (language, decoration or features) and interacting. Making a connection benefitted both groups. Ancient civilizations all had significant trust, cooperative and altruistic extra-familial generosity that contributed to the common good.

Concept of kindness and cruelty in creation of societies

Cooperation, helping and depending on others, promoted survival of the kindest and created the tribe, the community and the society. A cohesive group enjoyed enhanced immunity through better nutrition and lower stress levels that led to better physical and emotional health. Internal strife that led to anger, hostility, fear, jealousy, and hatred resulted in decreased immunity and increased sickness. The group even justified raiding, seizure from them and distribution to us, as a form of social order, with chief and followers, each benefitting from the other with a cooperative raiding group and receptive home group, all requiring social interaction. They were social with each other for protection, provision of food, emotional needs and development of sense of self and in relation to others. Lack of kindness devalued every other quality and could lead to disastrous consequences.

What drove the Europeans to kill the Natives they encountered? Greed, innate cruelty, evil, God? Why did they not "socialize", cooperate and share the resources they found? The Natives were social and programmed to accept, share and show kindness. (The Mashpee

Wampanoag tribe encountered the Mayflower Pilgrims in November of 1620 and provided the food and agricultural knowhow that saved them from starvation. They made a treaty based on trade. Where tribalism in some areas developed from a social life based on kindness, in other areas, it became something else filled with fear, hatred and suspicion of "others".

Vignette #17. In South Africa of 2020, a young girl of an Afrikaner family pulled into a gas station to fill her car with petrol before embarking on a long ride from Johannesburg to Capetown. A young Ndebele man was filling the tank and cleaning the windows when, in a frenzy, she discovered she had lost her credit card. Knowing the possible hazards ahead for her trip, without hesitation he paid the R100 fee and bade her a safe trip. Three days later she returned, paid him back and added a box of chocolates and a viral spread of their story made him a quasi-celebrity. He overlooked tribalism and instead expressed human kindness.

On the other hand, strict adherence to tribalism exists. In the 21st century, we may do business, interact, with others for mutual benefit, but the absence of trust in anyone or any group outside your own tribe can be devastating enough to ruin the whole deal. People fear what they do not know. The persistence of ignorance about others is unfortunate. Reduce this ignorance and you reduce the perception of threat. When enough connections are enabled, there will be a reduction in conflicts. When humans progress beyond fear and animosity toward others, to amicability through reason, logic and knowledge, more connections can lead to increased survival successes.

"The child who is not embraced by the village, will burn it down to feel its warmth." African proverb

In the absence of interaction and connection, the reaction can be devastating.

With the beginning of agriculture, (Neolithic Age 12000 - 9000 BCE) people attached themselves to the land and to each other (a dual sense of belonging). Burials nearby added to the sense of who belonged where. As groups spread out and land was settled, worked and "claimed", social life underwent change rather than simple expansion.

Belonging is a primal human need for safety, comfort, protection and sense of well-being. Acceptance or exclusion became the natural order. Through social behavior, connecting and bonding provides the basis for depending on one another for cooperation thru trust. Positive personality traits of openness, extroversion, kindness and cooperation developed that benefitted the group. The one who did not belong or was socially excluded, experienced low self-worth, low productivity and depression, high stress levels and subsequent poor health.

Human societies have members which we recognize, cooperate and socialize and against which we fight to eliminate as "threat", if for no other reason but that they are "different". Unlike the lower animals, depending primarily on instinct, humans can relate to strangers, process them as one of us and treat accordingly. Which of the DNA reactions will be expressed, kind or cruel?

With whom do I socialize and whom do I avoid.?

Since the Age of Discovery and Exploration and resumption of contact of practically all *Homo sapiens*, we used skin color and physical features as "markers", for exploitation and justification of genocide. In the 21st century we know that skin color derives from differing amounts of melanin associated with environmental differences in exposure to sunlight... nothing more, nothing less. Yet we continue to identify people of darker skin tones as enemies and act accordingly despite their character and intention. Skin color is not a race, it is an ID marker.

Besides appearance, we use culture, behavior, arts, crafts ethos of a group, to determine with whom we interact and we exclude those we feel do not belong. The development of hierarchy and status and ranking, determines who you are and with whom you interact. Communication skills and open personality increases your chances of encounters and interactions, while snobbery that feed the ego, greatly reduces one's social connections.

Group identity is based in the sense of belonging within the US and Them tribal mentality and is a combination of love and loyalty (US) as opposed to fear and hatred (Them). Your identity is how you fit into the social world, gives you the reason for doing things and gives others the reason to do things for and to you. Identity gives license for you to belong to group, to feel superior to others and to assume privileges over and above someone else. We base respect, both given and received, on identity. It shapes thoughts on behavior and affects the way others treat you. Identity determines who is in and who is out and with whom one can social and whom to avoid.

Children are DNA programmed to categorize others as like or dislike, depending on the reward. Little children reach out to all women for a hug and children of all sorts embrace and play together regardless of identity markers until we teach them this is not to be done. Our societies designate the population as insiders and outsiders. It is natural to favor one's own for kindness and show apathy or cruelty on those not included in the group. There are more human similarities of diverse societies than differences, as all have music, myths, daily routines, body adornment, language, art and a desire to have friends, so that the rejection and designation of others in an exclusionary manner are usually taught.

A society with complicated strict ranking and hierarchy that restricts interactions imposes higher stresses on its members. Reduction and loss of the opportunity for an encounter contributes to higher stress in all groups. Refusal to share (healthcare, social programs for those in need, food distribution and property) or to interact (building walls, barbed wire, prisons, closed borders) leads to higher stress and poorer health

Us And Them

Around 10,000 years ago in human development, some hunter-gatherers opted for settlements. Over ensuing years, land ownership, possessions and consumerism increased their fears of threats, and they abandoned egalitarianism for elitism, self-interest and inequalities. Hunter-Gatherers (Nomads) vs Settlers (Agriculturalists)

Pre-history saw the development of society through social interactions as essential to basic survival. For 100,000 years hunter gatherers were egalitarian, altruistic, social beings, with kind DNA being rewarded and cruel DNA, suppressed. Domestication of plants and animals, settlements, agriculture and possession of property generated self-interest as the primary form of survival over the next 10,000 years to the present where self-interest is destroying the planet. Why and how did humans slip so easily into the barbarity of murder and wholesale wars? With the abandonment of the principles of equality and sharing, aggression and self-preservation at all costs came to the forefront and man chose not to interact. He opted for demonizing "others" and willful acts to harm "them" while establishing his privileges. The prevailing principle became "Us good, them bad", which still directs social interactions today.

This social behavior had a detrimental effect on human health. By maintaining group conflicts stress levels remained high with constant fear of "them" which persists today. (local and global immigration fears). Ancient history saw the development and progression of the antisocial personality when we encounter someone who does not belong, or is not exactly like "us". The DNA ingrained "cruelty" turns on the instinctive reaction of fear and they see "others" as a dire threat to one's property, self-interest and cultural survival.

"Other"

Why is the concept of "other" so prevalent
in one place and not in another?

Consider Middle Eastern wars, territorial disputes and religious wars. Think about America's genocides and multiple invasions. What about the fact that opposition to migration is prominent in Hungary and Poland but not in Switzerland? Fear and hatred have displaced compassion and kindness, as antisocial reigns over social. At what point does a three-year-old "learn" to fear and reject someone who looks "different" or belongs to another culture? Are they given a choice? Options include dismissal, ignore "them" or competition, actively engage but maintain the antagonistic stance, or discrimination, actively oppose, exclude, and refuse any interaction.

How can the pleasure of kindness became the same pleasure as hating? Us and them led to human classification and cataloging to make it easier and justifiable to reject and oppose "other". The gratification from winning, whether using love or hate, became the same. Though it takes a lot more energy to hate than to love, we spend a lot more capital on widespread hatred than on widespread love. ("To Hate Like This is to be Happy Forever: a thoroughly obsessive, intermittently uplifting, and occasionally unbiased account of the Duke-North Carolina Basketball Rivalry", by Will Blythe.) Sports rivalries with utter triumph over adversaries in routing and sending "them" fleeing just fills one with glee. The utter happiness of the crowd at a lynching in the South. The satisfaction of a massacre of the "other", the larger the numbers, the better. These are the triumphs of cruel DNA, antisocial behavior over kindness and social.

Humans separated and solved conflicts with widespread murder and destruction. Wars of Europeans vs Natives, Catholics vs heretics, Catholics vs Protestants, England vs France, Christians vs Muslims, England vs the world, France vs Europe, Spaniards vs Natives, Germans vs Jews, everyone vs Germans, Serbs vs Albanians and white America vs Black America, have dominated human history over the last 5000 years. (*First recorded large-scale war was between Sumer and Elam, around 2700 BCE*).

In USA people in the same town, don't speak to each other, occupy separate bars, cafes, schools, restaurants, churches and vote differently on common issues. They promote their differences way ahead of their similarities and turn away from each other instead of facing. The resulting stress levels are high and the prevalence of chronic poor health is clearly evident in high blood pressure, diabetes, cancers and heart disease.

With whom do I socialize?

You socialize only with those of similar social status, abilities and patterns of consumption, You socialize only with those with which the social barriers are weak or non-existent. You socialize with those which society deems okay.

In the biochemistry of turmoil and conflict, the brain is wired to respond positively to those in need. The anxious infant cries to draw attention to those needs. The quiet infant joins the crying one in reaction to the sounds of distress. A mother feels compassion when seeing, hearing or touching the babies of others. Kindness is activated in the nucleus accumbens that releases dopamine in response to rewards. When we contemplate or harm others, similar brain networks are activated and light up. Cruelty either suppresses dopamine or is associated with an overproduction of dopamine, adrenalin, and cortisol. Anticipation of helping others triggers activity in the caudate nucleus and anterior cingulate, the reward and pleasure centers, which is the same reaction as personal desire, gratification and satisfaction. The brain responds to others' suffering by releasing "feel-good" hormones that prompt the individual to assist in easing their suffering. The heart rate decreases in preparation to approach and offer solace in response to the release of oxytocin and serotonin into the bloodstream. Though the meanness seen from the cheering for building a wall to keep out "others" and for the withholding of health care to those less fortunate, come from the same sources, the chemical content and amounts differ (meanness elicits flight or fight hormone reactions) and that antisocial behavior is more learned than innate. Though cruelty and kindness DNA are present probably in equal amounts, the environment of infancy elicits the feel-good hormones of kindness before those of aggression.

Oxytocin A released into blood results in compassion, nurturing, grooming activities, socializing, long-term bonding, warm smiles, and friendly gestures. Meanness, neglect, heartlessness, and other antisocial behavior results in and from low oxytocin, oxytocin B or copious amounts of cortisol, adrenalin and dopamine. The mental and physical damage of feel bad hormones result in high blood sugar and triglycerides, high blood pressure, and hormone imbalances that affect all organ systems. Hypertension, cardiovascular disease, obesity, diabetes, a chronically impaired immune system, high rates of cancer, and infections are associated with the stress response of cruel DNA.

The compassionate response of good-natured acceptance, engagement, social interaction, positive, inviting facial expression, touch caress and friendly pat, rewards for and from generosity, pleasure, warmth and good feeling in the presence of others, competes with the mean-spirited chants of "send them back", rejection, repulsion, shunning shying away, rough slap, social isolation and intentional harm. Both responses are DNA based and dependent on the genetic make-up and environmental expression, dependent on the quantity and quality of hormones released, programmed reactions, family and society behavior (tribal). "We are wired to be social" due to early DNA sourced motivations to connect with each other and stay connected for survival, growth, and reproduction. Development of the group into tribe into village, town and city favored antisocial behavior for the same ends. The romantic attraction of sweetness has been replaced by the strength of winner takes all. The bad boy jerk is now adored and the "nice guy finishes last".

Stress is a Major cause of disease and illness… and may be relieved and avoided by having good reliable social connections…

With altruism and cooperation on the wane, group survival looked to another source of sustenance for survival. They accepted "superiority" and paid "obeisance and homage" to those they believed would guarantee their safety and protection. The hierarchy set at hunting and gathering and campfire socializing built a society based at first on skills and contribution to the group, then on privileges, passed on from one to another. At first interactions were based on the same, like interacted with like, for cooperation to the same end. Who walked first, who ate first and best, who sat higher or in the best position, became the leader. Who stood, who bowed or stepped back, who acknowledged whom and with what gestures or words, became the followers. Survival remained the order of the day.

As the hierarchy grew further and further apart, more cruelty became established in the midst of kindness.

Religion

"Find the level of humanity at which we all connect, include morality and ethics and make this point the basis of all religions." (author's note)

How does one justify wars of religion? Or burning people at the stake? Inquisition and torture? Support for murderers in the name of religion? How is this Pro-Social and not Antisocial?

Religion is an observance, commitment or devotion to faith in an institutionalized system of beliefs. Spirituality is sensitivity or attachment to religious values. The hunter-Gatherers had cosmology, a relationship with nature and the known universe. With their transition to settler-villager life came increased famines, effects of floods on their crops, and diseases. They devised and adopted religion to explain causations and inevitability of the unknown. Gods and spirits, dreams and drugs, artwork, altars, sacrifices, burials and grave gifts, grew into idols, icons, priests, churches, and rules of morality to contain society. Either you belonged and agreed, fully, or you were ostracized and summarily doomed.

Why did Homo sapiens exchange life of leisure, togetherness & good health for life of toil, disease and poor health... didn't anyone ever think of going back?

Hunter-gatherers were peaceful, friendly, and healthy, without diseases or large-scale wars. Settlers were civilized, living in relative comfort in well-built cities, with organized labor, surplus produce, made wars, got sick and became mean.

Religion provided a belief system, and all who believed the same, social grouping were connected and belonged. Same belief was security, different belief became a threat. Different belief system, you move over there. If you come close or if you occupy space that we want, you are open to attack, raid and war. Religion cold function like a knife, do life-saving surgery, or use for murderous assault.

Until 1800, (the French Revolution), three quarters of the world's population were "enslaved". They worked for someone else, usually a wealthy lord or the state. The world still has slavery in the guise of low wage workers and the wealthy corporations. These inequalities, the determination of who is in and who is out, generates resentments and hatreds and are directly contrary to the teachings of every major religion. Wars, massacres, destruction of property are often propelled by religion, "Onward Christian soldiers, marching as to war…" and supported by cheering crowds. It was not quite social and not good for one's health, then or now.

Pre-history religion centered on and probably originated from ancestor worship. From Kwame Anthony Appiah's Asante libation pouring of spirits to honor his ancestors in Ghana to the dried skulls of ancestors on the mantle of an Andean home in the Urubamba Valley, this "identity" serves to promote belonging, as "connecting" to something greater. Besides the explanation of cycles of life and death, identity in tribal bonding, and rules of conduct, religion solves social problems by linking all to the supernatural as a solution. All have a creation story, all have faith, as a device for success of the tribe in facing natural occurrence, when competing with "others" in conjuring up hatred and fear, and in shaping the character of the society. Origin Humans instinctively need membership in a group to achieve happiness and survival. Once the group established physical security, the reasons for existence and core belief systems could be explored for the benefit of the mental stability. Religion connects to human awareness of self, links of past and future, and concept of death and an afterlife. Humans buried their dead with valuable items to support the belief that losing the body did not include the loss of the soul. Ancestor reverence connected with a belief in higher gods, supernatural beings, all knowing, all watching, all powerful and endowed with the love of the very ancestors that were now smiled upon by their presence.

Early religions rooted in small groups, produced painted caves and rituals with sacraments of bread, beer and wine infused with the products of psychedelic plants to give beatific visions that explained death, soul, afterlife and life. Psychedelic plants originated and evolved along with humans over millions of years and became the biological agents of religion and society by unlocking the meanings of life and death.

Ancient man used plants for sustenance, for religious connections, and for the process of social organization. (In Amazonia there are several plants deemed "teachers", with most containing powerful alkaloids and anti-inflammatories.) They organized social life into good and bad and issued rules for survival of a society. The "God is Love" is the basis of all religions and provides feelings of acceptance, belonging, mother's love, and the feel-good hormone release essential to life and survival. The major religions originated from similar mysteries. Moses and the burning bush bringing the ten commandments of how a society should behave, Paul blinded by a heaven-sent light and hearing voice of Jesus on the road to Damascus to set the basis of Christianity and Muhammed and the dictation of the Quran by the angel Gabriel during a series of trances, were all rooted in the supernatural, shared beliefs of the group. They all have the same purpose, the regulation of social behavior for the survival of the group. Socializing was at the very base of existence with the promise of salvation in the afterlife being conditional upon a life of social civility organized around the rules of religion.

In ancient religions, women were the leaders They were the most social. As the groups grew larger the level of distrust forced the need for a single entity to keep everyone in line. They needed gods to monitor everyone and impose the morality essential to the functioning of the society. Men took over and relegated the women to secondary roles, and installed priests to do the leading. We associated the earliest gods with Nature (fertility) and with Death (afterlife) and we connected to their social life, which centered on living in preparation for the afterlife. Human survival and what you needed to know was the main "purpose". The gods of society became linked to pairings, groupings, conflicts and catastrophes closely aligned with social practices to enhance and secure reproduction and survival. Human duties in providing offerings at temples, attending ceremonies, caring for the dead, praying and making penance, observing the rules and taboos were social activities designed for the good of the group and to ensure the afterlife. Social life and religion were interchangeable. Interactions between gods and humans were primary forces in the social life in places like Mesopotamia, India, Africa, Europe Meso-America and Native America. All religions have bizarre creation myths that justify their existence. The development of doctrine and spirituality (either self-conjured or drug induced) then justified the expansion and interaction with other tribes while searching for psychological security and physical gains. They acquired all this through group ritual and repeated obeisance that required extensive socializing.

Music: and drugs are closely related to both religion and the early social life. Flutes and rattles, chants and songs, produce sounds related to spirituality outside of human existence and are universal in all world societies. The wind rustling leaves, howling or whistling, creates harmony out of chaos which mirrors the aims of religion. Sounds associated with healing and with the dead. From early natural groans of mourning to hymns of praise that heighten the experience of pleasure, music used for worship was considered sacred. Anyone who has heard Gregorian chants or the Vienna Boy's Choir will attest. Singing in group worship enhances the union of one to another. Who has not been stirred by the music played on the organs of the great cathedrals?

Study: The Marsh Chapel experiment (Boston University, 1962) in which two groups of students attending services were given either psilocybin mushroom extract or niacin, vitamin B3. Following the service, the group receiving the psilocybin reported having had a profound religious experience compared to only a few of the placebo group. The experiment has since been repeated with the same results.

Hallucinogenic drugs have played a significant role in the development of religion, by producing otherworldly images and imparting meaning to life and death. All stimulate the release of dopamine (pleasure principle), relief of pain and anxiety, provide comfort and sense of well-being. The entheogenic theory of religion holds that "God is within the individual" and the psychedelic drug allows or enhances the encounter. Ceremonial use of *Cannabis sativa* among the nomadic Scythians southwest Asia in the 5th century BCE is suggested by hemp seeds found in the tombs in the Altai mountains. The ancient Greeks used wine in Dionysian rites and stronger hallucinogens in a concoction known as kykeon were used in the rituals of the Eleusian Mysteries. In Siberia the mushroom, *Amanita muscaria* was prominent in the ceremonies of the Neolithic people of 4000 BCE and kava was used in Pacific island ceremonies.

Moral beliefs and life security social purpose were supported by religious questions that brought inquisitive people together. Religion reinforced genetic kinship, language, and social purpose. For people during and after slavery in the USA excluded from all main community activities and denied access to opportunities, the church was an essential sustenance. Politics: Some kings used the gods to establish, secure and support their power and authority to direct and control society. Gods acquired responsibilities like justice, military, and food yield. Kings assumed divinity (pharaohs) and absolute authority (The Bourbons and Hapsburgs). People accumulated within boundaries as a country united by shared ancestry and religion. Community: Groups came together for information, direction and psychological support connected under the banner of religion. A common divinity identification and afterlife belief, earned them membership in a support group that reinforced belonging, morality and pro-social behavior. Religion was the expression of tribalism in which social connections played a vital role. Desert religions promote one god based on visions and divine doctrines. Jungle religions have many gods based on visions and variable doctrines. Both arose and developed to ensure survival. The Eleusian Mysteries was an annual Greek pilgrimage and festivities held in the town of Eleusis in the Fall equinox. From the Greek, "muo", meaning "to shut one's eyes", the mysteries captivated believers from 1500 BCE until the event was banned by Roman Emperor Theodosius in 392 AD. Were the belief systems of life and death revealed and then sworn to secrecy? "If you come to Eleusis, you will never die" was the mantra that drew a population that had survived childbirth, diseases, wars, in order to experience blessings and visions of eternal life. The Hadj to Mecca, the pilgrimage to the shrine at Lourdes, Santiago de Compostela and the sacred temples at Angkor Wat all attract and hold the attention of populations from around the world. Belief systems are powerful and the promises of salvation and immortality are supported by like-minded humans.

Religious support for health is clear in the strength of friendships seen between believers. The expression of creativity and thought is beneficial to health and wellness. Art expression and appreciation relieve anxiety and stress and reduces depression. Creative writing of religious literature directly increases the immune system response and the religious experience directly increases one's ability to interact with others. By relinquishing daily stresses to a higher power, one gains anxiety relief.

While shared beliefs were constructive and strengthened bonds of inclusion, human nature declared that those who did not believe were "others" and should be destroyed or refused the privilege of interaction. Every religion, in their own way, says to "love our neighbor as yourself", teaches tolerance and connection through interactions and yet, many humans do not do it. The basic principles are professed but not followed. Christianity and Islam, Catholics and Protestants, "Black" churches and "White" churches are not shining examples of healthy social interactions.

"Master, which is the great commandment in the law?" Jesus said unto him: "Thou shalt love the Lord thy God with all thy heart, and all thy soul, and all thy mind. This is the first and greatest commandment/ And the second is like unto it. Thou shalt love thy neighbor as thyself. On these two commandments hang all the law and the prophets." Matthew 22: 36-40 The two basic laws of humanity, as spelled out in every belief system, are respect and understanding of Nature and our being (God) and respect and care for our neighbor "as thyself". The beliefs are intertwined, interconnected and depend on mutual trust toward the end goal of survival. Jesus began his ministry at a Jewish wedding at Cana. There were days of celebration, drinking, his first miracle was turning water into wine, sharing meals, hospitality, approval of the marriage, and all the events that bring people together.

The 21st century is witness to walls, fences, exclusions, fear, hatred, cruelty of one group toward another, extreme wealth and deprivation in the same community. The behavior of humans to each other is atrocious, un-God-like and not religious in any way. Social interactions and connections are in a sorry state throughout the world.

"If you wish to experience peace, (then) provide peace for another." Dalai Lama

Health: A study done at Duke University revealed that having a stable religious belief system reduces blood pressure and lowers the risk by 40%. Believers have higher life satisfaction than non-believers, and social bonds are stronger within the congregation than outside. Religion offers a significant resilience in the face of insurmountable odds, such as in advanced cancer. Strong faith prolonged life in 7.4% vs 1.8% in those with low levels of faith. Religion has direct influence on the human immune system. Those with low or no faith had higher levels of interleukin-6 (inflammatory protein linked to cancers, autoimmune diseases and viral infections) than those with once a week services attendance, who had lower levels of measurable inflammation proteins.

Though other factors of lifestyle may have been in play here, those who attended services weekly added 7 years to life expectancy and had a lower early death rate than those who did not attend services at all. Faith delivers social and health benefits of a religious community. Religion is a powerful stress reliever by combining cosmic faith and like-minded friends to reduce stress, inflammation and disease.

The official origin of religion as a search for comfort and peace in the truth may be a bit too clean and tidy. Many religions are expressions of tribalism in which social connections play a vital role in survival through natural selection. It serves well to boost war beliefs in defense and protection of property, of principles and in acquiring possessions (mainly territory). It contributes to the organization of the social order of authority, priests, warriors, politicians, clerks, merchants, farmers and peasants. It assures personal security for the living and in the afterlife. All religions are based on teachings of submission to the will and good of the tribal unit with social behavior as the stabilizing principle providing a communal feeling of unity.

Religion provides a group experience with which to socialize and denies access in favor of one group over another, such as African Americans not being welcomed into white churches, Catholic declaration of elitism over all other religions, and separate services for Muslims, Christians, Jews and Buddhists. Conversely, as mentioned by a character in a café in Alexandria in Paul Theroux's travel novel, The Pillars of Hercules, "it is easier to be friendly without religion... you can have peace without religion". Religion both provides and limits the opportunities for social interactions.

Violence and benevolence are both a part of human nature. The dual nature of Homo sapiens is evident also in religion. Of God and Satan, good and evil, body and soul, man has a choice.

Quantum Physics

We may link consciousness in social connections to mechanics through quantum physics. A quantum is a discrete small packet of energy, the minimal amount of which may be involved in an interaction between energy and matter. In quantum theory, nanoparticles, the physical properties of nature on the smallest scale are subatomic, smaller than atoms. In Quantum chemistry, "feelings" are vibrations of feel- good and feel- bad hormones experienced upon encounter, interaction and connection. The feeling to connect or reject that we have come to know as "vibes".

We may examine social interactions in relation to the physical behavior of chemicals and matter. Human cells divide about 50 times, to give a life expectancy of about 100 years. The telomere length determines the longevity of the cell. The shorter the telomere the shorter the cell life. Telomere length is shortened considerably by oxidative stress. Contentment and lower levels of stress can reduce metabolism and cell division rates to extend cell lives up to 120 years. Stable social connections can contribute to this contentment.

Energy is linked to matter. Encounter, interaction and connection between individuals and groups is chemistry and physics. Magical thinking, mind-reading, love at first sight, miracles at shrines, and distance faith healing all draw social circles closer or tear them apart, as in cases of witches, druids, goblins, and devils.

"We are wired to be social" due to deep DNA- sourced motivations that urge us to connect, stay connected and be rewarded with growth, reproduction and survival. Being social requires a slower pace, less anxiety, more patience and less pace, which slows inflammation and slows the ageing process. Eat slowly and digest better. Not only have friends, but appreciate them. Make the time to experience true spirituality and examine its purpose. Be social. Where and when everything is done rapidly, fast food, eating alone, attending segregated churches, and avoiding your neighbors, is not religion, it is "clubbing" where status and material wealth are revered and people have little value. In quantum spirituality, the nanoparticles of honor and honesty is produced more readily than those favoring group treachery and dishonesty. If not, we would no longer be here.

When bacteria starve, they direct their own mutation to another state for survival. Can humans do likewise? Can we remain positive and create a new state of being? Can we evolve into supra-mental intellectual beings with body and mind connected to laws of movement of nanoparticles and chemistry of ultra-combined hormones (like experiencing and understanding the "aha" of love and the warmth of a sincere smile). Will there be total group recognition that we are all one race, one tribe, connected and the same with no need for forced separation, denial of resources to others by some, or exclusion from access to the full range of social interactions? Will religion develop to its full potential and with its true purpose?

"Beyond the subatomic world, is 'God'". Anonymous

CHAPTER TWO

PROSOCIAL INTERACTIONS

The interactions of ancient man with other human beings provided an exchange of members between groups, prevented inbreeding, promoted diversity, sprouted new ideas and enhanced the chances of survival of the group. Social activity is present in all species that range free, interact, and join as a genetic requirement for general health and sexual reproduction to enhance diversity, dispersal and survival. Possessing and using social skills, natural and learned, and the ability to elicit similar social reactions in others at the appropriate times, contributes greatly to the success of the species. Liking to be with and interacting with others; naturally inclined to companionship with others and reaching out across lines drawn by society that tend to keep people apart derives from this ancient pleasant, friendly, likeable, extroverted, and convivial pro-social behavior.

Sociabilis or *sociare* (to join), *socius (*associate) came into modern linguistic use circa 1511.

Sociality, the degree to which individuals in a particular population associate in groups for cooperation as a survival response for protection and good health. As groups grew into clans and tribes became communities, "societies" developed. The cohabitation of neighbors, arrangements of alliances through marriages, gifting, trading and sharing of news and knowledge all required adept socializing.

An encounter with eye contact, a greeting, a smile and a nod, could start an interaction that could lead to an engagement. A genuine interest in and reduced fear of others outside oneself could lead to a friendship, which with a firm basis in trust, could lead to a lasting connection. The purpose of any organism is 1. survival through protection in numbers and preferably with defensive skills, 2. procreation and 3. maximum comfort, pleasure through manipulation of the environment, which requires the cooperation of "others". From a simple greeting to an obsessive interest in a single person or a group... to ignoring the presence of others in a shared space run the gamut of social behavior. Most "normal "humans can find an interest in interacting, if only to read the intentions of others. In the abnormalities of autism and semi-autism, the brain is wired to ignore the presence of others. And then, there are the new millennials whose attention to electronic devices, ADHD, and concentration on their own specific space, render them relatively void of interactive skills. Why do some people interact, and others do not?

There is a human urge to belong to groups as opposed to painful solitude that borders on madness. When the game is survival, within groups selfish individuals beat altruists, but groups of altruists beat groups of selfish individuals every time. Such that in natural selection, the group with the most social behavior will have the most success. According to Edward O. Wilson, writer, biologist, naturalist and leading expert on myrmecology, "Social intelligence enhanced by group selection made *Homo sapiens* the first fully dominant species in Earth's history". Socializing is essential to human function and development. From a summary on animal social behavior in The Human Swarm, by Mark Moffett, "Chimps need to know everybody, Ants know nobody, and Humans need to know somebody." Socializing has been such an important part of humanity that it is associated with being "humane" as opposed to being inhumane.

The wealth of proverbs and adages in the literature that support social interactions are testament to the fact of their importance to the human body and mind.

Be grateful to people who make us happy; they are the gardeners who make our souls blossom.
Marcel Proust

Genuine friends: "To feel more agreeable in their presence, than in their absence."
Nikos Kazantzakis, Report to Greco

"The most beautiful things in the world cannot be seen or touched, they are felt with the heart."

"To forget a friend is sad. Not everyone has had a friend. And if I forget him, I may become like the grown-ups who are no longer interested in anything but figures…"
Antoine de Saint-Éxupéry, Le Petit Prince

"No road is long with good company." Turkish proverb

This is the recurrent theme of togetherness and friendship found in all works on love, wisdom and humanity. Kindness wins out over self-interest. We favor gratitude, fairness, trust, and cooperation over fear, hate, mistrust, and violent behavior. Understanding and embracing the intention to interact opens the mind and body to the value of social connections. When the initial encounter is supported by a genuine interest in being with others, social people make eye contact and acknowledge the presence of another. When we share the same space, we both have value. The least we can do is look at each other and acknowledge each other's existence. When you turn away, avert your eyes, and move away, you are saying that you do not trust me and I am not worth the effort of your attention. You are rejecting a basic interaction and blocking a social mechanism.

Social interaction is the second most important of the basic strategies of good health, after stress control. For social support you should have at least ONE trusted, reliable friend in whom to confide, and both must reinforce the elements of morality, compassion and cooperation encounter.

Science of Socializing

"The meeting of two personalities is like the contact of two chemical substances: If there is any reaction, both are transformed." Carl G. Jung

Once we realized that the benefits of compassion and cooperation for the entire group (and individuals within the group) contributed to the common good, we recognized socializing as the standard of behavior among hominids. Which developed first, oxytocin production from the expression of kindness or kindness from oxytocin production? Both most likely formed together with positive feedback enforcing the loop. The behavior of parents, availability of DNA specifying protein production and the reaction of the subject to the hormone all played significant roles. The difference between true compassion and basic selfishness emerged over centuries.

In anticipation of seeing or spending time with a friend, as in a tennis partner, there is a release of serotonin, endorphins, and alpha cortisol, all feel-good hormones. On the other end, when fielding repeated insults, humiliations, and enduring poverty, the release of beta cortisol, epinephrine, and other feel-bad hormones, damage all systems (Central Nervous, Gastrointestinal, and Cardiovascular Systems).

Teamwork and cooperation positively reinforced social behavior through feel-good hormone production, which led to a further increase in brain size and use. Social networks that got results promoted more social networks. Pains and pleasures raised cognition and awareness, which led to success. Increasing brain size made daily life easier and left time for thinking about and relating to other people. Wiring and re-wiring is what the human brain does when it finishes with motor tasks and naturally turns to the immediate social world and the pursuit of pleasure. We see this activation in newborns and infants easily smiling with pleasant strangers. The smiling baby is autonomic and contributes to the creation of conscious social interest and promotes interactions. The frowning, angry child is a learned antisocial behavior due to instructed fear or cultural custom, and its concomitant release of feel-bad hormones. Babies that cling to mothers and reject strangers usually have low oxytocin, and are reflexive of the parents' behavior and their low oxytocin levels.

The smiling baby/toddler shows an "interest" in ALL people, until we teach them to avoid, fear, hate and show disgust. The brain puts in "time" (10,000 hours) before age 10, in the social cognition mode of engagement. When finished with complex thoughts and activity, the individual turns on a "social thinking reflex", which becomes the brain's preferred state of relaxation. This social thinking involves "others".

After the initial encounter, engagement and interaction, individuals form friendships in which feelings of inclusion, warmth, safety, self-confidence and self-worth promote and result from the production of feel-good hormones (oxytocin, serotonin and dopamine) that give pleasure and associate with good health.

Socializing goes both ways. Time with friends, nature appreciation, and self-assessment all contribute to stress relief. A simple shared emotion emitting "feel good" hormones "I will see this person again", "I am about to see this person", the "we-click" feeling, promotes positive brain chemical reactions that lead to repetition. The resulting compatibility may be sexual or a non-sexual friendship, but the positive chemistry is beneficial to overall physiological health.

A positive rapport between individuals or sense of belonging between individual and the group, initiates pleasant feelings of excitement that may be emotional, physical or psychological, with the release of serotonin, oxytocin, dopamine and endorphins tending to euphoria which one then seeks to repeat. A negative rapport or bad chemistry arouses similar initial feelings of excitement with symptoms of rapid heartbeat, shortness of breath, increases blood pressure, skin flushing and weakness in the knees extending to a bad feeling when coupled with the cortisol and adrenalin rush of "danger". When prolonged or repeated, can lead to effects that are detrimental to health, which one then seeks to avoid.

The pleasure centers for reward responding with "like" are the nucleus accumbens, ventral pallidium, and para-brachial nucleus in the orbitofrontal cortex and insular cortex of the brain are the hotspots for hedonistic pleasure. The anterior cingulate cortex, ventral tegmental area, and amygdala are also activated in neuroimaging in response to pleasurable stimulation but are not hotspots. These feelings are natural responses that cannot be learned, taught, or synthesized in a lab. When we add or remove the appropriate chemicals, the feelings cannot be exactly simulated. They are natural relationship satisfaction reactions.

One may attain euphoria with reward centers activated through psychoactive drugs, but the natural reaction elicited by the feel-good hormone combinations are unique to friendships, love and human relationships. Social behavior with anticipatory excitement, laughter, music, and dancing, can induce a state of euphoria not duplicated by drugs. The neurological and neuropsychological components of the sexual response cycle and aerobic exercise are also euphoric, but friendship and romantic love are on a different plane.

The human brain is wired to think about the social world, our place in it, the threats and benefits of interacting, how we relate, and how we react. The processing of social information is fed by the knowledge and understanding of the minds of others. While general intelligence, problem solving, reasoning and basic cognition occur on the outer brain surface, social thinking is in the midline brain areas. Though socially challenged individuals appear to eschew interactions and connections, social intellect and analytical reasoning can and do operate together. (The inability to interact may be biological as in autism, or learned from the convenience of ignoring others.)

As the brain increased in size with more neurons engaged, humans could keep track of upwards of 150 individual members of a group. There was also an increase in neurons dedicated to "connections" between individuals and groups. As group sizes grew, so did the human cortex. Brain growth enabled increases in social relationships and the feedback stimulated more brain growth. More interaction increased cognition. More brain activity caused an increase in size and function. A larger amygdala and a broader seat of emotions opened the brain to more fear as well as more love, more aggression and more cooperation. A smaller amygdala produces less fear, proactive aggression and greater incidence of cruelty and contemplated murder.

How we think and act socially has a major impact on health. Physical nutrition is essential for the body and social nourishment is essential for the soul.

Health Benefits of Socializing

*True friendship is like sound health; the value of it is
seldom known until it is lost.*
Charles Cabeb Colton

Good health is being sound in body, mind, and spirit.
*The absence of physical disease or pain extends further to include
well-being, the state of being comfortable and content.*
(Merriam-Webster dictionary) 2017

Pro-Social behavior promotes emotional and physical health. Diet and exercise are good but social health is a foundation upon which to build and maintain one's health and well-being. Friendship with a reliable production of feel-good hormones and concomitant suppression of stress hormones, promotes good health.

*Being friendly, like giving or receiving a simple smile at the beach
or mall, is social. It is a basic interaction which may or may
not lead to a connection, but has a good health benefit. Turning
away, sneering or otherwise ignoring a greeting is antisocial,
unnatural unproductive and contributory to risk of poor health.*

From the first time a child steps onto the playground, he or she interacts with others in a meaningful way outside of the immediate family. They work out the processing of stress and process the benefits and risks. Physical confrontation directly affects blood pressure, heart rate and hormonal release. Physical activity enhances the endorphin release that adds to social interaction, facilitates connections and gives way to the emotional pleasure started by parental caregiving. Belonging, security, self-worth, are reinforced by the presence and acceptance of family members and others. Likewise, having trusted friends can extend your life. Study: A 2010 review of research found that people with strong social ties are less likely to die prematurely than isolated people. And that the effect of social ties on life span is twice as strong as that of exercise and equal to quitting smoking. Family and friends ward off chronic stress, which can switch on the pathophysiological processes of immunity and heightened alertness that results in wear and tear on the immune system and tissues and eventually to physical and emotional decline. Best friends can pull you through all kinds of difficult times... loss of love, job, finances and feelings of worthlessness.

Social interactions reduce the risk of Alzheimer's, heart disease, osteoporosis, rheumatoid arthritis, some cancers, depression, and anxiety. Friendship provides positive mental stimulation. Exercise through group activities is more effective than when isolated. When dealing with adversity, advice, encouragement and interaction with friends can avert the drinking, smoking and drugs to ease loneliness. Friendship reinforces feelings of acceptance and positive self-esteem. Social support gives a direct boost to the immune system, affords better sleep quality and higher productivity.

Having friends is one of the six best doctors in the world, in addition to diet, exercise, sunlight, and rest. Life is more enjoyable when all six are observed. A good friend is equal to one good medicine and a good group of friends is equal to a full medicine shop.

The best medicine of life is to have true friends. Anonymous

Compassion and trust seen as early foundations of social connections and lasting friendships, are on the decline in populations that perceive kindness as weakness and heartlessness as strength. Both exist as part of biology, and the development of each depends on environmental circumstances and experiences.

Giving and receiving are associated with gratitude, socializing and providing pleasant feelings. Society depends on gratitude for cohesion, advancement, and success. Gratitude is the foundation of social life in many cultures. This is nearly absent in a winner-take-all society that blames the victim, e.g. rape and accidents, and demonizes the poor for being weak and thus unworthy of compassion. Gratitude is humility, the recognition of life with the contribution of others as linked to happiness, good health and social connections. Being gracious and kinder, more pleasant to be around, welcoming, and inclusive all lead to better mental stability and a higher quality of life.

Nothing worse than doing a favor for a friend who did not appreciate it... and actually resented the obligation.

The Good Samaritan and repaying the kindness of others feed into well-being and inner sense of morality from the rules essential to maintaining a society. Pope Francis consistently and faithfully expounds and promotes goodness. "Follow the rules for the common good", he says, over and over and especially in times of crises. "Do not meet in large groups, practice social distancing, wear masks...for the common good". He opposed the Supreme Court's approval of open meeting of religious groups during the COVID -19 pandemic. "Social purpose and common good must come from sharing Earth's resources", he says, in direct opposition to the wealthy's promotion of taking all for themselves. (Brazil, Argentina, and Western Capitalism)

In a Guaraní tribe in Uruguay, the word for friend means "one's other heart". Indigenous people are always going somewhere, to meet, for ceremony, to trade, to socialize with family and friends. Their lives are full of joining and uniting. (One River, by Wade Davis). In the science of friendship, genes for kindness, compassion, and trust through social connections developed early, were culturally universal and passed on consistently because they were rational, got results and promoted successful survival.

Studies and Stats

Study: In a Gallop poll in 2004, 98% of Americans reported having at least one close friend, and the average number of "friends" was 9. The number of friends with which one could discuss important matters with—and trust—fell from 2.94 in 1985 to 2.08 in 2004. This was an indication of increasing social isolation in the society.

Study: Nicholas Christakis, an American physician-sociologist, found that friendship networks of identical twins were more similar in structure, features and formation, than those of fraternal twins... and mimic each other despite unique environments. This lent credence to the familiar sayings of "birds of a feather" and "blood is thicker than water". Some are born shy (introverted/antisocial) and some are more aggressive (extroverted/social). Humans selected the features of genes that specify bonding and social interaction and are passed on in the same way as genes that are specific for good health. Study: Yang Claire Yang, sociologist at Univ of N C, Chapel Hill, using biological statistics (blood pressure, body mass index, waist circumference and levels of C-reactive protein in the blood (inflammation) of those with friends and those in isolation between ages 12 to 91... found worse values in the isolates than in those with friends. The older they were, the worse the discrepancy and high the ill effects on health. National Academy of Sciences, Jan 2015. Study: The Netherlands followed 2000 residents, age over 65 and all dementia-free, for development of diagnostic symptoms and signs. Results: 13.4 with loneliness developed dementia, vs 5.7 of those with friends. Univ of Nijmegen. They concluded that having friends provide one with a longer, higher quality life. Friends can help one cope with rejection help you pick up the pieces and add value to your life. Getting left out (excluded) does not hurt as much when you have a friend. Study: A 2007 Harvard University research project found that the risk of obesity increased by 60% in those whose friends were obese or who also gained weight, because of sharing of habits and acceptance of consequences. Study: A Super-Ager study in 2008 at Northwestern University found that strong social ties promoted brain health as we age, through better memory retention. The effect in people over the age of 80, was as strong as not smoking and eating a good diet and exercise. The social side was equal to the physical side and supported the fact that psychological well-being prolongs healthy living.

Study: Rebecca G. Adams, at the University of North Carolina, Greensboro, found that friendship more than family relationships, had a bigger impact on mental well-being. Close friendships shaped lives and impacted health and well-being. The discussions of illness with friends were more important than with the doctor. Just having friends was protective and proximity was not a factor. Study: A Lancet editorial in 1989 reported that women with breast cancer assigned to support groups with other cancer patients had better quality of life and lived longer than women in a control group without similar support. Only smoking was equal to friendships as a risk factor in levels of importance. The reason was not entirely clear. *(The author suggests consideration of the levels of hormone release and lowering of stress levels. Do not discount the importance of stress in health).*

Hunter-gatherers with good vision, speed, strength, tracking, and social interaction skills, were selected to reproduce and pass on more genes for the same skills. Those with a high level of friendship genes further developed a penchant for popular friends, then a variety to make up a better social network that led to better hunting and produced more food that enhanced survival and passage of those same genes to ensuing generations. Those with gratitude, forgiveness, and social skills had fewer complaints, were better to be around and had better health. Quality traits with stable emotions motivated people to socialize and connect. When someone wishes us well, we do the same for them. That we recognize the patterns of benevolence and order in the world and behave in a manner that is "humane", became the normal productive way of life.

"All creatures that are not mad, need them." on having
friends from Circe, by Madeleine Miller.

Kinships, Acquaintances, Connections, Friendships

We learn that most social behavior is cultural and based on traditional habits and customs determined by genetics, competition, and what works in the society. It is influenced by the size and closeness of the group, the quality of communication and amount of labor. Cooperation and bravery strategies favor group survival, while selfishness and cowardice undermine the group and lead to failure. The infant/mother relationship of nurture and dependency was the root of the kindness and friendliness, which passed on to the siblings, father and extended kin.

Friendships occur in all species. When animals form friendships, males gain the competitive ability to acquire and provide food and for improved reproductive success. and females experience less stress, higher infant survival, and longer life spans. Kinships and tribalism forged deep friendships that afforded the development of important skills like communication and commitment that enhanced group and individual survival. The tribe was a small group organized on strong loyalty, conformity, cooperation, similar thinking, experiences, goals and purpose. A sense of belonging provided a sound basis for the survival of the group. When groups grew too large for individual tracking, or dispersed because of adverse events or diminished resources they broke off into smaller groups and moved on. The choices of who moved and who stayed were often based on established connections and efficiencies of members that would best ensure the survival of the group. Tribal perceptions of threat, both internal and external, were also a strong motivation to stay together or move on.

Friendships occur across species. Bonding forms between animals of different species where each benefits from the activity of the other (symbiosis) or simply each providing for the needs of the other. True friendships are usually seen in mammals like the higher primates, horses, elephants, cetaceans and camelids. All of these animals live in stable social groups.

The formation of friendships derives from shared interests and purpose requiring cooperation toward desired results. The emotional memory of these interactions serves to make connections for repeated successes. The ability to speak greatly attracted like speakers. As the best and brightest got together, reproduced and moved on, groups and tribes formed with like individuals with the best abilities based on social interaction skills. After dispersal, upon meeting and interacting with strangers, the ability to get along socially and learning together led to progress and success. Friends in pairs chose friends in pairs for larger group formation and social interactions led to connections into larger organized groups, with purpose, rules, relevance, trust, and cooperation.

Friendship ties to one another tend to be reciprocal and more numerous than the antisocial shunning of socializing, at least until the Industrial Revolution when materialism and possessions went full bloom. The mutual affection between people or bonding is based on displays and intentions of kindness, empathy, sympathy, honesty, trust, loyalty, generosity, genuine forgiveness, compassion and genuine enjoyment of each other's company. Why would someone socialize with person A and not with person B? It depended on the presence or absence of these qualities and the propensity for eliciting and maintaining the feel-good hormones. (Feel-good hormones also rise in cases of group antagonism against another.)

In the development of individual friendships, anticipation of what the partner is thinking, as to cooperate and coordinate, address and interact to get results and enable positive feedback for further bonding. In the camps of hunter-gatherers to the villages of the agricultural settlers, friendships enhanced the success of shared workload, avoidance of predation and protection from environmental catastrophes, alliances, food production and consumption, and reproductive rights. 10,000 BCE to 1700 CE, friendships developed solidarities flourished.

"A true friend is someone who is interested in your thoughts." Author

According to Aristotle's Nichomachean Ethics, friends enjoy each other's company, provide for each other's needs and share common moral and ethical commitments. Without these principles, members of a pro-social society will find it difficult to be friends with members of a cult that opposes every purpose, policy and goal and is bent on disruption and destruction. Friendships are the glue to a cohesive and eventually successful society. Hatred and fear disseminated by those who oppose friendships with particular people create anxiety and depression that can tear a society apart There are more sayings, adages, and axioms on friendship than on any other human topic.

"A true friend is someone with whom you spend quality time, share your heart with and then go to sleep knowing it is in safe hands." Author

*"A true friend is one who overlooks your failures
and tolerates your successes."*. *Doug Larsen*

*True friendship is when you walk into their house and
your wi-fi connects automatically. (internet)*

*Ultimate friendship is looking forward to meeting my
friend, Terrance, for tennis after a two-month hiatus and
grinning and giggling upon the encounter... the game
never interfered with the reunion. Author's experience*

*Oil and perfume rejoice the heart so doth the
sweetness of a man's friend by hearty counsel. A sweet
friendship refreshes the soul. Proverbs 27:9-11*

*"Lots of people will ride with you in the limo, but a friend will take
the bus with you when the limo breaks down". Oprah Winfrey*

*"A true friend is one who gives you his best bottle of wine and
expects nothing in return, except that you enjoy it." Author*

*"A true friend, loves what you love, admires what
you admire, in music, art, literature, and in matters
of the soul." Orlando Figes, The Europeans.*

*"A true friend would never turn you in or on
you, for any reason whatsoever." Author*

Hold a true friend with both hands. Nigerian proverb

*Walking with a friend in the dark is better than
walking alone in the light. Helen Keller*

A real friend is one who walks in when the rest
of the world walks out. Walter Winchell

"Ultimate friendship is being able to sit with your bestie
and in complete silence, yet each understanding the
other exactly." Author and his friend Frank Cook

Friendship is not about who you've known the
longest __ it is about who walked into your life, said
"I'm with you," and proved it. Unknown.

"Friendship is when you steal my chocolates from my bag every
day... and yet, I still keep them in the same place." Anonymous

On the power of friendships, "I got your back" gives the speaker good feelings of responsibility and the recipient good feelings of security. The connection of man and pet is expressed beautifully in the movie, Hatchi; A Dog's Tale, in which the relationship and bonding reveal a depth of spirit and loyalty unmatched in most human connections.

"There is nothing on this Earth more to be prized than true
friendship. Love no matter what." Thomas Aquinas

On men and women relationships, from Donna Leon's, Earthly Remains, "Casati had been the only man with whom his father had never quarreled, the man his father had always considered his only friend...men have companions, pals, buddies, colleagues, but very few "friends"... a best friend is usually their wife." Men rarely trust each other. Betrayal is easy and often, over a woman, over money, over principles, competition for dominance access to reproduction, rivalry, and envy. Women forge and maintain friendships easier and longer and hence are more social than men.

The German army (Hitler's Wehrmacht) fought so hard and desertion was almost zero. They stuck together, not because of training, equipment, ideology, beliefs or country, but due to loyalty, solidarity and a friendship with each other so deep that it brought out cooperation and trust to fight on beyond any hope, so as not to disappoint the others. Camaraderie was the army's strength and in most successful wars: Alexander's Greek army (until they stopped trusting each other, split up and chose sides), Roman legions (until they divided into us and them, immigrants), Genghis Khan's hordes, Bolivar's rag-tag army of "independentistas". Brutal violence is terrifying and difficult to endure when alone, but much easier when done with someone you trust and love, a comrade. (theme from Band of Brothers, TV episode 1) The recruitment of jihadists is not for ideology of religion or conviction of principles but often done between best of friends and for friendship's sake. This loyalty gives meaning and purpose to an empty life and becomes a basis for being social.

> *"I may not be the most important person in your life... I just hope when you hear my name, you smile, and say "that was my friend". Anonymous*

The true value of friendships lies in trust and loyalty. There are real friends and fake friends. A real friend is sincere, supports all your endeavors, forgives you for anything, always has your back no matter what the cost, provides encouragement, maintains contact and keeps your secrets as sacred things. A fake friend discourages you, easily holds a grudge, sides with the enemy behind your back and is only present when needing something for themselves.

*Friendship, like phosphorus, shines brightest
when all around is dark. proverb*

Only a real friend will tell you when your face is dirty. Sicilian proverb

True friendships are born of social connections.

*It is a good thing to have a friend, even if one is about to
die. I, for instance, am very glad to have a fox as a friend."
(24.8) Antoine de Saint-Exupery, Le Petit Prince*

****As people mature, they realize it is less important to have
more friends, and more important to have real ones.*

Friendships generate feel-good hormones. One of my defini-
tions of a true friend is someone you look forward to seeing and
spending quality time without conditions… the thought of which
gives you a good feeling. *Friends make you smile, laugh and live a little
better.*

*We crave and cherish closeness with other human
beings, just sometimes have trouble recognizing them.
Friendship is never anything but sharing.*

These are all expressions of loyalty and trust, the base of
friendships.

*"The language of friendship is not words, but
meanings." Henry David Thoreau*

When an interaction becomes more than just words, it becomes
a connection.

"Anyone can sympathize with the sufferings of a friend, but it requires a very special nature to sympathize (and applaud & support) with a friend's success." Oscar Wilde

We tie friendship to a sense of belonging and origin, both to place and self. Friends connect you to a comfort zone, give you a sense of purpose and make life worthwhile. If you can be comfortable with yourself, then you can develop the social skills to be comfortable with others. Learning to use basic manners can carry you far in transforming acquaintances into friends. Communication is the main social skill in forming relationships. Kindness and compassion are the essential ingredients.

"Sometimes Me think. What is friend? And then me say. "Friend is someone to share the last cookie with". Cookie Monster (Sesame Street)

"Kindness and politeness are not overrated at all. They're underused." Tommy Lee Jones

Communication and basic manners are seriously lacking in some societies, especially between a dominant group and "others". Some people deemed different are excluded and considered as not being worth the effort of having a conversation.

"Kindness is a language which the deaf can hear and the blind can see." Mark Twain

"No act of kindness, no matter how small, is ever wasted." Aesop

Friendship forms and receives support from natural family care and the kindness of individuals and groups. Physical and psychological support can morph into extreme support, as in brotherhoods, fraternities, blood bonds and mafia. Superficial friendships can be based on material goods, giving and taking, and perceived reciprocity, but deep connections are associated more with kindness from the heart that is natural and real. What matters most and lasts the longest are human emotions and actions that uphold a sense of purpose.

Cultural friendships depend largely on tradition, with social parity and power dominance, taking a lesser role. Why do island-based nations seem more friendly than continental-based nations, like the Pacific Islands, Greece, Ireland, and Iceland. Warmth and "easy living" tend to boost the human social condition and behavior. Ancient encounters of Babylonians and Assyrians gave us the hand-shake. See and feel that I have nothing threatening in my hand. I greet you in peace and bring you safety with good intentions. Along with hands on the table, it became a ritual gesture, a pledge of trust and friendship. A hand on the hilt of a weapon, or below the table had the opposite connotation. The 17th century greeting of touch, embrace, and cheek kiss, indicated no threat, no domination and no violence. Chivalry was one of the earliest social mechanisms giving way to the modern version of eye contact, nod, and a smile (ECNS).

"What glory can compare to that delight of conversing with friends on a sunny afternoon." Epicurius

Friendship has value. Acquaintances made across cultural lines expand one's scope of knowledge and experiences. Having a friend from a different culture expands your range and perspective, stimulates and exercises your brain to a better level of health. Even reaching out across town or state to others not normally in your vicinity is a positive step in expanding your range of interaction Exposure to new information different lifestyles, perhaps new technology can only be helpful and enhancing to life. Turning to each other is always better than turning on or away from each other.

Alfred L. Anduze, MD

Convenient, pick-up-the-mail friends may become come-to-dinner friends, then got-your-back- friends, may become into take-a-bullet friends. Or acquaintances may go no further than superficiality or may become direct enemies, friend in need, throw you under the bus friends. When an interaction becomes more than words, it is a connection, with loyalty, trust and security.

"A true friend sees the first tear, catches the second, and stops the third." Anonymous

"It is less important to have lots of friends and more important to have real ones." Charlie Brown & Snoopy sitting lakeside) Peanuts: Charles M. Schulz:

The definition of a true friend, is "someone who says pleasant things about you when you are not around." Having a friend like this is a rare and valuable asset. Be sure to treasure it.

The ultimate connection of friendship is love, the intense feeling of deep affection. It is like an addiction, withdrawal, depression and even death when unrequited or lost, and euphoric when secure.

"Love is not about staring at each other, but staring off in the same direction." Antoine de Saint-Exupery.

"Two things you will never have to chase: true friends and true love." Mandy Hale

A brief review of how friendships form begins with the initial encounter, the interaction, and the connection. Depending on the quality of communication, respect and trust, the relationship progresses to a friendship. In 1980, my quality of friendships was high in time spent together, with in-depth letters written, shared activities (camping, sports, trips), trusted face-to-face interactions, wide circle of trust, Deer Hunter type to-die-for friendships, and deep core discussions. In 2020, the quality and quantity of friendships have diminished substantially, now relegated to Internet interactions with established friends, zero trust in new encounters, posted pictures on social media, Facebook friends, rush to cut the time spent, diminished circle of trust and still less use of people skills.

With the Internet, the diversity has widened as foreign friends are easier to reach. My range has expanded from 5 countries to 25 in the past ten years, from Mexico to China, each in contact at least on a weekly basis. The quest of all social behavior is comfort and happiness.

> *"Happy people are not those who have the most, but those who are grateful for what they have". Guatemala quote*

There are different types of friendships. The most common type we think of is the long-term, non-reproductive relationships with others, with reliable interactions, and within the safety of the group. Banding and bonding together, teaching and learning in groups, is the type that enhanced survival. Friends with collective interests, individual respect and a common purpose, instinctively connect and maintain. These friendships are controlled and somewhat limited to proximity and similarity.

Animal friendships depend more on amount of time spent together; relationship of a maternal relative and at least one unrelated individual as seen in chimpanzees, baboons, and dolphins. With hands free, primates use of touch and language to express emotions greatly enhanced the forging of friendships. Through interaction and cooperation with others, morality, reproductive partners and useful friendships developed that further ensured survival. Society's success passed on the beneficial genes. Similarities of friendships across cultures bear witness to the process. Friendships provide stable bonds, create social networks, help develop people and creative skills and positive feedback for successes based on interactions.

Friendships in old age are the greatest source of happiness when all else is shrinking and disappearing. Good friends link the present with the past. When you lose a friend, you lose part of your past. Old age friends are no longer interested in reproduction or competition, but in providing collective health and comfort. Leonard Anduze, in his book, Drinking with the Gods, about life on a cacao plantation in Trinidad, in the 1930s, illustrates the concept of the essence of friendliness with this excerpt: "My father and (Leong) Poi (a shopkeeper) were roughly the same age, and had known each other the greater part of their lives: he never went to the district without going to see Poi. The evident mutual pleasure with which they met showed me the affection they had for each other, and when I went to live at El Perial, I inherited that goodwill from Poi."

"Good friends are like quilts; they age with you and yet, never lose their warmth." Anonymous

There are friendships with minor risks and no discernible benefits, like when elephants, dolphins, and lions, help humans who are in trouble, and accept the innate release of feel-good hormones. Perhaps, all good deeds are not based solely on reproduction and survival. Plants make chemical attractants for friends and toxic repellants to avoid being eaten by enemies. Both kingdoms sound the alarm to warn their own that benefits all, then join the run that increases chances of survival. Social groups reinforce positive social behavior when it works.

Friendship is a useful mutual aid, an innate sense of duty and a feel-good comfort, more valuable than ostracism.

*"Greater love has no one than this: to lay down
one's life for his friends." John 15:13 NT*

This is the basis of war, of defense of the group, of acts of sacrifice on and off the battlefield, of sharing scarce food, and of risking organ donation. Friendship is a powerful factor in promoting good health, both mental and physical, and appreciate in times of extreme stress. Friendships may be imaginary in covering the impulse to make and have friends. In my three-year-old mind, "Gregory" my life-size plastic doll, my best friend, was quite alive.

"We are lucky in our friends. Two of them seem almost of mythological quality_". Lawrence Durell (Corfu 1949) Travel Reader

Even if a friendship is imaginary, it is worth more than none at all.

We organize tribal-based friendships on loyalty, conformity, cooperation, similar thinking and experiences, similar goals and objectives, a strong sense of belonging, and pooled activities for survival of the group. Mass society breaks off into tribal groups within the greater whole, sometimes natural by choice or forced by an event, such as size of the group relative to its needs. More often, tribal perceptions of threat from "others" are the strongest motivational force to break off or stay together. Tribalism reinforces friendships, creates enemies and fosters betrayals. We should have evolved past it by now.

*Basic Tenet of Human existence: "All human beings are born free
and equal in dignity and rights. We are endowed with reason
and conscience and should act toward one another in a spirit
of brotherhood." Spanish philosopher, Miguel Unamuno*

This comes from a country that provoked one of the greatest betrayals and genocides in human history, the conquest of the Americas. The "Us vs Them" and "Others" concepts are not conducive to the formation of friendships. The company you keep influences your social behavior, as well as your dietary fare, exercise regimen, stress levels, mentation and risky habits. Your tribe determines your traditions, hospitality, or aversion to strangers. On the ECNS scale, the people of the Czech Republic, Poland and Hungary with little experience in showing hospitality to tourists, appear to be cold and detached, while the people of Greece, Denmark, and Netherlands is warmer, more open and more welcoming.

Then there are extreme friendships. The Japanese have set up social networks based on the concept of Ikigai, "a reason for being", within the society, but excludes strangers or anyone not homogenous or 100% within their circle. There are blood brothers, males, either siblings or those with sworn loyalty to each other. The practice of Laotong in China, where girls are bonded as kindred sisters for eternity, as more than best friends.

In some areas of the United States, gangs or just plain folk can be hostile whether you belong or not. Unfortunately, not everybody or anybody is capable or willing to be your friend. Some people actually find it easier and more comfortable being anti-social.

"Lots of people will ride with you in the limo, but a friend will take the bus with you when the limo breaks down." Oprah Winfrey

People pretend well. At the end of the day, real situations expose fake people. Of migrants, prisoners, the homeless, jobless, disabled and all discarded people, it could be said, why them and not me? Why the harsh judgement, treatment and willful neglect directed towards that don't look like me? We are reminded almost on a daily basis, that we need each other, that none of us is independent, or can be separated from the other. The rancor and hatred displayed when countries close their borders to people in need or people refuse to cooperate with requests to benefit the common good, will only hurt and make friendships impossible.

"The future is made of you, it is made of encounters, because life flows through our relation with others. Quite a few years of life have strengthened my convictions that each and everyone's existence is deeply tied to that of others: life is not time merely passing by, life is about interactions… The only future worth building includes everyone." Pope Francis: The Future You, Ted Talks April 25, 2017

Social Skills: Basic Kindness, Manners, Openness and Trust

Being social is interacting with other people, living in communities, enjoying being with others, and/or living and gathering in groups. Spending time with and/or talking or doing things together with others; liking to be with others, relating to people or society and being aware that dealing with one another affects their common welfare. Sociability, the noun, socializing the verb and sociable the adjective are all ways of describing the positive interactions between individuals, as friendly, cooperative, altruistic and parental. We recognize that actual interactions to superficial friendships and deep connections are essential to the health of a society.

Welcoming the Stranger

Of all the countries I have visited, none is quite as good in welcoming the stranger, as is Greece. (Of course you may differ in opinion but the underlying basis would be similar.) The Greek "phi-lotimo" is the pride in having something to offer a stranger. Is it innate, imprinted in the DNA or did it develop because of location at a crossroads of travelers plus years of tradition? Is it religious?

"For I was hungry and you gave me food, I was thirsty and you gave me drink, I was a stranger and you welcomed me," said Jesus of Nazareth. Do Greeks adhere so strongly to his teachings? Note that the Delphi Oracle's "Treat everyone with kindness" pre-dates the New Testament.

Do the Greeks feel so secure in their relationship with themselves, with others, and with the world that they can show kindness and compassion without fear? Do they really adhere to Agape, the show of love expecting nothing in return? Are they so secure in their history, their ruins, their past glories and failures, wins and losses that their sense of belonging is strong enough to offset any fear of "others"? Sharing with strangers is not only not a a problem but it is a custom that is spontaneous, expected and appreciated. *"You are a human being. So am I. That's enough,"* said an old lady upon being asked "why", after giving 2 honey-dipped figs to a stranger she passed along the path; from Report to Greco, by Nikos Kazantzakis). In the "Song of Achilles", by Madeleine Miller, Achilles expresses his Greek mind, *"No man is worth more than another, wherever he is from…Is a stranger worth the same as a brother or a friend? A stranger is someone else's brother or friend. So his life is just as important."*

In Greece and many Middle Eastern countries, impoliteness to strangers is not allowed. How a country treats strangers is an excellent gauge of its character and its value Greek mythology has countless references to kindness to strangers. Homer's Ulysses on the way home from Troy, encountered a swineherd who fretted over getting him food. Dionysius, the god of wine, and his wife Ariadne, toured the Mediterranean recruiting strangers for their festive events. The benefits of talking to strangers included acquiring news, gossip and sharing news to carry.

Aristotle described the Celts as barbarians who went naked in cold weather, were huge and terrifying, wore bright fabrics and were *"hospitable to strangers"*. He found this to be an admirable trait not readily found in many other places...even back then.

The welcoming of strangers in modern times and in certain countries is weak. In the United States, United Kingdom, Australia, Scandinavia, Russia, China, and Japan, the population seems not to care about the lives of "others" especially visitors who do not look like them and who may or may not be interested in staying. There is very little communication nor wish to interact much less connect with people they perceive as a threat to their possessions and their "way of life". They appear uncomfortable" in the presence of strangers from another country.

In a survey done on commuters, reply to a conversation open-ing by a foreigner in USA cities was 40% positive and 60% negative. In Greece it was 90 and 10%.

Even when travelling in other peoples' countries, some go in groups and avoid the "locals" as much as possible. Even the so-called ex-pats, when given the opportunity, will seek out their own kind for interaction and entertainment. Besides being rather insulting, it is counterproductive. Why visit a foreign country in the first place if you refuse to interact with its people? Strangers are people too, with thoughts, feelings, and something to offer.

Welcoming strangers is also strong in the Middle East, Mediterranean and African nations like Senegal, and Morocco. The people in these countries appear to be at ease with and accustomed to the movement of strangers. They recognize "others" as a part of basic humanity deserving of respect and basic interaction. For them, finding and making a good friend has value.

"One good friend is equal to one good medicine. One good group of friends is equal to one full medicine store. And the best thing is I have that group of friends." Anita Nehra

There is great comfort within those who welcome social interactions with strangers. Security and trust in their own capabilities makes connections possible. Inclusion is innate, a part of society, while they frown upon exclusion and consider it undesirable. The combination of happiness (joy and contentment) and health (freedom from disease) contribute to well-being and appears to be associated with the source of the tradition of care and concern for the stranger. *"The 'I' in illness is Isolation and the crucial letters in wellness are 'we'"* is a quote in The Heart Speaks: A Cardiologist reveals the secret language of healing, by Mimi Guarneri. It links friendliness firmly with wellness.

In some regions, a wider range of communication is available. People speak several languages and are able and willing to communicate with others, strangers. Some 92% of Europeans speak a second language, compared to 20% of Americans. Another language expands your "social" range of contacts and interaction opportunities. Besides enhancing cognition and focus, languages contribute to empathy and patience in communicating.

Meeting and interacting with strangers online in today's modern social networks can be risky and have undesirable outcomes. Antisocial behavior is more frequent and more intense when originating and being conducted behind closed doors, with false and harmful intentions. Humans are social animals, happier and healthier when positively connected to each other.

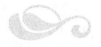

CHAPTER THREE

ANTISOCIAL BEHAVIOR

Actions or conduct that harm or show inconsideration for the well-being of others makes up anti-social behavior. The first principle of all organisms is survival. Ancient hominids' survival rates soared when being social and fell when being competitive and antisocial. Negative, reduced or lack of social interactions between humans gained favor in and between societies long before the present pandemic. Certain people just do not like other people, feel they are a threat and have no problem expressing their dislike or simply pretending the other does not exist. After settlements and the elevation of possessions to the highest level, greed and selfishness made headway in the human condition.

Humans are the nicest or nastiest of species / both social and antisocial.

Nobody adopts antisocial behavior unless they fear they will fail if they remain on the social side of life. Alfred Adler

Being antisocial can also mean that you're aware of how annoying it is to be social. Dov Davidoff

*"If you don't go to someone's funeral, they
won't come to yours." Yogi Berra...*

*Humans are naturally social. It is civilization that
causes us to be antisocial. Kirk D. Sinclair*

*You might be an introvert if you were ready to go
home before you left the house. Criss Jami*

Diversity is a key feature of Nature. Those who follow natural patterns should be successful. Those who defy should fail. Nature has a duality, and humans display the classic capacity to create and to destroy, often at the same time. Kind and cruel DNA gives us good and evil within the same genome. The initial social behavior that gave success in the advent, gave way to the antisocial behavior of modern times.

Movement is a feature of human nature. It leads to migration, travel and intermingling, and socializing, which were major reasons for our success. Around 10,000 years ago, when humans began to settle down, grow their food and choose material possessions over humanity as a main purpose for existing, antisocial behavior emerged as a major factor in the determination of human history. Interactions and connections carried a different influence.

*"Islands were dangerous places. You met monsters
as often as friends."* Circe, the prophetess

We were going along quite fine as "social animals". Compassion was an instinctive behavior sourced in infancy between mother and child, and extended to kin and friends. So when did the heartlessness arrive? It too is an innate, early defense mechanism sourced as an aversion to pain. But avoidance and disdain for other humans is manufactured and then leads to antisocial behavior. The child learns to hate. Both social and antisocial behavior are DNA derived, abuse and counter- abuse, love and hatred, the duality of Human Nature. The infant is born social and the child chooses to be antisocial.

The Paleolithic hunter-gathers were social, capitalizing on kind DNA to promote cooperation for protection and essential survival skills. Upon encountering others, they interacted, assimilated, and formed social networks that benefitted whole groups.

About 10,000 years ago, the Neolithic nomads decided to settle down, grow their own food in one place and collect materials. These became possessions, land, food storage and valuables. This started the concepts of "mine" and "get more" and "belonging", which needed even more protection particularly against strangers who would take them. The hunter-gatherers' innate social kind DNA and cooperation included the settlers' antisocial, cruel DNA expressed as fear and reactive aggression.

Aggressors welcome tough leaders to confer feelings of security. ("Build that wall!") With the accumulation of possessions, the hospitality of the nomads led to reduced interactions, xenophobia, and reduced sharing. Bonding rose to ensure the numbers needed for success at making war. We started as social cave dwellers and became antisocial hierarchal *Homo sapiens* in modern times. Nature provided hunter-gatherers with time and incentive to socialize, settlers worked to produce and took time to store and hoard, and socializing lost much of its importance. Paleolithic people observed all six strategies of good health, movement, diverse diet, low stress, low exposure to toxins, mental stimulation in creativity and interactions, and healthy social life. Neolithic people had a limited diet, less movement, high stress, exposure to animal diseases and a segregated social life. For the nomads, the friendliest survived while for the settlers, the cruelest hoarders flourished. They kept the toughest as rulers, and war became the instrument of success. (Support for the meanness and cruelty towards others generated by the administration of Donald Trump between 2015 and 2020, actually increased as the "normal" in the USA.)

Anti-socials replaced people with things, conjured up as "others", those with whom they had little or no contact, and toward which there was great fear and animosity, and developed a military solution to everything. The expression of DNA depends on circumstances, as in the response to fear and threat and a desire for dominance and greed.

"In all cities, it is easier to hurt a man than to help him." Plato

The reasons for antisocial behavior range from inherent shyness to deep cruelty. The primary driving force remains the survival of the group (individual) with procreation, reproduction and extension of the family line at the forefront. The individual need and capacity to socialize moves down in importance as a useful instrument. The natural DNA wiring expands to include antisocial behavior, which highlights differences over similarities.

"All animals are equal, but some are more equal than others." George Orwell

Vignette #18: Onlookers at a whipping or lynching of a black cheered with each lash, hurled epithets at the slumping body, then applauded the broken neck. Cruel behavior was common and acceptable well into the 20th century. "So it is the fear, weakness, selfishness, and cowardice of onlookers that permit evil behavior to persist." Laura Schlessinger

And descendants of these same onlookers recently gathered at rallies and screamed "lock her up" and "send them back" with the same fervor and malice of intent. Is it coincidence or predictable results of the antisocial dictum, "Us vs Them"? Can there ever be any genuine equality and social interaction between us and them? When abhorrence and hatred are the main emotions elicited from one human being toward another because of their differences (social status, history, skin color), there can be no social interactions and certainly no connections. Social health suffers when one group shuns and inflicts cruelties upon another.

Vignette #19: The Erik the Red Sagas on the encounters of the Norse with the Native Amerinds in North America, emphasize heroism and ingenuity of the voyagers and highlight the "differences" of the natives. This is a clear incidence of Us versus Them. In the first encounter, Thorvald, brother of Leif Erikson, immediately and without hesitation, killed 8 of the 9 people he met. The 9th escaped, returned with reinforcements and did away with Mr. Thorvald. It was not until years later that Thorfinn Karlsefni and his crew met and traded with the natives. And still the Sagas highlighted the differences not the similarities.

Materialism breeds privileges that generate inequality as the fuel for antisocial behavior. To be effective, social interaction must be repressed, social environment reduced and social feelings rendered insignificant. This increases self-satisfaction and removes any guilt from proprietary gain. As the concept gains popularity, pro-social behavior that is no longer needed is easily replaced by anti-social behavior, which takes less effort and provides a greater reward. Anti-social behavior got results and enhanced survival. It is rare that the wealthy got their wealth by playing fair. All had and made use of advantages in access and opportunity. Then they oppress and suppress the less fortunate to maintain that advantage and pass it on to their heirs. Normal people do not go around destroying other people, unless it is for material and egotistical gain. How one treats those who can do nothing for them, shows what genuine character is all about. We often find antisocial people lacking in real character.

The human capacity for making friends is the same as for making enemies. Kindness, compassion, competition, animosity, dislike, bullying, and negativity have roughly the same values. The key is to recognize and distinguish between the two.

"Keep your friends close, and your enemies closer." Sun Tzu, The Art of War

In the modern world, we forge some friendships for gain as in what can you do for me, and not for meaningful relationships, as in I'm doing this because I really like you and want to help. Socializing relies on trust and cooperation to bind us together and motivate us to depend on one another for survival, In "modern times", the need for reliability for survival is no longer valid. We have replaced it with self-interest. Anti-social behavior is highlighted by the severe level of distrust and breakdown of the social structure into tribes based on class, skin color and nationality. African Americans and European Americans living in the same area speak differently. They hardly speak to each other and socializing together is at a minimum. They live in different worlds. There are two different Americas. When one group tries to exclude the other group as "not belonging", antagonism arises, heading towards a tribal war.

Refusing to socialize, interact, or share space with fellow human beings is severely compromising to one's health. Social anxiety and pain of isolation are real and detrimental to emotional and physical health. Both sides suffer. The social brain is wired to make and keep social connections, such as with the mother-infant- family-group. A high level of social pain results when we threaten to remove these relationships. Both sides live in constant fear, resentment, anger and anxiety, with cortisol levels on constantly high stress alert.

The United States was less social in 2019 than in 1985. Antisocial behavior in the form of gang attitude, demonization of others, hostility and aggression, blatant cheating and outright theft is an integral part of societal behavior. When the population glorifies a celebrity who only backs winners and ridicules losers, we accept anti-social behavior as the normal. We no longer exile the alpha male for the good of the community, we elect him to lead.

Antisocial behavior is fueled by and causes more antisocial behavior. Working a job you do not love, daily stress (excess cortisol) building tension and abusive habits and feeling forced to interact with people for whom you care little, all provide damage to body and mind. Undervalue and under-appreciation produces adverse hormonal changes and directly affects the cardiovascular system to influence blood flow, perfusion of tissues and quality of blood. The anti-social person feels unworthy, struggles to interact, fears connecting and comes up short in achievement. Once failing at happiness is established, reactions turn to jealousy, anger, fear of change, loss of control, blaming, and bad choices.

Currently, we appear to be going backwards, with loss of communication and storytelling skills, ignorance of cultural histories and geography (especially our own), loss of appreciation and creation of the arts, of connections between each other and with nature. Anti-social behavior is fueling denial of climate change, abuses of energy sources, environmental waste, poor health delivery systems, where material profits supersede the welfare of the planet. This rise in meanness and selfishness is damaging to all of us.

When bacteria starve, they direct mutations to another state. Will we do the same, change, or stay the same course?

Science of Social Anxiety

The primary cause of antisocial behavior, the trigger mechanism that turns on the cruel DNA, is lack of contact, which generates fear. When I walk past you, make eye contact, smile and nod a greeting and you turn away and act like I do not exist, that is antisocial behavior, pure and simple. This behavior damages your health (and perhaps mine, depending on my reaction). It releases bad hormones within your system. Upon seeing me, your choice to ignore me and reject a simple encounter denies my identity in your mind. This rejection is subconsciously harming yourself.

Your cortisol levels burst upwards as you get a sense of dread and fear. Your pretense that I do not exist is not healthy. You shall have no social peace if you refuse to acknowledge my presence or existence. In the same way you ignore the homeless or the destitute, pretending they do not exist, or you give them some change but refuse to look them in the eye. The energy used in disgust and hatred promotes poor health. At a higher level, that of indifference, consciously ignoring someone is derived from the energy used in "hating", which releases a constant wave of cortisol, the stress hormone associated with fear and hatred. From either angle, as an anti-social, you harm yourself mentally and physically. Limiting the range of one's interactions to only one's group (tribe) due to learned ignorance and false superiority, may increase feel-good hormones initially, then the resulting isolation and deprivation eventually lead to the release of feel-bad hormones and chronic anxiety associated with maintaining the blockade.

If one knows it is wrong, depression, social isolation progressing to dementia, heart and neurodegenerative diseases, hypertension, diabetes, stroke, and obesity are the eventual outcomes. With the antisocial mindset, the biochemical release of stress hormones when challenged is always present. The people in a restaurant who avert their eyes at the presence of "other", will not have complete digestion and absorption of their meal. The physiology of the gastric system remains "on edge" and both body and mind suffer.

The ancient medicine of Hippocrates proposed that human health rested on the status of the four humors, or temperaments. Black bile, represented by the spleen, indicated sadness and depression. Yellow bile came from the liver, was hot, and signified choler, anger and neurotic behavior. Phlegm came from the brain (and lungs), and meant coldness, aloofness, and introversion. Blood associated with the heart and indicated emotional stability. A balance of all four was required for proper physiological and mental function. An imbalance in one or any combination led to mental and physical illness.

In the Latin American world, those who make eye contact with a nod and a smile and say *"Buen provecho"* to fellow diners when entering a restaurant, have low stress hormones and high levels of feel-good hormones, which all contribute to good digestion, absorption, and later elimination of essential nutrients. It is simple, try it.

Emotional pain and physical pain use the same neural wiring in the Central Nervous System. The pain that one experiences from social rejection and humiliation is equivalent to the pain of gastritis or a migraine. A threat of damage to social bonds elicits a physical pain response. Upon exclusion one heads to depression and compensates with an anti-social behavior similar to the original insult. A positive response is acceptance or immersion in video games, fantasy world, drugs, comfort food, big win lotteries, hoping to create a new identification, one that is invulnerable to similar attacks. A negative response leads one into depression, prolongs and intensifies the effects and ends with social isolation. Anxiety and depression contribute to dementia-type brain dysfunction, a compromised immune system and stress-related systemic diseases. The choice of participation or subordination, of fight or concede rank, leave or remain within the pecking order, move from pro-social cooperation, food-sharing group to an excluding, antisocial, selfish, competitive group, from equality to inequality, social comfort to social anxiety was made which often led to frequent migrations, re-locations and group reformations. They based social status on self-worth and valued the group according to appearance and level of acceptance of anti-social behavior, Status was attached to material wealth in a "what are you worth" fashion and whole societies were affected positively and negatively.

With whom do we socialize?

We choose our friends from within equal networks, out of expediency and proximity. The French aristocracy had few friends in the peasantry, the tsars and the serfs, American slaveholders and slaves, and American "blacks and whites" rarely socialize. With the upward movement of "us", we leave "them" behind. The higher one climbs the further away from "normal" the lower the ability to respond positively to human suffering, especially of "others". There is wholesale disregard for the suffering of any group we deem inferior, as the fact that they suffer makes them inferior, and it is not worth the effort. We develop and stick to markers for socializing, such as wealth index, social status, skin color, and manners and appearance. Anything that diverges from this model may lead to social anxiety. In the book, Post Mortem, Patricia Cornwall describes her serial killer as one of the "social misfits, the ones who don't fit in with the in crowd; the ones who never got a second glance because their fathers had dirt under their fingernails; because they were common."

Social anxiety may have initially appeared as "shyness", a vulnerability in ancient man, that manifested as blushing, heart palpitations, and butterflies in the stomach as lack of confidence in approach to a potential friend or mate. This initial reaction was a real stressful chemical reaction that was quite unpleasant. After having done something considered as immoral and negative by the group, the anxiety response of blushing indicating "shame" influenced the thought processes to avoid for the next time. If not replaced by confidence and success in a positive result for the next time, then anxiety and depression ensured.

Psychological avoidance of anxiety is deliberate and learned. To avoid anxiety and social isolation with associated mental instability, we developed and honed our social skills in keeping with the norms of the society.

Stats: Mental illness in USA in 1980 at 2% increased to 12% in 2010 and 20% in 2019. (NIMH health statistics.gov)

Physiologically, a negative hormonal coupling of oxytocin and testosterone occurs from a "ganging up" on a weaker group. When one group can ostracize and terrorize another the hormonal reaction is intense, prolonged and damaging. In a state of perpetual fear and on alert in preparation for aggression or defense, large segments of some societies remain under clouds of distrust and fear. This is even worse when the threat is perceived as coming from within the society, such as with police brutality, gangs, and one community against another. The outcomes cannot be good for the health of either group.

Social anxiety, with its variable moods and movements, affects health through the dopamine pathways, with both excesses and deficiencies. "Normal" amounts of dopamine dilate blood vessels, excrete excess sodium, regulate normal levels of insulin, maintain good immune and cognitive function, and provide ample feel-good hormones. High dopamine release from sustained antisocial behavior links with agitation and aggression and manifests as feelings of dread and threat, anger and hatred directed at external sources, eating disorders and insomnia. This state of chronic stress can lead to neurosis and psychosis. High dopamine with alternating pleasure and depression can sustain prolonged fear and anxiety, resulting in irreversible neuronal damage. Low dopamine in the circulation leads to a reactive rise in cortisol and a concomitant drop in serotonin, resulting in depression. Antisocial personalities derive pleasure from being mean, bullying, shunning, avoiding, demonizing, and dehumanizing "others". (Note the crowds at recent political rallies cheering for hateful behavior). With dopamine excess, the initial pleasure is short-lived. As the object of their hatred persists, the release continues to excess and feelings of dread and threat, become full-blown paranoia. Sometimes, dopamine goes extracellular, increasing the number of receptors available for uptake, and the individual needs to use "drugs" to get and maintain the same dopamine boost.

When anti-social hunter-gatherers became settlers and found that no bolt of lightning would them if they stole, lied and murdered and that hoarding, cheating and self- interest, actually enhanced their status, that the feel-good hormones came back if they suppressed their conscience and ignored their shame. They could express the mean, cruel DNA freely and were well on the way in the construction of modern man.

To justify antisocial behavior, the perpetrators work at the erasure of history and denial of conscience. The denial works to neutralize some negativity and reduce the effect on health, but conscience is innate, and some vestiges remain. The sociopath exhibits antisocial behavior, but grudgingly participates in society. The psychopath is more egocentric, has no remorse for his actions, no empathy for the suffering of others and often has criminal tendencies. When a large group supports a doctrine that is psychopathic, it will break off to ensure that its behavior remains the standard and is expressed normally.

The rise of anti-social behavior is directly influenced by the growing inequality gap in the United States. This gap is created and sustained by practices like exclusion zoning, opportunity hoarding, and blatant discrimination that ensures separate housing, schools, churches and workplaces, which reduce the range and frequency of interactions across ethnic and class lines.

A very small amount of anti-social behavior was linked to lead toxicity. Researchers found that between the decades of 1920 and 1970, exposure to lead in early childhood was associated with anti-social behavior. ... March 1, 2002. I hardly think that this is of any significance today. (Children's Hospital Medical Center of Cincinnati: Chemical causes of antisocial behavior.)

With whom do we interact?

Social sorting determines access to and range of encounters. By keeping communities deemed "different" apart, there are fewer encounters, interactions and almost zero social connections across classes and ethnicities. A nation divided into tribes, with little or no positive interaction between any of them, has antisocial behavior on display as its "normal".

Some anti-social behavior is self-induced in those without the social skills to interact. Some of these people prefer to be alone and do not attempt to make friends. We all saw these personalities in High School and College. Some of this behavior is environmental. The layouts of many American cities are not conducive to provide for or stimulate the interactions of people. The construction of "neighborhoods", gated communities, sealed off buildings, protective fortresses, suburban lock downs, and isolated rural, most surrounded by keep-out barriers, is not an invitation for people to get together. The lack of open meeting places (café, pub, brauhaus, market) is a clear sign of division and separation of the society from within itself.

Active Antisocial Behavior

Once we accepted anti-social behavior, it thrived. There are those who enjoy humiliating and insulting others. And there are those who simply ignore others. Whether it serves a purpose such as to elevate one's own ego to take comfort in ignoring or mocking another, to abnormal levels in either case, none of this behavior is compatible with good health. Satisfaction at inflicting hurt or humiliation on others sets off the feel-good hormones that are incompatible with normal physiological processes. Taking or getting pleasure at having the upper hand or at the perception of being better than someone else leads to an array of hormonal reactions that are inappropriate and detrimental to good health. (see Snobbery)

The antisocial personality disorder includes disregard for right and wrong, persistent lying and disrespect to deceive and exploit others, manipulation of others for personal gain, arrogance and aggression, sense of superiority, heartlessness and hostility with a lack of remorse about the harm done to others. These are features of the "sociopath". However, most antisocial behavior borders on just the amount needed to get desired results that are acceptable to the society and are without consequences.

When the exclusion of others is deliberate and widespread, it narrows the field and reduces the availability of those with whom to interact, hence fewer chances of connections and reduced success. Exclusion often results from low self-esteem producing the need to instill a false sense of security by demonizing and ostracizing others. There is a tendency for the active antisocial to hyperactivity with a release of bad hormones (cortisol B), which associates with further lowering of self-control, erupts into sensation seeking that manifests itself as violence. The promotion of

hate originates in the brain's cortex and subcortex and generates aggressive behavior. The planning and execution of anger and hate take a lot of energy. This is especially significant if there is any aware-ness of moral right and wrong. If there is no guilt or shame present, the hormones stay in abeyance. If there is one ounce of morality/ethics internally the promoter gets eaten up by the chronic cortisol B, the mental and physical poison, bane of the antisocial behavior.

The victim of hate goes into survival mode within a state of constant stress, chronic release of cortisol, persistent anxiety, insom-nia, and depression. Poor health all around.

"When you hate and seek revenge, prepare to dig two graves." Confucius

A boy has two wolves inside his teepee. One is peace, love and kindness and the other one is fear, greed and hatred. He asks the Chief, which one will win? Whichever one you feed." Native American

Feelings of hatred use up energy and are destructive. Political rallies of rabid followers shouting obscenities, name-calling and cruel slogans are stressful, unhealthy gatherings, both physically and men-tally. Antisocial America feeds off hatred, discrimination and sep-aration. We allow our government to issue calls for extreme anti-social behavior against other tribes by magnifying differences and issuing open threats of aggression. We allow ourselves to get riled up and convinced that the only solution is to inflict harm upon "oth-ers" we perceive as a threat… when no realistic threat exists (Iraq, Iran, Venezuela, Cuba). And just by making this statement, there are groups that will go ballistic in accusations of embracing the enemy, which is equally absurd.

Hate is stressful and seriously reduces the range of social inter-actions while driving up the fear factor. It is a neurosis, promotes conflict and is a direct risk factor in diseases of anxiety, tension head-ache, heart disease and hypertension. Negative emotions produce chronic stress with unnatural release of cortisol, which disrupts hormonal balance, reduces happiness hormones and impairs immune system function by damaging white corpuscles through deprivation of activating hormones and bombardment with destructive proteins.

The extreme is the psychopath. Devoid of conscience, remorse, guilt, blame, shame, he or she is a loner, clinically sane (functional), able to lie without blushing, and capable of planning and killing without remorse. Usually has violent sexual fantasies, little grip on reality, and slips easily into serial killing. Although many kill for the thrill, their defenders assign the blame to the family and ultimately the society. Inability to interact and connect, having been shunned and abused, it is not their fault.

So where does this destructive behavior come from? A study done using brain imaging at the University of Southern California, Department of Psychology, by Adrian Raine, April 2002, revealed that a combination of prefrontal cortex deficits, low autonomic functions and early poor health factors contribute to anti-social and aggressive behavior beginning in adolescence to early adulthood. Low resting heart rates promote reduced noradrenergic functioning resulting in fearless, stimulation-seeking behavior with lack of control over emotions and inhibitions leading to aggressive, often violent thoughts and actions.

Passive Antisocial Behavior

The introvert is deficient in functional social skills. We confine his or her comfort zone to small groups, cliques, gangs and solo activities. People go mad in crowds, then recover their senses slowly, if at all. The individual gets lost in a crowd and ceases to think for himself. We transform intents at morality and skills in communication into raw aggression. Interactions like these do not lead to connections except for a nebulous cause. The production of excess hormones for antagonism and anti-social behavior easily replaces the capacity for empathy and compassion, as the reward system has changed. When groups polarize, they do not interact in a healthy manner. We make connections only to "reject others". You can't love your own group without hating "others". This anti-social behavior based on fear and competition promotes social identities (skinheads, Nazis, white nationalists) is a strong determinant of who interacts with whom. Conflict outperforms cooperation. That withholding interactions makes them strong becomes an identifying feature.

Agoraphobia is when social anxieties induce panic when in a group. Depression and outright avoidance may ensue or turn to alcohol and drugs for relief. This reaction may be accompanied or influenced by other disorders, bipolar, eating, and/or drug dependence. The underlying basis is h*ow we feel about ourselves and how we get along with others.* Our sense of self and of how others perceive us control our social well-being and determine how we interact and with whom. People who lack self-confidence and have low self-worth are less likely to interact multiculturally with "others or them". Fears of threat to physical and mental affects both physical and mental health adversely.

Brain Scan studies identify particular regions of the human brain devoted to social organization, xenophobia, and friendliness. The antisocial person's brain reacts differently than the social person when presented with issues of morality. In the absence of self-awareness of right and wrong, stories around the campfires of original sin, blushing as a signal of conscience and acceptance of good over evil, social interaction is no longer essential to survival. morality

A lonely person is an unhealthy person. He or she requires companionship, trust, a modicum of dependence and a dash of reliance in order to be truly healthy.

Socializing Drugs

Some socially challenged people seek company and acceptance by taking mind-altering substances. Stimulants like Adderall and Mydayis of the amphetamine group can help you pay attention, stay focused and control behavioral anxieties. They boost dopamine levels that enable acceptable social behavior. When the effects wear off, dopamine levels plunge and one needs higher amounts to achieve the same effect again. The artificial social behavior can turn ugly fast and become profoundly anti-social.

Beer was the first fermented drink laced with psychedelics, for the purpose of gaining access to the afterlife in rituals linking the individual to the ancestors and gods. (Temples at Gobekli Tepe excavated in Turkey). Chewing coca leaves in the Andes and riverbank communities of the upper Amazon River, was used rather freely for thousands of years during social encounters in a practice that still survives today. Besides enhancing stamina, reducing hunger and neutralizing altitude sickness, it reduces shyness and timidity during the interaction. Mind-altering plants added to drink (wine) increased cohesion among participants in rituals and Ceremonies of all the world's major religions in much the same way as in pubs, bars and cafes today. "Those who drink together, stick together."

Using drugs to ease social tensions is universal and as old as mankind itself. Opioids substitute for the absence of the warmth of acceptance and inclusion, assuage rejection and eases depression. When the culture of social interactions that should come from families and friends in communities with purpose and dignity is absent, a drug-use society arises, which can result in poor social, physical and mental health.

Sugar in tea and coffee make them inviting drinks for sharing in the process of socializing. Alcohol in the bars and cafes provides similar opportunities and even greater effects.

Medicalizing social anxiety as a "disease" that is then treated with pharmaceuticals like Prozac and a long list of antidepressants is counterproductive and unhealthy. Self-diagnosis of social anxiety proceeds to self-treatment with easy access to pharmaceuticals, like weed/ cannabis/ marijuana to get the "edge" off, loosen up, reduce inhibitory restraints; removal of social anxiety. The delta-9 tetrahydrocannabinol (THC) affects how brain cells communicate with each other and with the outside world, slows things down, "relieves/ reduces" social anxiety, alters sensations, induces euphoria and makes everyone "happy". The benzodiazepines, Valium, Xanax, "the bennies", and "benzos", depending on the generation), reduce anxiety by hypnotic, anticonvulsive sedation. They act at receptors for the neurotransmitter gamma-amino-butyric acid (GABA) resulting in a calming effect, a "mellowing out". In making the situation appear less threatening, these drugs enable an artificially "sociality" in which one is able to do things not otherwise probable under natural conditions. Sooner rather than later, like with sleeping pills, the socially challenged individual cannot function without them. Addiction.

Cocaine is the master social drug of all time. The enabler for removal of inhibitions, the provider of energy and intense feelings of happiness, mainly from a high dopamine effect, was and is very popular as a partygoer's drug of choice. The ticket to the road to the unconscious is also a primary reducer of the discomforts of awkward social situations.

Alcohol, probably the most damaging of all social drugs, as taken in large doses, increases brain chemicals that slow things down, stimulates the dopamine effect that increases pleasure center activity, then tips over into combativeness and meanness or stupor and sleep. By reducing the behavior regulators in the brain, it lowers inhibitions, and releases the "table dancing", clothes stripping, pool diving with clothes on, blatant sexual advances, "social" behavior.

Social Isolation and Health Effects

The power of people connecting lowers harmful stress levels and boosts immunity for both physical and mental health and well-being. With a narrow field of contacts and severely reduced interactions, the socially isolated are open to anxiety and depression disorders that frequently lead to full sickness. Many of these conditions occur in our elderly, who have lost family and friends, have few acquaintances, live alone or apart, and suffer a high prevalence of chronic illness. The risk of premature death in this demographic is roughly the same as that of obesity, smoking and physical inactivity. The risk of dementia in this group is upwards of 50%.

Historically, humans were egalitarian, cooperative, hunter-gatherers, not competitive, aggressive, individualistic, antisocial aggressors or frightened, secluded hermits. Human nature was consistent with altruism and equality. True meritocracy served the entire group as those with natural ability used their skills for the benefit of the entire group and not to move up and leave the rest behind. This upward mobility led to more separation, less communication, and less connection. Genes evolved for both social and antisocial behavior, with expression dependent on life situations and environment. Brain function changes occur during brain development. We know that the rich do not think like the poor and that men are more likely to exhibit anti-social behavior than women. Besides chemical and hormonal differences, factors include levels of exposure and reaction to violence, abusive conduct as "normal" and neglect from both internal and external sources.

Social isolation is a relatively modern phenomenon, which may not be a direct cause of poor health, but is a huge factor in the development of depression, which is directly associated with heart disease, anxiety, and psychosis. Being expelled, ignored or ostracized from the group is worse than quick death, and sometimes elicits the same.

The dominant group helps to create social outcasts by forcing the disabled, the unwanted, the not-like-us, into social isolation. Some prefer to be isolated, away from the scrutiny of the dominants and others just lapse into the "feeling lonely" realm. Because of the inner pain, they prefer not to be with other people. Contributing factors include physical disfigurement, childhood trauma, mental illness, physical dysfunction, strangeness, ineptitude, poverty or being homeless, unpresentable and drug addicted. Others, like writers, thinkers, and those wishing to embrace unconventional behavior may seek solitude and safety away from distractions. Study: "How social isolation is killing us." New York Times article by Dhruv Khullar, MD, Dec 22, 2016. On isolation leading to loneliness to depression and the biochemical reactions invoked. There is a rise and fall of dopamine, which affects body metabolism and decreased function, similar to that experienced during grief. The sadness of isolation is more profound than that of death, and the suffering is worse when one is in poverty. Between 1980 and 2016, social isolation affected 20-40% of the population of those over 65 years old, and 50% of those in the 80s. Those who were uneducated were more likely to not have someone to talk to about personal matters and were even more isolated.

Social isolation is a condition of loneliness with feelings of being marooned, alone, spurned, lost and worthless, with nowhere to go or to turn. It leads directly to mental and physical sickness, weak to zero relationships, no friendships and reduced life expectancy, all of which the recipient is acutely aware. The effects on health start early. Socially isolated children have poorer health some 20 years later, impaired development and poor social skills. They exhibit low sleep quality, dysfunctional immunity, high inflammation indices, high levels of stress hormones, and high chronicity of symptoms.

Study: National Institutes of Health (NIH) report 2017, that social isolation raises the risk of heart disease by 30%, stroke by 32%, cognitive decline (dementia) by 30%, and risk of death within seven years by 30%. Loneliness has the same risk factor for premature death as smoking and obesity. Though there is firm evidence that prevention can and will improve these statistics, the society does very little to fix relationships and attitudes toward interactions, the medical profession prefers to throw ever stronger potions and therapeutics at the problem. Social isolation requires societal repair, not medications. America, for one, refuses to fix its social interaction problem as it continues to allow and even promote a foundation of hatred and class division. The rich see the poor (them) as evil unfortunates whose only wish to take from us. They have succeeded in spreading this view nationwide and perhaps globally. The promotion of staying in your place and with your own kind is on display daily with the mass media's continued separation of Americans into "black and white communities", and "majority and minorities" as if they are different species of human beings. This is a fact, and if nothing else, in the interest of health, it needs to change. We require social connections for the acquisition and maintenance of good health, and we are responsible for promoting humane social behavior.

The disruption or absence of solid friendships and access to relationships has the equivalent effects as smoking and obesity. Hostile relationships have the additional effects of reducing the efficiency of the immune system function. (This is perhaps a factor in the inability of the nation to make sufficient headway in the control of the Covid-19 pandemic.)

Stress, Depression and Heart Diseases

The list of diseases associated with negative social behavior, include mental stresses, depression/ anxiety, dementias: Alzheimer's, heart disease, cancer, and neurodegenerative diseases, like Lupus erythematosus, Multiple Sclerosis and Amyotropic Lateral Sclerosis.

Kinships, friendships and quality interactions of the Neolithic, hunter-gatherer times generated hormones that supported good health and the principles of survival. Good cortisol A released in acute situations, absorbed and disappeared when the threat was over. The accumulation of possessions and self-interest principles of the Paleolithic farmer-settlers promoted antisocial behavior based on anger and fear of a threat from others, released bad cortisol B continuously, which contributed to the stress diseases, heart disease, hypertension, diabetes, and cancers we see in modern times. Deprivation of feel-good hormones when coupled with reduced exercise, limited nutrition, chronic stress of anxiety and depression, lack of purpose, and high exposure to toxins, all associated with inflammation, which is linked to diseases, both infectious and non-infectious.

High cortisol levels over a long period may cause behavioral and physiological changes similar to those seen with exposure to a harsh environment of cold and heat, prolonged darkness, and exposure to pollutants and toxins. We associate exposure to lead, mercury, aluminum, and cadmium with cognitive decline and inappropriate behavior. Chronic stress wears down the body, mind and spirit. The primary system affected is that of **immunity**, especially in its response to viruses. Excess cortisol weakens the production of T cells, renders interleukin-2 producer T cells unresponsive to interleukin-1 (IL-1) and the system cannot produce T-cell growth factor required for proper responses. High cortisol prevents the production of cytokines, thereby reducing the capacity to fight infections and carry out cell signaling. B cells that produce antibodies and T cells that attack intruders become dysfunctional, affecting signals to the brain that the body is sick, and it suppresses the ability to fight illnesses. (Only natural killer cells are not affected by cortisol levels.)

The negative effects of stress associated with antisocial behavior related to fear, anger, frustration, arrogance, greed, envy, and selfishness as expressed by religious sectarianism, sexual repression, social and racial oppression, are allied with poor health. These bad feelings and inappropriate behaviors are energy draining and destroy the fabric of social connections. Chronic stress speeds up ageing, degenerative diseases and cognitive decline. Low frequency and quality of social interactions and few connections are directly linked to mental illnesses in all countries and cultures, especially in those with high inequality indices, where both rich and poor are less likely to help neighbors, the elderly, immigrants, the sick and disabled. Those with physical stress of living, eating and being alone, lacking support, under constant tension, fear of social situations that render them more vulnerable to humiliation are more likely to be stress-related diseases. Those who are easily annoyed and react aggressively or those who internalize the reaction until it explodes into full- blown sickness, are also likely to become victims of heart disease, cancers, stroke and dementias.

Lack of social interaction leads to anxiety and/or depression. The chronic stress that results in signs of weakness, fainting, chest pains of terror, shortness of breath of anxiety, dizziness and rapid heart palpitations result in health damages because of the release of excess cortisol at the wrong times and in excess quantities. One can measure the cortisol levels in the saliva and blood, and the levels of fibrinogen, which are increased in the presence of stress hormones.

A Cambridge University research study on student well-being showed differences in brain chemistry in youths under stress and a difference between acute and chronic levels of cortisol. In acute stress, cortisol levels were high, focus increased, regulated and returned to normal in the short term. In chronic stress, cortisol was high, character became aggressive, heartlessness, and sustained over a longer term or until the source of the stress was removed.

Jenny Tung of Duke University, Durham, NC, and Luis Barreiro of Univ of Montreal, Canada, through an analysis of gene expression and immune cells before and after alteration of the social status of the macaques, found that their ranking alters immunity. The low social status monkeys with infrequent access to interactions (lack of grooming partners) and lack of intimate contact, had multiple health issues (apart from inaccessibility to adequate food and other resources). Chronic stress is a cause of disease susceptibility.

Working at a job you do not love or like the Japanese "Karoshi", sudden death on the job from overwork, are both subjected to stress with excess cortisol, resulting in tension, feelings of worthlessness, under-appreciation, all of which affect the cardiovascular system resulting in reduced blood flow and perfusion irregularities. Anti-social behavior, active or passive, with its core belief of heartlessness, and its constantly high levels of damaging cortisol B, may cause stress-related diseases.

Depression is the most common disability in the world. Linked directly to poor self-esteem and feelings of loneliness, we associate it with low social interactions and weak social connections. Feeling "disconnected" appears most often in the teens and worsens with increasing age. Defined as an inability to take care of oneself due to lack of motivation, lack of caring, and lack of emotional drive, it is characterized by high levels of cortisol, high social anxiety, abuse of multiple medications (as a temporary cover), frequent and lasting distress, increased risk of heart diseases and eventual mental illnesses. Of depression and heart disease each can lead to the other. Depression raises the levels of inflammatory cytokines and stress hormones and associates with increased risk of coronary heart disease, myocardial infarction (heart attack), cardiac arrhythmias, congestive heart failure, hypertension and stroke. Depression also associates with type 2 diabetes, dementia, chronic inflammatory arthritis, and suicides. On a cellular level, the inflammatory chemicals released damage the endothelium of blood vessels and impair function. There is science behind a broken heart.

In Japan, there were more deaths from suicide in October of 2020, than from Covid-19 infections. (2153 to 2087). The global average of suicides from depression and social isolation is 10.6 per 100,000 persons. In Japan, it was 18.5 per 100,000. With the pandemic putting additional pressures on women to work their jobs and take care of the children, the suicide rates soared. Heightened sensitivity, fear, anxiety, powerlessness and high cortisol levels lead to depression and directly to suicide. At risk markers include a positive family history of schizophrenia, aggressive behavior syndromes, smoking during pregnancy, early traumatic abuse, compromised immune systems and antisocial behavior.

With both social isolation and anxiety at the core of depression, symptoms include a marked decrease in activities of daily living (ADL), ability and willingness to care for oneself, and a reduction in cognitive activities. Causes may include genetics, reaction to medications, environmental changes like recent moving, loss of friends and family, recent abuse, conflicts, and grieving response to death. Signs persist as sadness, weeping, loss of interest in previously enjoyed activities, sleep disturbance, change in appetite, change in weight, fatigue, low energy, sudden anger and anxiety followed by loss of concentration and focus. These features may be mild to moderate with a minimal effect on normal activities, or serious enough to impair mental and physical function.

According to SC Griffin, it is the reaction to social isolation, not loneliness or cynical hostility, that produces a cognitive decline in older Americans. (Journal of Ageing and Health, 2018). It is the reaction to being without adequate stimulation that leads to the lower cognition. It is the condition of retirement, with no further purpose, loss of independence, often accompanying hearing loss, absence of spouse and friends that leads to poor health and premature demise.

A study following 1200 male students at Johns Hopkins Medical School over a 40-year period, found that those with a history of clinical depression were twice as likely to develop coronary artery disease as those without a similar history. (Audiey Kao, MD, PhD. Depression and Heart Disease/Journal of Ethics/ American Medical Association, Sep 2005).

The most common management of depression in modern times is with antidepressants, like citalopram, fluoxetine, paroxetine and sertraline (Celexa, Prozac, Paxil and Zoloft). Success with psychotherapy follows with confrontation, understanding and control. For loneliness depression, a genuine friendship may be all we require for healing.

"To get yourself out of the pit, climb, don't dig." First Law of Holes

The effect of obesity on one's social life includes humiliation, low self-esteem, discrimination, reduced quality of life, high susceptibility to depression, and more poor health risks. Body shaming, social isolation and social anxiety with withdrawal into loneliness are expected but not always clear. We associate obesity with all-causes of death from hypertension, hypercholesterolemia, dyslipidemia, type 2 diabetes, coronary heart disease, stroke, gallbladder disease, and osteoarthritis. However, with one in three Americans being obese or overweight, and the numbers increasing to include the rest of the world, the shame is being diluted and obesity is fast becoming the "normal". Though the physical risks of obesity remain, the mental humiliation appears to be fading.

Inflicting Antisocial Behavior on Others

"We may not be able to stop evil in the world, but how we treat one another is entirely up to us." President Barack Obama 2018

The core belief system of the anti-social person comprises fear, detachment, and comfort in isolation as well as hatred of everyone designated as "other". Why behave in an anti-social manner if it results in discomfort and illness? Initially there is elation from the release of feel-good hormones related to the pleasure of inflicting pain on others, which, in the normal" person, soon changes to feel-bad hormones (guilt) because of the chronicity and having a conscience. The active anti-social person is always looking over his/her shoulder for the threat of someone doing the same infliction on them.

We are introduced to anti-social behavior in childhood, where it is either diverted or left to thrive on its own. All the inappropriate behavior is then reinforced in early adulthood. Refusing to engage or speak with someone from a different background or rank is taught and learned as the natural order of things. Defiance and deviant behavior emerge and take root at this time. We adopt patterns of anti-social behavior directly from distrust of others, which we use to further the goals of self-interest and immediate satisfaction. Life concentrates on me and my possessions, which must be safe-guarded at all costs. We shed the reciprocity that was built into social relations in favor of competition and gain against other groups that more often than not, cannot be of any threat to our well-being. Anti-social behavior, initially programmed into our DNA as a defense against cruelty and possible harm, grew into an offense for gain and dominance. Developing from protection of possessions to this is mine and ours, not yours, and we will fight to keep or take it, antisocial behavior transformed humans into the most war-loving creatures on the planet. As nomads tended to avoid violence and used friends for cooperative efforts to enhance comfort and increase chances of survival, settlers used violence to protect and acquire materials, which would eventually set them aside and apart from their neighbors. The kind oxytocin portrayals of animals and religious motifs in cave paintings became the heartless testosterone of wars, weapons, horrible wounds and mass burials seen with the aggression of the settlers. Anyone previously unseen and unknown became an enemy, to be eliminated.

The Tower of Babel story, Genesis 11:1-9, is an attempt to explain the existence of different people and the profound misunderstanding that comes from speaking in different languages that was divinely inflicted upon the population of Biblical lands... that ultimately prevented people from interacting. When they, the Babylonians, tried to build a tower to reach the top of the heavens, extreme cooperation, the Biblical God punished them by inflicting the misunderstanding that continues to this day.

Besides limiting the pool of social interactions, this behavior increased the negativity in human relations, caused acute and chronic stresses and harmed the health of all parties. Each act of refusal, denial and antagonism releases chemicals into the mind and body that have long lasting toxic effects.

Caste and race in modern society remain powerful factors in blocking social interactions. Refusal to socialize with a group (tribal aversion) with different identity markers (skin color, mode of dress) results from ingroup assignment of stigma to the out-group, which is then locked off from contact. In the USA, people identifying as "white" limit their social interactions with those identified as "black". Social ties that could promote productivity and good health are lacking and the resulting antagonism is leading to poor health on both sides. The costs and detriments of not connecting far outdo the costs and benefits of connecting.

Where gain through reciprocity is the only reason for engaging someone of a different rank and status, the range of interactions is severely limited. A well-connected individual with a wide range in a well-connected society is more likely to be successful than a well connected individual in a poorly connected society. "You scratch my back and I'll scratch yours." I expect something in return. "I'll scratch your back because it is the right thing to do; it makes me feel good and it is good for society."

Instead, many societies are full of isolated, aloof, cold, distant, unsociable people. Anti-social behavior starts with a basic lack of manners, usually not learned in childhood and promoted by parents and adults by extension. There may be a lack of opportunity for contact, but the hallmark of the behavior is being unable or unwilling to take part in a basic social interaction. In one society, people of differing skin tones do not talk to each other, which leads to a lack of genuine interaction on an equal basis. They live in the same place but are so full of fear and distrust, that they do not care to know each other.

This refusal to interact is not only not human, it is insane.

Antisocial Behavior of Rudeness, Disrespect, Hostility, and Humiliation

From the passive, "They don't know better", to the active, "they are mean and cruel to the core," encounters that make us feel uncomfortable with each other pushes social contact into an ordeal. Nothing raises social anxiety more than the belief that some people are worth more than others. Both low self-esteem and a sense of high worth can lead to shameless behavior.

Basic courtesies and socially acceptable manners originate in the home, around the campfire, in the school and throughout the village. Kind treatment of family and friends as well as heartlessness and rejection of those outside the tribe start and are promoted by the behavior of the dominant adults in the group. Lacking in or bad manners reduces one's encounters with others, adversely affects interactions and reduces connections. Blockages range from one family rejecting another, to entire groups of people refusing to interact with another group of people, such as the animosity that persists between groups of hyphenated Americans, based on skin tone, ethnicities and /or religious differences. Hence, interactions are few and superficial, while connections are almost non-existent.

Does a rude personality increase with increasing age? Neuroimaging studies on Alzheimer's patients showed damage to cells in the frontal lobes. MRI revealed a direct connection between brain volume and adverse personality changes associated with violent activity, psychopathy, and aggression. They linked structural and functional brain disorders to certain abnormalities in the fronto-limbic brain areas, amygdala and hormonal chemical imbalances. (Neuroimaging studies of violence and antisocial behavior. Matthew J Hoptman. J Psychiatry Pract)

At what point does a child in one of these groups realize and accept that social interaction is limited to like persons? And that the expression of this antagonism is to be done with rudeness and disrespect. That putting people into categories of "off limits" reduces everyone's humanity, and capacity to socialize. Cooperation barely exists, production suffers, and the basic tenet of survival is hampered. Everybody suffers.

Social interactions are stifled by antisocial behavior of those unwilling to share, to engage and to include others who are not in their tribe. Current antisocial behavior erroneously designates sharing as weakness, greed as good, hoarding as strength and lying as truth. Acquiring and having wealth is the goal and purpose of life. Anything that deviates from this line is "socialism", undesirable, and subject to suppression. Modern society has dealt a serious blow to social connectivity in its highlighting of differences and promotion of separation.

Human goals of self and tribe stifle social interactions

Though in the book, "To Hate Like This is to be Happy Forever", William Blythe explores the live and let die rivalry of Duke University vs University of Nevada Las Vegas basketball, this level of allegiance can apply to American racism. For one group to hate an entire people is to sustain a defective integrity just to keep the ego intact. With self-interest at the helm, threat and fear ascribed to defense of possessions is one thing. But the "I am flawed but I am better than you, not because of what I am doing or what I did, but simply because of the color of my skin" is another thing. There is a human tendency to categorize and organize into groups with specific connections within the group. This phenomenon is widespread across the species, but has no basis in biological facts. One group has convinced all the others that separation according to skin tone is logical. This deduction strongly influences "with whom we socialize".

To exist in groups is natural, to live alone is not.

Humans evolved to form social networks to live in groups with specific connections to other individuals whom they know, like and love. This is normal, but the separation into us vs them, black vs white, friend vs foe, good vs evil, severely hinders the effectiveness and range of social connectivity

An offshoot and close second disrupter of social connections is the "me-first", self-interest behavior of the individual over the social well-being of the extended community. Turning into and focusing only on oneself generates fear and hostility toward and lack of consideration for the well-being of "others". In his book, The Selfish Gene, Richard Dawkins highlights the prevalence of self-interest in the survival of the shrewdest, most clever and most ruthless. (This behavior is showcased in the plethora and popularity of reality shows.) The biological need for participation and communication with others, the morality of pro-social behavior, and the selection of friendly over antagonistic for reproduction have all but vanished. Of both selfish and altruistic genes, the expression of antisocial behavior appears to be firmly established in the 21st century. So many refusing to contribute to the welfare of the unfortunate are perfectly content with being inhumane, anti-social and selfish. Though the capacity to band together is instinctive, the trend toward exclusion over inclusion and hoarding over altruism is more attractive and productive for some more than others. Social groupings and spaces have changed the ways of interacting, opportunities, frequencies and qualities of encounters. The pandemic simply magnified the situation. The **disconnection** that has occurred because of antisocial behavior is the new normal. (Emersion into the use of electronic devices is only a small part of the disconnect).

Inclusion provides more opportunities and rewards than exclusion; participation and cooperation is more productive; kindness is healthier than heartlessness, yet antisocial behavior continues to gain ground. "What's in it for me" and the "greed is good" of Gordon Gecko in the 1980's, legitimized and promoted "let the cruel genes rule", "I'm better than you", and "you are not worth the effort and time of interacting with", "an enemy must be eliminated at all costs" and "a lesser being is simply to be ignored". The anti-social person struts about with airs of superiority induced by not having to speak to or acknowledge a "minority", someone less than himself. Only humans can walk by each other with total indifference and without a fight. (Chimpanzees, dogs, ants and lions don't pass each other without sharing something, seeking sex or starting a fight.) We root this aversion to interaction in a deep fear of threat of harm, which has morphed into a lesser fear of being exposed as similar or tainted by association. This behavior leaves a sizeable portion of the population unable or unwilling to engage and associate with other people in a normal or friendly way. The initial release of feel-good hormones is then overcome by "feel-bad" hormones released in response to the dread. Together they wreak havoc on the immune system and nervous system.

One of the earliest and most classic examples of antisocial behavior in history was the encounter of Christopher Columbus with the Lucayan people on the island of Guanahani on October 12, 1492. While expressing amazement at their niceness, docility, and unfamiliarity with guns, his inner impulses had no problem declaring, "they would make fine servants". His antisocial brain launched the Trans-Atlantic slave trade, the almost total annihilation of 50 million people, and the promotion of the "Us vs Them" policy that still stands today. Cruelty built on differences and craving for profit through exploitation became the pervasive human purpose and goal of the day. Societies built on the recognition of individuals as "humans" became fixated on separation by exclusionary tactics of promoting fear and hatred of immigrants, LGBT citizens, hyphenated Americans, and "others". The antisocial person who has replaced social relationships with inanimate things, video games, fantasy worlds, drugs, and comfort food as a "way out" from the effort of socializing. Ironically, the chronic stress generated by lack of socializing, creates depression and anxiety that lead to poor health. The excluded person suffers a chronic release of bad hormones of low self-worth that takes a similar path.

Modern humans developed a selective focus on recognizing and getting to know only a few social connections in order to survive within a society, excluding the rest. Knowing no one leads to social isolation, loneliness, illness and premature demise. The homeless immigrant with lost connections, subject to mistreatment (victim) becomes angry, despondent and doubles down on antisocial behavior. Gangs and organized crime groups provide the social connection and physical dependence of belonging. We characterize them as "bad" people, when some just want to fulfill their basic needs. "Pauli, Mickey, Johnny the Reb are terms of endearment intended to provide inclusion to those having previously been excluded from the mainstream.

Anti-social behavior is mainstream. Free riders, cheaters, white collar thieves, opportunists all those who take without giving are heralded, celebrated as "winners". The public opinion that used to tear them down is no longer in the forefront. The anti-socials take the lead, their policies of denouncement of sharing and promotion of selfishness dominate. Predatory seizure of advantages is applauded and rewarded, so that a single individual can amass $136-billion in assets. A total breakdown in the system of social selection allows anti-social behavior to be passed on in genes. Conscience, altruism, empathy and generosity are replaced with self-interest, greed, exclusion, limited social interactions and few social connections. Relationships are confined to spouse, mate, partner, family, less than 50 friends, a smattering of acquaintances, with society, tribe and nation off in the distance.

Inequality and highlighted differences promote emotional separation and distrust putting people further from one another's lives. Few socialize outside their immediate small like-minded, like-sized social group. Rural with rural, white with white, black with black, they do not speak to each other. It is as if association is harmful to their purity. They see life as a competition with the goal being to amass as many possessions as possible, while totally avoiding the hassle of interacting. Gated communities, heightened security, avoidance and hatred of people you do not even know are all expressions of the pervasive fear in social reality. Total neglect of the emotional and psychological rewards gained from togetherness, meeting new people, experiencing new cultures and traditions is the dominant behavior in many modern societies.

Friends are essential to mental and physical health. Small exclusive circles appear to fill the bill. Today we take our iPads and laptops to café or luncheon to be alone. We use headphones to signal, "do not speak to me". We have poor social skills and no desire to improve on them. We disconnect from each other, and this is considered as "normal". Family ties are weak, unreliable and tenuous at best utilized only when help is needed. The collective release of feel-good hormones is replaced by the enormous prevalence of societal loneliness. The coffee and tea together shared experiences with their additional advantages of providing antioxidants protective of several metabolic and neurodegenerative diseases, already in decline in quality and quantity, have drastically been reduced by the pandemic. Sickness incidences are on the rise and a sick person is not very sociable. Energy levels and mental stability determine degrees of socializing. Toxic behavior along with bad habits, like cigarette breath, uncleanliness and poor social skills are deterrents to socializing. It is difficult to be successfully social when one is stressed out.

We keep hearing and using the mantra, "Stronger together", then totally ignore it in pursuit of material possessions, a process which pits each one against the other and puts a damper on socializing in any form. The antisocial is ignorant of other cultures or just does not care and continues in the collective quest of acquisition of wealth and power, along with its concomitant fear and anxiety of failure or loss.

On the receiving end, there are groups that are under constant stress of defense and humiliation. It takes a lot of energy to be "unfriendly" and a whole lot more to absorb or attempt to ignore the intentional hostility. Avoiding and dodging "Unwelcome here" signs and signals use up a lot of energy that could be directed toward more productive projects.

The distrust of strangers is a built-in protective mechanism for survival during the Neolithic Age. With the exposure and knowledge of today, there is little excuse for the wholesale rejection and exclusion of strangers or any other group of people. Spain's expulsion of entire groups of people followed by the extermination and subjugation of even larger groups should have been lesson enough. Today we know who, what and where they are and their capacity for production of destruction. There is no excuse for the mistreatment of "others". The rejection and punishment of modern refugees in the 21st century by countries that know better, is a wholesale expression of serious antisocial behavior by a large swathe of their citizens, (attention, Brexiters, USA immigrant-bashers, Poland and Hungary).

Distrust invented racism, disrupted natural social mechanisms, promoted erroneous classifications that separated humans into different "races", which though scientifically disproven, holds sway to this day. This behavior that led to untold atrocities against and the extermination of millions still lingers in the persistent dictates of the news media and policy makers in decrees that continue to separate people into "blacks and whites", promoting fear and maintaining hatred needed to keep the status quo. Fear provides the stress hormones that lead to immune system dysfunction, which damages the cardiovascular system, with interrupted blood vessel flow dynamics and nerve transmissions. The gastrointestinal tract responds with excess gastric acid release that causes indigestion, ulcers, irritable bowel syndrome and cancer. There is decreased fertility, accelerated ageing and premature death. Hatred is a poison that eats you up from the inside releasing both acute and chronic stress hormones in the giver, and rage and reactive hatred in the receiver. Negative body responses increase the risk for the same immune system dysfunction, heart disease, hypertension, anxiety, and depression as seen in the perpetrator. Antisocial behavior promotes toxic emotions that adversely impact one's health. The antisocial personality by not only just not saying hello when greeted or failing to acknowledge the presence of another human being, feels that he/she is normal. That fear and hatred are acceptable emotions to display. If you get hit on the head, suffer brain damage, and survive, you are likely to be incapable of being social. You become impulsive, rude, self-centered, reckless, arrogant, less attentive to others, no interest in other perspectives, "don't blush" and don't feel shame. There is a high probability that you have low feel-good hormones, low kindness DNA and will be uncomfortable in the presence of others.

In his book, "Talking to Strangers", Malcolm Gladwell states that antisocial behavior is largely a matter of distrust. We do not trust each other, and rightfully so, as so many of us are subject to harm from our fellow human beings. Even when faced with a friendly stranger, many of us see the offer as a threat rather than as an opportunity. The antisocial is forthrightly unwilling and /or unable to associate with other people in a normal and friendly way.

Vignette #20: The following is an example of anti-social behavior in full bloom. On a pre-pandemic three-hour flight from City A to City B, my assigned seat was 18B. The 50ish year old gentleman in seat 18C, on his cell phone, got up to let me in, no pause, no eye contact, no further acknowledgement of my presence for the entire flight. The 17ish year old in seat A (window), behaved no better. He watched the same video game for the entire trip. Upon arrival, he called his father to pick him up, stumbled through the call, got up as if in a hurry. I moved aside in the aisle to let him pass in front. He hurried off, no thank you, no nod of the head, never making eye contact with any of his fellow passengers.

Why? Un-interested? Fear of interaction? Lack of social skills? What effort would it have taken to offer or return a simple hello?

And where was a thanks? Who taught him manners? We will never know. Hopefully, I will probably sit next to his father on my next flight.

Vignette #21: Negative interaction; expressions of hatred and disdain by one group toward another. The purpose is to inflict humiliation through name-calling and insults. Someone in a group will call out a jeer, then look to the group for approval and support. Demonizing and demeaning others to gain approval, reassurance and recognition is a common antisocial tactic.

Antisocial Tactics

Refusing to make eye contact, turning your back on someone, or otherwise ignoring their presence, constitute negative body language. The Magellan penguins in Patagonia, turn their backs on humans with cameras to make themselves invisible and/ or to make humans "disappear". Coldness, no smile, aloofness, and scowling are forms of punishment, humiliation, criticism, and expressions of disdain intended to inflict pain on those deemed not worthy of attention. The "I'm too busy to notice you" is a vital tool in the anti-social kit. It is a lame tool as it takes little effort to smile and nod as you encounter another person.

How did we become Antisocial?

Status and ranking came with the advent and importance of possessions, and their uneven distribution. Some took more than their share and, leaving nothing for others, blamed them for their inferior status and deliberately avoided contact. Upon encountering "others" the differences in status were noted, similarities ignored, and dominance established. Brain chemicals of good feeling and primary survival merged with those of separation and self-interest to provide the stimulus for antisocial behavior. Like attracts like into "comfort zones" of safety, security, and lack of fear. Seclusion became the normal as repulsion superseded the need of others. The Puritans/Pilgrims encountered the Native Amerinds and used them for survival. Once they were established, they discarded their benefactors and waged a ruthless campaign to eliminate them all together. What kind of people behave in this manner?

The **Disconnection** within humanity we see in modern society, has its roots in antisocial behavior and lack of basic compassion, understanding and knowledge between groups. Adolf Hitler fooled the British diplomats and leaders of Europe for years as no one really knew him or what he was capable of doing until it was too late. The CIA lost much credibility and valuable information when its officers, unable to understand 'strangers', recklessly allowed disinformation to be disseminated within its ranks and no one knew the difference. No one knew who to trust and who not to trust. Some voters chose Donald Trump not knowing who he really was and what he was capable of doing. They were all willing to be "antisocial" in their dealings with "others" and harbor a dangerous inability to distinguish between truth and misinformation just to boost their own importance at the expense of "others". Neo-Nazis marched openly in American cities, un-hooded and blatantly alt-right racist, chanting "Hitler was right", "Jews will not replace us". This is antisocial behavior on a national stage. Their anti-immigration, anti-diversity, and segregationist views in promoting isolation on a global scale whittles down to personal levels. The demand for and acceptance of separation is a huge disconnection that defines the national character from how people interact or refuse to interact.

We promote antisocial behavior on the airwaves when popular talk show hosts indicate that we need to hate, greed is good, fear is necessary, exclusion is good, inclusion is bad and diversity is ruinous. Free expression morphs into a troll heaven of vicious hate talk providing a toxic haven where insults thrive. Antisocial behavior promotes class differences or rich vs poor, white vs black and class vs classless. We discourage interactions and block connections.

The Internet provides a forum for freedom of speech in promoting voluntary separation, refusal to acknowledge the presence of or associate with others. Loss of the intimacy of in-person socializing (the pandemic contributed here), lack of opportunities for bonding, and loss of intimacy all contribute to the disconnect effect. Human kindness and compassion giving way to heartlessness and cruelty are an integral part of antisocial behavior. Facebook "brought us closer together". It also brought us unfettered hatred and magnification of differences that has torn us further apart. Facebook changed the way people interact, yes. In college communities, towns, cities, countries, the internet makes or breaks relationships sometimes without ever having met face-to-face or touched or interacted. "We connect people" yes, and also provide bullies, terrorists, haters, name-callers, liars, fake news promoters, and antisocial people with a forum on which to peddle their hatred and fear. Informal laws of the Internet pose that antisocial behavior is conflict, conflict is attention, attention is influence, influence is power, and power is good. Antisocial promotes materials, as in what I have is what I am. Antisocial promotes beating another person bullying, name-calling and lowering their social status raises your own. Antisocial makes one appear strong. Walking by or into someone's space and ignoring them makes one look important. Having no respect for others reflects as no respect for self. Modern humans have neighbors and do not even know their names. "Then I have to say hello to them every time I see them, and maybe they would want to be friends. Nah! It's not worth the effort." Facebook changed how and why people speak to each other, and think. It provides an open forum for the expression and acceptance of antisocial behavior to flourish. On the Internet one can find all the pages or groups you need to become and remain antisocial. Meanness is power and appeals to innate bigotry and expression of cruel DNA.

The solution? Identify the root of the problem, the belief in "separate" races, that "others" are not as good, neither of which is science. All humans are genetically the same, with slight environmentally directed variations. Eradicate the idea of separation and incorporate the fact of togetherness. The idea of a true multicultural, multiethnic democracy in a society rooted in dignity & equality of the individual as a reachable goal, is a noble goal that this country (USA) has never come close to reaching and few ever have."

Antisocial behavior produces sociopaths with an inability to understand or just not care about the feelings of others. They can break rules and make impulsive decisions without guilt of the harm it will cause to others and then brush it off as nothing, deny it or insist that it was right. The antisocial personality often has a superficial charm, manipulative skills, and a grandiose sense of self. With emotions that are shallow, they display self-serving behavior, incapable of loving or caring, and lacking in guilt, remorse or shame. They are usually irresponsible with a tendency to instability, and move around.

Why do we remain antisocial?

We have lost trust in each other and eliminated conscience. Once humans realized that we could get away with meanness, cruelty and even murder, (wars) and that this behavior actually brought us more materials and more power, the antisocial behavior was grounded and compounded. Our choices and lifestyle strategies determine levels of health and are themselves determined by levels of trust. When humans realized they could release and enjoy feel good hormones by being antisocial, still survive (i.e.no bolt of lightning from above) and even flourish, we changed the dialogue to being "mean is strong, greed is good, uncooperative is easier, conflict brings great gains and wealth is pleasure." With antisocial behavior on full display, I can go to a trump rally and not wear a mask. I can infect you because I can. I have the power to kill you, and it makes me feel good. I have the power to hurt you, to cheer when you are vilified and called names and it makes me feel good. I have the power to put my foot on your neck and kill you and it makes me feel good. I have access and opportunity and I will deny it to you. It's competition, unfair, but it makes me feel good, so I will continue to do it.

There are practically no relationships across class divides. Socioeconomic contacts and mixing is within the confines of strict boundaries. The mass murderer worked in a building for years and nobody spoke to him, nobody "knew" him. He came one day and shot them all. And then they wanted to know "why". Neighbors who fear each other will not interact socially. Fearful people remain strangers at work, at play, at home, they do not interact. There is no place of welcome. Separate churches, separate schools, separate communities, bars and saloons in which "injuns" are not allowed, parks, pools and beaches that cater to separate tribes. Not allowed. Lives based on high material capital, and low social capital continue to promote antisocial behavior. The hunter-gatherers and early farmers had cooperation, community, and reliance on each other for survival. In the modern world, we have lost the need to be needed. We have replaced the community with a world high on drugs, alcohol and technology obsessed with financial gain and oblivious to the loss of family, friends and higher purpose. There should be no surprise that this behavior leads to a high level of loneliness which promotes poor health.

People come together when there is a common enemy. We created and demonized the "other". We named the evil, feared it and despised "them". We declared "do not socially interact with them".

The reduction in socializing in this atmosphere has led to poor social habits, less friendliness, and the rise of bad manners.

Entering a room full of people while wearing electronic headphones over your ears, is bad manners. Deliberately avoiding eye contact upon entering an occupied elevator is bad manners. Failing to acknowledge others in a shared space is bad manners. Failing to give or receive initial greetings when sitting next to someone anywhere and in any situation, is bad manners. Acting only in self-interest is beyond bad manners. We share space on this planet, but fail to behave like it.

Hostility and Humiliation

In modern times, the hatred, division, "them" and "others" determine with whom we interact. Humanity has yet to grasp the reality that all humans are equal, have the same DNA, all have value and all are worthy of social interaction. Life itself is social.

"And the Kingdom of brotherhood is found neither in the thesis of communism nor the antithesis of capitalism, but in higher synthesis." Martin Luther King, Jr. in a speech to SCLC, Atlanta, Georgia, August 16, 1967.

All influential thinkers, philosophers, successful rulers, scientists, religious leaders, postulated that social interaction is good and required for success of the society. A society that ostracizes, demonizes, and blocks the activities of certain groups, does not move forward or survive. One would think that by now (2021), we would see that the acceptance of a "higher synthesis" of social behavior bringing all people together for the common good, regardless of minor differences offer natural advantages. That better health, less poverty, suffering, despair, stress, rage, hatred, and violence against each other would be advantageous. That the world's population would at last accept the fact that we are all the same. That two rich men in Wisconsin should not have value above one billion people in India. That poverty is cruel, and restricts with whom the poor may socialize and has no place in an "advanced civilization". That restriction of socializing is detrimental to the health of the individual and of entire communities and nations.

We accept and promote that antisocial behavior is rooted in basic fear, hatred and disrespect for others. "I am better than you, so you are not worth interacting with, not worth a greeting." I cannot engage as I never developed the social skills". "I don't care." Apathy, lack of compassion for others as in the entire group opposing "the caravan" invading from Mexico, mocking immigrants and condoning the taking of children from their parents as a punishment for being poor and desperate are deeply rooted. Heartlessness consists of inherited and learned meanness. There is an initial release of initial release of "feelgood" hormones, soon overwhelmed and followed by a release of bad hormones. The moral sense of protection of homeland, self, and group from others as expressed in the act of spouting and spewing hatred, leads to a bombardment of cortisol that damages organs, nerves, blood vessels causing stress damage that is real and lasting. The science of hatred and fear leads to intense mental health issues and chronic poor health. Sick populations exhibit genocidal behaviors, negative ideologies (Naziism), mob behavior, disrespect for life, and chaos.

Study: Acute social and physical stress interact to influence social behavior: The role of social anxiety. von Dawans B, etal. PLos One 2018, 13(10) (Germany). Stress (mental and physical) has detrimental effects on physical and mental health. Antisocial behavior leads to social anxiety on different levels, that range from not saying hello in an elevator full of people, to snarling and sneering at "others". Both raise bad cortisol levels that lead to increased heart rate and blood pressure.

Feel-good hormones makes the bully "feel good" in being mean. The initial satisfaction may make him/her feel protected from real and imagined threats, but the chronic release of cortisol in over-whelming amounts that follows is never healthy. In the bully's chem-istry, the amygdala in the brain reacts to fearful/ threatening facial expressions, by releasing more cortisol that infuses one's body and mind with anxiety, a constant level of alert and alarm. Paradoxically, the oxytocin receptor gene (OXTR) is also involved in aggression and social affiliation. When activated in the presence of cortisol, it intensifies the aggression. (OXTR and deviant Peer Affiliation: A Gene-Environment Interaction in adolescent antisocial behavior. Fragkak I, etal. J Youth Adolesc, 2018 Oct 12.

Inequality in which people are ranked in terms of monetary value, plays a huge role in the determination of with whom we socialize. The inequities in social life, lack of access to essential goods and opportunities, different levels of schools, churches, workplaces, access to nutrition, less knowledge, less trust, reduced life chances, poorer health, lower life expectancies, all reduce the range of social mobility. According to an Oxfam report in 2018, the richest 26 peo-ple had more wealth than the poorest half, 3.8 billion, of the world's population. "I am worth much more than you." It is impossible for one to socialize with the other without the involvement of high levels of social anxiety. Kings and peasantry, CEO's and workers do not communicate on the same level. Some people have more value than others.

Antisocial behavior originated in the agricultural society that no longer needed cooperation for group survival. It had food storage and possessions that led to status and societal separation. They divided open houses for sleeping and for physical separation according to status. Room dividers morphed into house dividers and neighborhood dividers, which essentially separated humans into superiors and inferiors. The need for a wide range of social interaction gradually lessened. As lords and servants increased so was the contact between them reduced. Material accumulation produced status and class, and the need for group interactions was diminished. Where in egalitarian societies, outrage and ostracism was the reaction to one who took too much, in the 1970's the dominant CEO was celebrated, applauded, emulated and rewarded for successfully demolishing the "competition". While often relying on cheating, greed, and acquisition of income by illicit means, by 2016, we elected them to lead major countries. Wealth acquisition is not only a common goal, it is the most coveted and imitated behavior of humanity today. Outward wealth gives inner comfort and pleasure. Greed overcomes altruism, but comes at a price. Guilt and moral fortitude have been assuaged by feel-good hormones, but they come with an essential requirement of anti-social behavior.

In many Amazonian tribes there is little evidence of high blood pressure with increasing age and very little cancer. People live together in longhouses, sleep, hunt and socialize together. They follow rules and activities that benefit all. In modern rural and urban communities, there is marked increase in blood pressure with advancing age, and in younger people from the stress of daily living and inadequate human relationships. Italian nuns in a convent have no high blood pressure with ageing. They live in a stress-free environment, out of status race, and in social harmony. Status and social anxiety, how we are seen and judged, leads to chronic stress and decreased health.

In the Theory of Mind #2, in which the awareness of self, thinking about others, thinking about self and what others think of you that led to establishment of identity markers, the intentions of faces, poses, gestures and behavior, determines whether or not to engage. Ranking based on status and outward appearance determines whether to engage or reject. Debasing others in order to lower their rank and justify not engaging also serves to elevate oneself.

"There is no need for a truly noble person to denigrate another." Author, 1974

A society that equates material wealth with high status, can expect low self-esteem and social anxiety when some have and others do not. This inequality results in low self-confidence of the latter that leads to the chronic release of stress hormones, depression and poor health. A natural reaction is one of self-promotion, self enhancement, use of drugs, alcohol, boosters, and appearance building. Apathy results in a similar anxiety, consumerism stress, and reduced social interactions. Those at the top level have anxiety related to maintaining and keeping their wealth and position.

Snobbery

The Art of Snobbery is a pure form of Anti-Social Behavior.

"The eye cannot rise above the eyebrow." Arab proverb

"I don't need to wallow with the pigs, to know that it stinks in the pen." Anonymous

"I am not a snob. I am just better than everyone else." Anonymous

"I'd die first, before associating with those people." Caribbean declarations "I may be a snob, but I am not antisocial." Anonymous

Divisions of social class, political and economic, are major factors in the expression of antisocial behavior. "Us", with letters after our names, wealthy zip codes and hefty saving accounts, do not mix or mingle with "them". The other side of the tracks that are poor, unattractive and dangerous to visit, much less live in, is the epitome of modern snobbery. The 18th century lexicon recorded the word "snob" as a term for a shoemaker or his apprentice. It was then adopted by English students at Cambridge to refer to students who lacked a title or were of humble origins, and later used to refer to anyone who was not a student. Another origin is that the notation, "s. nob" was used to refer to one "sine nobilitate", as a person not belonging to the upper classes or one who was not an aristocrat. (Norman DeWitt, The Classical Weekly, Pittsburgh, PA, Oct 1, 1941)

The art and practice of snobbery were around long before that. It was a lifestyle established from the differences in lifestyle resulting from wealth disparities from the Neolithic Age of agriculture and settlements. Those who lived in silks did not rub elbows with those who lived with pigs, a relationship that still holds today. Though the implication of the word has changed from shoemakers and students to those who imitate and admire their superiors, while rebuffing and denigrating their inferiors.

Snobbery is the need to elevate oneself above those among whom we live…to get and maintain the edge over someone else. The human sense of superiority over and relative status to others carry with it the confidence that enables and ennobles self and members of the same group while devaluing others as mentally, physically and socially inept. The negative snob, lacking in self-esteem, imposes their preferences and status upon others by diminishing their existence. The positive snob simply ignores everyone.

"Don't get huffy. Everyone is a snob about something. Snobbery, like snoring, is universal." Gina Barreca, Great Falls, Mt 2016

Between 5000 and 3000 BCE, human social dynamics changed from egalitarian to hierarchal and did so in several areas simultaneously. (Nile delta, Indus Valley, Mesopotamia, Meso-America, Northern China, and other locations.) We stopped living in small communities and expanded into larger towns and then cities. Settlement and farming brought surplus food, more reliable protection and expansion of the population well beyond the 150- limit per group supposed for tracking and recognition. History accompanied geography in that the land and climate probably changed to accommodate agriculture and a reduction in animal population made big game hunting a secondary occupation. A stable food supply led to larger populations which then required specialization within the group into leaders and followers. Further division into occupational levels, complete with rules, regulations, competition and status was inevitable. Each level or rank on the scale was capable of producing a snob. The one who thinks of himself as superior to another seeks recognition of status. He requires and makes good use of this reference point, then designates "other" as inferior, and by refusing "interaction", establishes a viable pecking order. Though other animals have ranking systems, snobbery is a unique human contrivance.

The inner source of snobbery developed from an insecure need to offset the threat to ones standing. It arose from the practice of "ranking others" through the determination of worth, based on superficial traits like wealth, academic credentials, beauty, and class. Are you worth my time and effort to engage? Are you worth the risk of exposing my rank and status?

Internally, the fear of being overrun by strangers, losing privileges and possessions release powerful emotions and results in imposing permanent inferior status on and rejection of those perceived as being the threat. The efficient snob categorizes, ranks and designates as "them" anyone below his/her own rank ordained to be treated with contempt, heartlessness and neglect.

Feelings of superiority release tremendous amounts of feel-good hormones into the blood- stream. Snobs "feel good" whether the source is true or false. The release of the "I am better than you" hormones lift the spirits, feeds the ego, stabilizes one's status, and supports one's purpose and meaning. Looking down on social inferiors and expecting little or no social interaction, though limiting the range of acquaintances, establishes one's ranking and base from which to aspire to greater things, like moving up on the hierarchy. The separation of groups into caste-like sections would be the first blow to social interactions. Aristocrats demanded and expected demonstrative "deference" from their social inferiors while exhibiting admiration for their superiors. This active behavior at both ends released feel-good hormones that nourished their egos. Whether with or without conscience, in order to maintain this posture and position, built on fear that some awful contagion will rub off and cause untold damage, eventually the "feel-bad" hormones of fear, isolation and hate will manifest, resulting in symptoms of anxiety and depression. Being a snob initially provides comfort, pleasure and security. Maintaining the position takes work and effort. Making someone else feel inferior adds to feelings of self-worth and the dread of being on the receiving end. The active snob exalts in and inflates his/her position by constantly reminding his inferiors that they are not on the same level. The passive snob simply ignores his/her designated inferiors. The truly superior person does not need to display either behavior. ....

A newborn initially interacts with the provider of nourishment (mother or nurse), and later with the environment. Yet, some respond and interact more than others. Does the degree of interaction depend on the level of social and antisocial hormones released and used? What role does the parent or nurse play? One may have social babies and antisocial babies in the same family. Some babies focus on their food source and some only on self —and totally ignore others. Some reach out early and interact with others. Some baby behavior goes on into childhood and adulthood. Are snubbing and socializing linked to kind and cruel DNA? In some cases, the parent exhibited similar behavior at similar stages in age. In most cases a combination emerges depending on the environment of openness or closure. An abundance of feel-good hormones available from parents, the environment and experiences combine with feel-bad hormones in a constant state of release, under stress, fear and poor health. Some babies cry and twitch in terror and others smile and rest in content.

Studies on feral, "wolf-raised" kids with total lack of human interaction reveal individuals lacking in all forms of social skills or experiences. Some can learn and some cannot. A study on the role of natural DNA in determining degrees of snobbery vs friendliness: Kid A willingly goes into the arms of receptive strangers, makes eye contact, smiles and interacts. Kid B cringes, draws back and refuses any form of interaction with someone other than parent. Is this learned behavior or innate? Results are pending.

Active snobbery imparts feelings of being "with it". Keeping up with best friends who are rich, and influential is physically and mentally expensive and accompanied by a profound dread at the prospect of losing status and rank. It requires time and effort, up to date appearance, communication technology and knowledge expansion. Being "out of it" creates anxiety at being left out, left behind, and out of the mainstream. A good "with it" snob changes with the times but never lowers himself to his associates with an "out of it" minion. The anxiety resulting from active snobbery is detrimental to immune system function and results in poor health.

Ancestors acknowledged socializing as an essential tool of survival. It paid to know everyone. It made good sense. It released feel-good hormones. It provided safety and comfort within the group. Whether inherited or learned from parents and peers, it became acceptable behavior.

As the group grew into a society, snobbery replaced egalitarian behavior. Feeling superior to someone else bathes the passive individual in self-generated feel-good hormones, based on social position, status, rank, lifestyle, and material wealth. Expressing that position compounds the good feeling, while the individual on the receiving end is sometimes flooded with feel-bad hormones, especially if he or she does not "know their place". Snobbery initially releases feel- good hormones by stoking the ego, but by being antisocial its envy, hatred, and belief in inequality eventually produce emotional anxiety. And when a snob is "outdone" or ignored, the rush of feel- bad hormones can lead to serious anxiety and depression in itself. Individual A's BMW is better than individual B's Cadillac, but individual C's Bentley puts "shame" on them both. A snob wavers between releases of positive and negative hormones and is seldom content.to see the world in relation to "others". The snob is not at ease with self-esteem. Continuously balancing superiority with inferiority, forever envious, and afraid that one's pretenses would be revealed, his/her position is always under threat. When coupled with the constant urge to acquire more materials as a badge of station, the snob reaches for higher ranking, while making sure that the lower ranks are sufficiently stifled, and rises to a state of constant stress. He/she sits on a mountain precipice of social status, wealth acquisition up and the threat of losing it.

It is human nature for people to look more favorably on those who are like themselves, but They enhance the separation when snobbery is employed as a primary tool and rarely seek interaction with those they consider below their station and rank. Is this natural? The apes have ranking and status. It must be okay. But what do they do with it? Hierarchies exist in nature. But in and of themselves, they do not obstruct socializing.

There are many types of snobs. The material snob believes and invests in income and wealth accumulation to establish social status. And associates exclusively with people of like stature. The intellectual snob rests on laurels of education and accumulated knowledge. The personal snob bases social rank on personal attributes, like clothing, language, manners, and tastes. The occupation snob flaunts his rank as ruler, clergy, official, clerk, and artisan. Rank and status are natural products of an organized society, but setting up barriers to socializing across strict lines according to identification markers and confinement to place, are uniquely human. The Merlot wine snob does not mingle with the Thunderbird drinker. The classical music snob remains in chambers and does not venture out into the heavy metal arena. The cuisenaire would rather dine alone than share culinary flavors with the fast- food chef. And not to mention that clothes make the man. The world of fashion is a perfect place to study the art of snobbery.

Snobbish behavior established the "I am more important than you" doctrine. The snob exalts in his/her accomplishments, items owned, names dropped, and places visited. He/she sticks stubbornly to claims of self-achievement though the facts reveal that no one rises alone without the assistance of others. The snob exalts in contact with celebrities and superheroes and repeats the event (s) as a claim to their own status and position. Time is money and greed is good, are the prevailing mantras of the consummate snob. When approached by a lower ranking individual, they assume a "how dare you contact me" attitude or react with a "what's in it for me to interact with you" mien. Arrogance in on full display by "charging" you for the conversation. You will pay one way or the other.

To be a snob, you must have a target, a reference point, someone to compare with, to identify as inferior. Conspicuous consumption needs an audience. The snob is content only when both levels accept his/her worth. Any challenge or inquiry to his position on the ranking scale leads to anxiety, distress, anger, resentment, and perhaps depression, all detrimental to physical and mental health. Inflicting gives pleasure, receiving brings despair.

Cultural snobbery is discrimination based on social class. True snobbery draws its origin from the social structure system of royalty versus everybody else. The lower royals, the professionals, educators, established middle class, new affluent workers, traditional working class, emergent service workers, and the poor, all hold their specific places in the society, with little mobility in either direction. At this system, Victorian England was the best. *Their country is open but the houses are closed"* was said by the German novelist, Theodor Fontane on an 1880 visit to England. *"Hospitality had become extinct and replaced by English stuffiness, due to the horrid weather and deprivation of any contact with the continent".*

Stiff, stilted and cold in this society, snobbery was the major feature. The British did not look to anyone else for "culture", they expected to be sought out as an example and delighted in looking down their noses on everyone else. The aristocracy did not regard servants as man and woman, only as "servants", one step above non-humans. In the practice of snobbery, there was a total disassociation from those deemed as "unworthy". Turning away from those considered as lesser beings or of little usefulness, was perfected by women as a natural defense against attack by aggressive men which then became a habit. Men used snobbery to isolate and separate potential rivals, and by belittling them it reduced the competition.

The English class system and the Indian caste system, originated separately then grew side by side. Snobbery served both societies to limit the association or interaction between "betters and lessers".

Americans, finding the English class-based status of royalty and peerage most amusing, turned against it from the inception of the country. They replaced it with the worship of money and those who had it. Property and possessions brought power and influence, and effectively partitioned the society.

"But Glory be, I don't have any friends you see, and whom am I to marry?" In the American South, there was very little to choose

from, because you refuse to associate with anyone who was not at the same level of society as yourself. As the "friend pool" was effectively whittled down by snobbery and too small for consideration, often the only recourse was to marry your cousins. Snobbery hampered the range of interactions and hence, the results of reproduction were often yachts, mansions, and cars may denote status, but not "class". Education and wealth on paper may have value but little "class", unless one has connections with the world and its players. Donald Trump could not converse or interact on the world stage without insulting someone. Incapable of interacting or connecting in a civil manner, he forfeited the influence of his position. He has no class.

Class is not only about occupation, income and where you live, it is about how you live, your health, daily routine, entertainment choices, availability, access to interaction, and exposure (travel). Development of the ability to interact with a wide range of human beings, to socialize freely, openly and successfully, this is "class".

Class is the knowledge of and respect for other cultures, the ability to interact through communication and connection with others. Most Europeans speak 3 to 4 languages and can communicate with a wider range of humans than other countries limited to one language. Economic and social rank is when one group has a status that confers advantages that another group lacks. "Class" is more than that. It is the ability to interact with character, knowledge, and experience, elegantly. It is the quality of the interaction and one's personal behavior at a high standard, with style, skill and appreciation. Class involves connecting with others. One may have all the money in the world, but cannot converse with a king or a pauper, because he/she has no "class". Though many travelers have wealth and education on paper, the inability to communicate with and disinterest in the local population limits the range of possible interactions.

"With whom do we interact?"

Vignette #22: " '*He greeted me like I was somebody', said the indigenous guide about a European acquaintance. "most are rather arrogant, loathe to make friendships with the local people and prefer the company of their own kind' ". The Unconquered: In search of the Amazon's last uncontacted tribes. by Scott Wallace.*

Upon eye contact, nod and smile (ECNS) testing or on presenting a basic greeting upon encountering another person, a negative or less than positive response can be interpreted to indicate an antisocial or asocial personality. Possible causes may relate to pure, true fear (hormonal deficiency or learned response from parents and peers or the expected reaction of the societal role, do not interact with "them". For some the failure to respond is just bad manners, a cultural lack of "class", but for many it is willful snubbing, a holier than thou reaction, "I am better than you so I don't need to acknowledge your presence; you are too far beneath me to be worthy of a response; you have little value, so my responding is a waste of my time".

All societies harbor and express layers of snobbery. With whom, where, and when to socialize are unwritten rules. Some societies take it to extremes with physical separation to ensure that there is no interaction between class units. What does it accomplish but to severely limit the numbers and types of people with whom one is permitted to socialize. If snobs were truly superior there would be no need for the pretense and the status stratification. Snobbery is driven by fear, of loss of possessions and rank, of being tainted in some way, or of finding out the that "we" are just like "them".

Snobbery is the voluntary and/or involuntary, direct activity of excluding others from the scene or in-group, with internal and external motives of self-interest, involving envy, exploitation, and a need for separate levels of human value.

In some Latin American countries, the friendliness, warmth and manners of the people are on display on a daily basis, and ironically, so is the Arte de Comemierdaria. Certain segments of the population are adept at holding their noses so high in the air as not to smell the presence of those they do not like. There are several variations on the translation.

"I wouldn't be caught dead with anyone from there," is a statement referring to poorer communities, inferring that one is way too good to associate with anyone of a lower class. Taking measures not to socialize with anyone considered as being "below" ones assigned station, takes on the air of behaving like a "comemierda". Under the veil of entitled narcissism, the snob is adept at not giving value to others, while displaying a sense of self-assigned privilege often beyond reason. All are sincere and genuine about this behavior.

Vignette #23: At a high school reunion at a small private academy in 2019, a remarkable number of 48 out of a class of 70 were in attendance. What was even more remarkable was that they proceeded to separate into smaller groups as they had done when back in school years before, and once again they did not even know each other despite spending 4 to 12 years together in the same grade in the same school. Snobbishness and reverse snobbishness filled the dining hall. As amusing as it was, the barriers that snobs build and reinforce, keep people apart and prevent them from connecting through similarities rather than separating due to flimsy differences. The practice contributes nothing to the health of the society.

The dissolution of social connections involving snobbery, was based on fear and pleasure. The fear of being contaminated by those below created a deep anxiety. The caravan invading the southern border leading to certain infection by brown people that would incite such a reaction as to justify the expenditure of billions to close the border. The same event elicited extreme pleasure at rising to such a height that looking down on others provided a rush of feel-good hormones and lasting satisfaction of intense snobbery. Without or with a damaged conscience, the snob totally ignored the fact that he/she had climbed the wall and crossed the same borders in the not-too distant past. The social climbing snob reaches what he/she sets as the limit, then turns to stop others from climbing as well. The one most adept at erecting and enforcing the obstruction, usually the ones most familiar with the process and most recently in the vicinity. The new-be snob suffers from the "uncertainty" of his/her new position, the reality of true status and the possibility of losing it. Social interactions play out according to group ideology.

Extreme forms of snobbery can lead to injury, both mental and physical. "Whites only" is an extreme form of snobbery, a deliberate limitation on social interaction between groups separated by skin tone. Privilege, derived from "private law", is the assumption of rights of social superiority as delegated by and to oneself and requires constant reinforcement. The thought of sharing privileges with others is akin to a fate equated with social and physical death. The Europeans, faced with loss of income and social position, had titles to fall back upon, with station and rank having more rigid stability. Americans had no titles, so could fall more easily, more frequently and further. The constant anxiety about money and social status added more strength to the barriers erected to prevent social interactions between "unequals", resulting in both sides becoming socially inept. Americans do not make or keep friends as easily as Europeans. Socially challenged, less communication skills, less breadth and range, they live further apart both physically and intellectually, in distinct communities ideally demarcated for separation, stratification and resultant low interactions. Snobbery determines who interacts with whom, to the degree that is decreed by the society.

No one can make you feel inferior without
your consent. Eleanor Roosevelt

This dictum sounds good but does not work in the real world. Hundreds of years and thousands of miles trekked by people of the Jewish faith suffering under the weight of Anti-Semitism (and the same Jews that suffered under the Nazis, treat Palestinians in the same way) castigated as being inferior and resented for being superior, American racism, systemic and institutional, featuring lynching of 3900 individuals since 1890, and Anti -LGBT activism thrust into the mainstream all provide social anxiety at the highest levels. Active snobbery depriving entire groups of people the chance to prove their social value.is the worst injury of all. African-Americans subjected to chronic stressors on a daily basis, never being allowed to exert their full value, never a part of the whole, results in serious mental and physical anxiety.

Seen at a recent march for the homeless, were signs proclaiming, "We're human beings, acknowledge us" and "Help us, please". Billionaires pass poor Roderick, who is sick and dying in the street, and never acknowledge his presence. In the 1970's, Washington, DC office workers driving through Anacostia on their way to work in the Capitol in the 1970's, look straight ahead, deliberately ignoring the extreme poverty existing at their doorsteps. Sick, starving migrants beg for alms in church doorways in posh European cities, as lines of healthy visitors enter and exit without so much as a glance. Not only does total disavowal exist, but the refusal and in most cases the inability to interact prevails throughout our societies.

We humans live on a planet that is shared space. Though our numbers may have exceeded the limits of peaceful productive existence, there is no excuse for some of the atrocious behavior exhibited by our species toward each other. It may seem trivial but think about it carefully. When one enters and sits in a common space and no one acknowledges your presence, what is the significance? A smile directed and a warmth offered and it is totally ignored, as with most Americans, Spaniards, Italians, and Asians. What expenditure of energy does it take to smile and give a simple greeting? Aloofness indicates self-importance, establishes and reinforces dominance, and indicates a lack of basic human decency. With antisocial behavior avoidance may be "human", but insults are "inhumane". A society separated into multiple parts that do not communicate with each other, is doomed to fail. It does not make use of the full potential of all its citizens.

Of the possible solutions to curtail the practice of snobbery with the aim being to enhance social interactions, knowledge, cultural familiarity and good social skills come to the forefront. Only the truly intelligent can attain the level of security needed to overcome snobbery. Ageing is another solution. As one ages, you no longer have to look up to someone, so why still look down on someone? Hopefully, you will have acquired the knowledge that everyone has value, has a right to communicate and that refusal to interact may miss your opportunities to expand your knowledge and self-confidence. Treating everyone equally no matter their apparent rank or status is another solution. Humility and decency win. Social behavior, the manner of conducting oneself, comportment especially in relation to others is positive and benefits all as well as the society as a whole. Tribalism, as a fundamental human trait, in defense against rival group and an offense for gain, is passe. Clinging to old rules of social interaction detains its progress. Social testing, checking out one's status (usually by appearance) before interacting, their fitting in, their belonging where, how, and with whom as a determination of granting a license to interact. Social barriers by race may be slightly lowered compared to 50 years ago, but "class" barriers have widened. Diversity has been accepted, somewhat, but class still matters. Money, wealth, status and rank still determine *"with whom you interact"*.

Accepting diversity may expand the number and kind of encounters and interactions, but not the connections. True connections indicate long term commitments, and people who still place so much importance on "social class" as conferring privileges are not about to give this up just to expand the range of interactions. Blatant discrimination and antisocial behavior will continue.

Us versus Them

"Everywhere in the world, kids cry the same, there is no difference between them." *Nenad Stajic, a Serbian teen basketball player*

Children are social and naturally move to play together, until they are <u>taught</u> to separate and employ antisocial behavior. Is it at puberty that the separation occurs? Competition for reproduction and perception of threat to survival? (If they just realize that all are the same and survival involves the entire human race together, instead of just pieces). Early in childhood, around 3 or 4 years of age, they are taught by parents and peers to recognize the differences between "us" and "them", and that we are good and they are bad. When backed up by the society on a daily basis, the concept is deeply ingrained. In blocking the possibilities of familiarity through interactions, usually based on appearance, proximity and societal lore, one group successfully ignores the humanity of another. When they don't count and have value only as useful tools, this justifies the implementation and maintenance for slavery, discrimination and even wholesale elimination.

The designation of "them" was never more evident than in the history of the Americas, when the indigenous peoples were designated as "them", savages to be used to gain wealth, stripped of the land they had occupied for thousands of years, then denied access to a decent living share. When one group was wasted another was brought in to take their place, and similar antisocial rules and activities applied to "them". When slave labor produced more wealth, the only way to keep it working was to separate, deprive and despise "them". The level of hatred that still exists toward and between these two groups, is an inexcusable expression of inhumanity.

Antisocial behavior is evident in elevators, upon entering a room, building, in parks, on the street, in restaurants and wherever people gather, Encounters are superficial, sterile and fake. Differences between groups of people are highlighted and similarities ignored. *The reds don't interact with the blues.* In all American cities, the black and the white communities exist separately. The fact that their speech patterns are so different indicates that they do not speak to each other on a regular basis, enough to initiate and sustain viable social relationships. The deliberate lack of sincere interaction and connection is a major impediment to social and physical health. With high tech medicine, the life expectancy in the USA is low and falling. Comparatively low levels of social connections contribute to the prevalence of heart disease, cancer, obesity, diabetes and dementia as causes of premature death. The fact that a sizeable portion of the population lives in poverty and apart from the mainstream, contributes to the same prevalence. In addition, the practice of blaming "them" for disparities in health and productivity is not a viable solution. Shutting off access to genuine interactions and any form of positive connections are not viable solutions.

"They are different from us." Sarah Palin,
Vice President candidate, 2008

Gated communities are designed and intended to keep "them" out. Safety is listed but not wishing to engage, to interact with "them" as an act of extreme snobbery is the primary reason. The Haves with access to education, employment, and earnings refuse to share, with those without access. We move away from each other socially, physically and mentally and pretend that it is normal. I have lived in a few gated communities, and attest that this is so.

Hating and Being Hated are very powerful emotions.

Snobbery between and among groups is one thing, but hating your fellow human takes it to a different level. The amount of energy expended; the amount of stress hormone released, the amount of lost creativity and productivity from lack of cooperation, provides a huge contribution to poor health of the community. Observe the way one's mouth curls up into an intentional snarl when talking about people they don't like. See the way one reacts when being insulted as the pit of the stomach feeling responds to the rush of bad cortisol. The daily practice of us against them reduces the number of encounters, interactions and connections possible in separated societies. ...

Exclusion

Humans tend to discriminate against those they do not consider their equals, even if no history, no prior communication, no apparent differences or no logical reason. To exclude those we don't feel comfortable with, to prevent them from entering our space, our sphere, we lower their social status, peddle hatred and immorality stories about them, categorize and label them, then set firm criteria of identification according to ethnicity, education, background, passions, income, address opinions and social class. When we are satisfied that they are firmly in their place, we erect barriers to ensure there be no interactions that lead to connections that might taint our self-exalted social class. *Hatred directed at Mexicans and Asians based on hearsay and outright lies, and directed by someone tapping into the fear and hatred that was already there, shuts off all social interaction and is bad for the health of both groups involved.*

Antisocial behavior thrives on disgust, a sensation that promotes mean cruel behavior that promotes separation and distancing of self from the object of disgust that raises negative emotions. This social threat leads us to exude hostility, reject deviants, and build walls.

Study: In 1990, the Yale University Infant Cognition Center found that babies at 6 months old preferred good over bad. The majority choose the good puppet over the bad puppet. They chose familiarity over strangeness, thus displaying early xenophobia. They showed aversion to the unfamiliar. As adults, they would be more likely to be nice to their own kind and horrible to "others".

After 5000 BCE, humans living together as equals were increasingly seen as being weak, and vulnerable, and easy prey for materials and dominance. They chose leaders to protect and provide them with security and comfort. Depending on the environment and on the nature of the individuals comprising this group, egalitarian became despotic societies. DNA hard-wired for compassion and empathy, learned meanness, hostility and exclusion as a means of control and survival. From the warmth of inclusion, we see a middle-aged Mediterranean man patiently waiting his turn to join the group of boule players on a small field in the town of Ponte Vedra, France and the coldness of exclusion of an old man sitting alone and being ignored at the end of a long bench occupied by a group of chatting, laughing elders in Plaza Loreto, Milan.

We show kindness to our own and cruelty to "others".

Exclusion is the tool we use when empathy towards others becomes wrath. We went from feeling another's pain to inflicting pain on others, from noting the plight of victims to making them into enemies, and from including, sharing and protecting to excluding, hoarding and exposing others to harm. Exclusion draws its action from intolerance and negativity resulting in a constant load of bad hormones (cortisol) in response to chronic stress of disdain which intensifies and prongs its effects on the immune system that leads to dysfunctional illness. Those with the strongest negative attitude toward "others" also have lower thresholds for things that cause personal disgust, and are more prone to use exclusion as a formidable weapon against their "enemies". In 1874, barbed wire was invented to keep people out of large tracts of land, (Texas), then used in wartime trenches (WWI) and morphed into razor wire at prisons and government buildings, and along the Berlin wall. Not exactly a social tool. This meanness is evident in the display of extreme antisocial behavior against immigrants, refugees and poorer citizens, falsely held responsible for all the ills of a society or just to keep "them" away from the land you occupy.

In 2000, the Israelis built a 400- mile- long wall of cement and barbed wire surrounding the West Bank and intended to separate (and protect) themselves from the Palestinians. Almost all the occupants inside agree with this tactic. The power of group negativity in social behavior to influence the direction of society is overwhelming, despite its resulting unproductivity, destruction and inhumanity. A striking feature of antisocial behavior is the refusal to share (land, food, profits) and preference for fighting to take or hold what is perceived as possessions. This dispute has been going on for the past 4000 years and is a glaring example of extreme antisocial behavior.

The disgust-based, mean-spirited mocking of the poor and disabled and the expressed hatred of "others" is of such magnitude that the collective health of the society and the individuals are severely in question. What if, every time you have a positive experience with friends or strangers, social health notes are deposited in the bank, like bitcoin. Hating, snubbing someone, mocking them, supporting someone who revels in this behavior or otherwise having a negative exchange, 9like killing them, is spending those social health notes from your bank account. A negative balance is the equivalent of poor health.

Extreme Antisocial Behavior

How did "they" change from being the "others" at encounters of early *Homo sapiens* to being the objects of such intense hatred at political rallies and designated battlefields? How did anyone not like me become the objects of murders, massacres, and wars? The hunter-gatherers needed each other and "others" for creativity and productivity. The settlers viewed encounters as competition and rivalry. Antisocial behavior developed as a substitute for inherent perceived weakness and was expressed to appear strong externally. When own identity was not strong enough to stand on its own, the humiliation and blaming of others was a useful tool in establishing control and power. One could gain power by taking it from others. Being antisocial as a show of "strength" became firmly established in one's own mind and in the minds of companions who also saw it as a strength.

For the recipient, to be actively humiliated, one feels a loss of self, a dehumanization that elicits either submission or a rebellious response. Extreme antisocial behavior is present every time a person encounters another, looks right past them and totally ignores their presence. A good friend told me that his father remarked on that look of indifference, as treating someone like a piece of furniture, to be used only on occasion. (Such was the look on Derek Chauvin's face while he was ending the life of George Floyd in May of 2020.) The attitude that entire groups of people do not matter, cannot lead to peace, much less to a modicum of social interactions.

War is an extreme expression of antisocial behavior. It is the dominant side's response to conflicting ideas and physical differences. It is the ultimate solution for those who oppose cooperation, collaboration and social connections War exposes the natural evil, makes it legal and glorifies the destructive side of human nature.

Leonardo DaVinci, the consummate Renaissance man, did not reveal the entire design for his submarine, "on account of the evil nature of man, who would practice assassinations at the bottom of the sea by breaking ships in their lowest parts and sinking them together with the crews who are in them." Albert Einstein's opinion of the atomic bomb was that "we thus drift toward unparalleled catastrophe." In 2020, in possession of one billion small arms and over 13,000 nuclear warheads in the world capable of destroying humanity many times over, are we social or antisocial? Since 5000 BCE, we have yet to a full year of zero conflicts, worldwide?

World War I mobilized 70-million Germans and French to fight on several fronts. Entire societies geared their economy to the war effort that would kill 20-million of which half were civilians. It destroyed the European infrastructure and dismantled empires. Yet they sang as they died in the trenches and went after each other with a vengeance after the treaties were signed. World War II promoted the manufacture of 286,000 tanks, 557,000 combat aircraft, 11,000 naval battleships, and 40-million rifles and humanity gathered together, socially, with the sole purpose of killing one another, extreme antisocial behavior.

It appears that when groups grew large enough and there was enough distance between them to declare different identities, they waged organized war on each other. (Sumerians and Elamites in Mesopotamia, 2700 BCE. The purpose was presumed as being to acquire more possessions and territory. If one includes the antisocial urges (cruel DNA) and compulsion (hormones of aggression) to assert dominance by killing fellow humans, the first principle would have been the dehumanization of the enemy. The tactics would have been the same that continues today, kill, massacre in groups, torture, beheadings (eliminate the head), starvations, and rape, all designed to maximize effect and satisfy extremely swollen antisocial egos.

Spaniards killed 70-million Native Amerinds in a very short time and never showed an ounce of remorse, ascribing the events as being God's will. European Americans massacred the same Amerinds and worked Africans to death, then lynched them for looking askance or staring and continue to kill them today merely for existing. Group killing for pleasure is the ultimate antisocial behavior and expression of cruel DNA.

Within the German Schutzstaffel (SS) military police unit, charged with the killing of Jews, some did it with pleasure, and some, as a job. Very few refused to kill. They wiped out entire towns, killed everyone, justified it and continued doing it until they were finally stopped by external forces. Evil atrocities contrived from within and openly committed can be found throughout human history.

War is a balance between controlled killing and overcoming natural inhibitions on killing. The choice is between compassion and empathy and heartlessness and compulsion. When it is overdone, sacking cities, execution of prisoners, killing everyone, burning churches with refugees inside, and shooting unarmed black men pleading for their lives, it calls into question the very fabric of the human psyche. War is rules, laws, honor, glory and pure murder. The organized massacres at Wounded Knee, My Lai, Nanjing, Austerlitz, Treblinka, and the killing fields of Cambodia. War as annihilation of "others" occupy a large part of recent human history. War grew from the mutation of moral strength through the suppression of conscience and shame, into the much stronger, more pervasive strength generated from heartlessness. Fear, mistrust and hatred, separation and taboo of socializing with others seeded ancient wars. Principle, honor, and glory with displays of courage along the way, fueled the middle wars. And fear, mistrust and hatred whether real or contrived support the wars of today.

"He looked like a demon, so I shot him", said the officer who shot Michael Brown, in Ferguson, Missouri in 2018. There was and is no way that officer had or was ever going to sit anywhere, have a friendly chat and a beer with anyone who looked like his victim at any time. The US Caste system is effective in limiting the extent of social interactions and there is no understanding of intent or conceptualization between groups perceiving themselves as rivals. Fixed ranking of human value determines with whom we socialize, whom we avoid and who deserves to be eliminated. Hate and war can only lead to destruction of "other".

War has some redeeming values. At times it is a dance, a march in cadence, attack or retreat together, move and think in unison, all with discipline. War, according to Pete Buttigieg, in his book Trust, promotes the same in others, placing your well-being and life at the mercy and in the hands of your comrades. Trust must be validated by experience. If everybody is good, trust holds up. If there was one out of kilter, or too many known to be bad there is distrust all across the board. Practical trust in 2020 in any vicinity where there are groups of people is relegated to the background as the mantra is "keep your valuables close, others cannot be trusted."

War is considered to be part of human nature. As a legally sanctioned human activity, it is an alternate expression of cruel DNA, reaction to fear and threat of others. Violence is an instinctive reaction and expression of greed, drive for dominance and satisfaction of ego. The male chimpanzee's primary drive is to eliminate other males. Food and sex as rewards for violent behavior is the ultimate expression of antisocial genes. Wars or threats of war prevail in the in the 21st as a major activity to procure and secure access to oil, energy, possessions, and power over others.

In The Goodness Paradox, the anthropologist, Richard Wrangham, proposes that humans underwent domestication by suppressing their cruel DNA and using war (their violent side) for protection in such a highly organized manner as to get what they wanted in resources and possessions and status. These good/bad impulses were more prevalent in some groups than in others. As time and evolution progressed, humans became nicer (more diplomatic), got better at killing (more efficient and effective) and justified their urges as defensive maneuvers. Instead of sporadic chimpanzee-style free-for-alls, we organize great battles for food, sex, religion and politics and designate it as anything worth killing and dying for. The nomads were adept at moving away from conflict, but with agriculture and homes to protect, settlers went headlong into wars, enjoyed the feelings, and proceeded to create more unequal societies where the strong got ever better at exploiting the weak.

War is organized aggression of one group against another with the intent of changing an undesirable situation, obtaining possession or eliminating the enemy altogether. Peace is interacting or existing on a plain of kindness —civilized and engaged in the embrace of fellows without regard or desire for material gain. Both activities are innate, instinctive and expressions of genetic and environmental conditions. Upon encountering the Europeans on their shores, if the Taino in the Caribbean had more cruel DNA and better weaponry, they may have repelled Columbus and his men instead of welcoming them (1492). If the Wampanoag had let the Pilgrims starve instead of sharing and showing them how to grow corn the history of the North American continent may have been quite different. If the Incas had managed to avoid the smallpox epidemic, stopped the Pizarro brothers and sent them back to Hispaniola, South America would be a different place. Greed was the initiating force in the Conquest of the

Americas, but jealousy, snobbery, and cruelty were all capable of sustaining the conflict. Continuous war proceeded from social unrest, lack of trusting social connections and resentments that resurfaced on a daily basis. Differences continue to fuel conflicts, with access and possessions of resources as the main causes.

As we continue to evolve, culture and environment play a larger role in shaping human nature than biology (genetics), and the antisocial dominates the social.

"War is to man what maternity is to a woman." Mussolini 1938

Play your role in society be strong as a man not weak and emotional like a woman, notwithstanding the fact that many women are capable and have waged war as good as or even better than men. When the Iraq war broke out no matter how wrong and insane it was, all segments of the society were thrilled and burst into cheers. The Roman society, as were many before and after, was obsessed with the art of war with its skill and discipline lording over everything else. War provides a shared identity. The drill of soldiers marching in unison, disciplined formation, gives an emotional thrill, pleasure and sense of well-being at being a part of the unit. The march is music and dance, the satisfaction of moving together and the skill and pleasure of muscular bonding. (William McNeil, historian, 1945)

Wars identify and clarify "us" versus "them" as a derivative of those with whom we socialize and those with whom we don't. Aristocracy, nobility, professionals, issue the ranks that determine not only with whom one interacts, but where, when and how. Deference is still demanded and expected by social superiors, but is less and less on display.

War can act as a social glue that binds people together in a common cause, hatred of the enemy. Civilian support for the war effort often depends on the collective hatred of "other". War infuses life and energy into a society that is dominated by its dark side of cruel DNA and aggressive hormones. Where strength is equated with the ability to kill the most people and destroy the most property in the most efficient manner, victory and domination are strength and peace and kindness are weakness.

"The French should be shot and stabbed to death, down to the little babies". Johanna von Puttkamer, wife of Chancellor Otto von Bismarck

General Sherman's march of destruction to the sea through the American South in 1864 (Civil War), "We are not fighting hostile armies, but a hostile people..."

The Jim Crow South emerged from the ashes and has yet to change its antisocial habits Jean-Jacques Rousseau's Social Contract championing the rights of people to associate freely with each other has somehow morphed into chants of "kill them", and more recently, "lock her up" and "send them back" indicative of the persistent racism and specific antagonism toward women in power.

Vietnam War atrocities begat more atrocities. Death and destruction the in the name of Capitalism. Killing Vietnamese was easier when they were "gooks" is another line form Other. America has yet to "socialize" with Vietnam and anti-war proponents and veterans alike are still being met with scrutiny and punishment. Modern wars are supported by the entire society and any that are not present serious social issues and misplaced blame.

The 1813 Battle of Leipzig between the French ad the Prussians produced 150000 casualties over a span of four days. The 1916 Battle of the Somme, WW I, saw 1-million casualties over four months. In the six years of World War II, there were 50-million casualties of both civilians and soldiers from mass murder, bombs, starvation and diseases. One bomb killed 80000 people at Hiroshima in 1 day and thousands afterwards. Where are the kindness, compassion and empathy? This annihilation of "others" through heartlessness and hatred is beyond antisocial. We have a society in which winning at any cost is everything, the lottery is at the top of every wish list and gun violence is the solution to every problem. Such a society is bound to have low social interactions, lack of trust, minimal time allotted for socializing, and interactions of poor quality. When money is more important than people, (recent choice where opening the economy took precedence over control of a pandemic) social interactions are null and void. When profits preempt people, social interactions become meaningless.

Who benefits from this disruption of a healthy society? The sociopaths come out in droves behave antagonistically and violently towards others, feel little or no remorse and take no responsibility for their actions. The poor health that follows is directly associated with the stress that is produced. Sociopaths make perfect war machines.

War with justification is fine-tuned antisocial behavior. Engagement designed for killing and eradication of others, through belligerence and cruelty, is very much alive and well today. Shakespeare's Henry V soldier, "we are the king's subjects: if his cause be wrong, our obedience to the king wipes the crime of it out of us."

War is the organized expression of the cruel DNA and the comradery of men is the ultimate expression of kind DNA. Even war can be "social" and can bring out the best in human cooperation, friendships and loyalty. There is no greater sacrifice or honor than to die for your fellow warrior. Soldiers band together and sacrifice for own kind can be ultra-social and ultra-cruel to the enemy in their treatment of victims and prisoners. Social Darwinism interprets its survival of the fittest to suit its own prevailing ideology between us and them; that every human society has a natural enemy that must be eliminated so that military values can be promoted and a strong society can be built.

In the chemistry and mechanics of extreme antisocial behavior, after the rise of agriculture, each member of the caste system perceived the "other" as a threat that instilled fear resulting in high levels of chronic cortisol circulating in the bloodstreams of Neolithic man. A reduction in social interaction coupled with weakened immune systems resulted in a myriad of mental and physical illnesses. Oxytocin, the love hug hormone within your own group is also a rage hormone released in copious amounts upon one's encounter with distrusted strangers.

When the antisocial is involved in an encounter, and refuses to acknowledge the presence of another or engages with negativity, it is only a few steps removed from dehumanizing and demonizing and then depriving them of life.

Possible Solutions

To avoid sinking deeper into the mire of antisocial behavior, the first order of reformation is to understand the situation and expand your rational self. There is a difference between right and wrong, Certain people are better at some things than are others. Your rational self understands the situation, identifies the underdog, recognizes that he/she has some value, and acts accordingly within the standards of humanity.

We know that being kind to others as to your own is the worldwide maxim. We love our own kind but fail to realize that others have loved ones too. Instead of pushing away and rejecting others, get closer understand their culture, engage, interact and try to connect.

Others are not so different from "us". Work together to use the same DNA, of kindness and compassion for the whole community, not just the few who can help you.

Try to follow the teachings and example of Jesus of Nazareth, New Testament, Instead of antisocial behavior, try to engage, include, interact. Try to understand, use reason, intellect and rational thought, instead of self- interest emotions… (especially in a pandemic). We need to come together and act as one in solidarity to change destructive behavior, implement rules and policies to curtail diseases, avoid starvation, alleviate the suffering of poverty, and neutralize climate change, or else our antisocial behavior will doom the society to failure.

> *If you greet only your brothers and sisters what*
> *more are you doing than others? Do not even pagans do that?*
> *Matthew 5:47 Solution to Others.*

Why can't you be nice to everyone? Why must you be cruel to strangers?

Receiving Antisocial Behavior: Loneliness

Some days you are the pigeon and some days you are the statue.

Loneliness, the perceived lack of meaningful relationships, stemming from social isolation, living alone and feeling alone, often results in mental and physical damage to health. Subjectively, the inability to find meaning in one's life and the negative reactions that follow, leave the individual feeling disconnected and associated with poor health.

The introvert turns his/her concentration inwards and directs the antisocial behavior outward. We usually describe them as being shy and comfortable in being alone. We associate alone time with high levels of creativity and productivity, and not necessarily linked to "feeling lonely", so is not a major factor in poor health. Monitoring of "alone time" reveals high levels of feel-good hormone release.

"Where are the people?" resumed the little prince at last.
"It's a little lonely in the desert." It is lonely when you're
among people, too," said the snake.
Antoine de Saint-Exupery, Le Petit Prince

"Loneliness does not come from having no people about
one, but from being unable to communicate the things
that seem important to oneself" Carl Jung

"Introverts are word economists in a society suffering
from verbal diarrhea." Michaela Chung

"People empty me. I have to get away to refill." Charles Bukowski

"Be a loner. That gives you time to wonder, to search for the truth.
Have holy curiosity. Make your life worth living." Albert Einstein

Loneliness differs from being alone. Feeling lonely is the pathological misery, feeling the absence of others who were once close, homesickness, the grief of lost love, and feeling lonely in the midst of people. Being alone, voluntary down time, may be positive and necessary for recharging, rebalancing, sorting out memories, being creative, and planning for the future. The loneliness that profoundly affects one's health is associated with feelings at having failed at life, missed out on belonging to anyone, place or worthwhile cause; and a failure at love, connection and lasting attachment. Some loners absolve themselves from all fault, and move from refusing to acknowledge the problem to refusing to do anything about it.

Loneliness is involuntary solitude that can be associated with low self-worth or a perceived worth too high to risk being with others, inability to communicate or get along with others, or desire to be only with the perfect companion, oneself. The loner is usually a complainer with a negative outlook Internal: self-created sources of social stress associated with poor social skills are very prevalent in the 21st century, as well as external sources of social stress, like overt hostilities and racism. Sometimes, exclusion is a source of satisfaction, the belief that you are unworthy of happiness, love and good health. You replace vulnerability, uncertainty and deficiency with acceptance and fear of connection and of change. You use system blaming to transfer responsibility elsewhere, on bad friends, betrayal, or the past, to justify overwork and immersion into ignorance.

Currently we are going backwards in removing many of the activities that brought us together in the past. Removal of history and geography from curricula that served to expose us to other cultures, decrease in poetry and storytelling skills, lack of connection between each other and with nature (electronic device use), increased sports for profit, bizarre entertainment that we observe then try to emulate, all lead to mental problems. We downplay or ignore the importance of global warming to the entire planet, energy shortage, nuclear warfare, environmental waste and toxicity and our inadequate health care delivery systems. Our dismissal and diminution of our innate urges for social connections, is leading to higher incidences of poor health.

We directly associate loneliness with stress-related diseases, hypertension, cardiovascular dysfunction, diabetes, depression and cancer. Having companions and relationships associate with less risky behavior, better diet, more exercise, better access to healthcare and preventive measures, and less stress.

The chemistry of loneliness is punctuated by the almost continuous release of cortisol, resulting in increased blood pressure with damage to the heart and blood vessels, with concurrent increase in norepinephrine release that shuts down the viral defense and deregulates the defensive inflammation response leading to reduced immune system function and higher susceptibility to illness. IN 2005, a study on loneliness found the condition associated with a low antibody response to the flu vaccine resulting in higher risk of contracting the disease. Since emotional pain uses the same neural centers as physical pain, loneliness results in higher risks of suffering, fibromyalgias and neuromyalgias, dementia and premature death. Loneliness for early hominids was a warning system of high alert to get with the group to avoid predators. The sense of threat activated the brain to seek group protection. Modern man interprets the threat differently and remains in solitude or pushes others away. Opting to remain in a state of chronic inflammation leads invariably to tissue breakdown, impaired dysfunctional immune system, and high susceptibility to disease with feedback as irritability, suspicion, fear and heightened social anxiety pushing him further into social isolation. As the body and brain mull over the processes and consequences of feeling lonely, stress hormones and brain peptides signal the immune system to reduce the production and manufacture of white blood cells. Further triggers and signals link dopamine metabolite HVA and serotonin metabolite 5-HIAA to impair the regulation of dopamine activity, thus unleashing aggressive impulses. When presented with the suffering of others, the centers for empathy and concern for others fail to engage or connect to processing and decision making. They cannot imagine the pain of others.

Loneliness often occurs in the later years when friends die or move away, with family and community abandonment, or loss of trust or confidence in what was once a friend. Low opportunities for social interactions, onset of poor health with impediments, actively preferring not to share life with another person, and active avoidance of others. Many people reside in single unit dwellings, choose not to associate with others or limit themselves to small groups. When ousted or shunned, they have nowhere to turn. Many pass days on end without speaking to another human being. Biochemical results of loneliness recycle to become causes of pathology, such as poor digestion and absorption, nervous anxiety, allergies, autoimmune disorders, all related to dysfunctional chemical enzymes and unbalanced metabolism.

Some loneliness is self-imposed, due to lack of ability to make and keep friends, low desire to interact, low availability and quality of time with friends and family, and lack of commitment to "connect". Some loneliness is accepted due to unwanted interactions, denial of opportunities, and exclusions that limit the range. Loss of self-confidence, low self-esteem, lack of regard for others and refusals to expand are some internal causes. Frequent changes in location, loss through distance, divorce, and attrition are some external causes of loneliness. Contentment with small social networks of the same individuals and weak social relationships lacking in diversity and depth, offer little consolation.

In ancient times, the brain needed friends, and the body saw foes and moved away to protect itself. With large expanses and few "people", physical disconnection was likely and well-tolerated. In modern times, social disconnection within a dense population is in concert with antisocial behavior. In a research study by Professor Holt-Lunstad at Brigham Young University titled "Lack of social connections and disease risk, found that some lived alone and were not lonely; and others lived close to and with family, but were not connected. They surmised that loneliness has a strong internal mechanism.

In the socially isolated, subjectively lonely and physically lonely, the risk for premature death was similar. The socially connected had lower disease risk and higher life expectancy across the board. These results were from a pool of 70 studies, with 3 to 4-million participants followed over seven years.

The internal mechanism, the drive that determines how man relates and connects to and disconnects from his fellows, has been on display throughout our history. It was mentioned by John Fowles in his opus, The Magus, of the famous psychopaths, Adolf Hitler, Josef Stalin, Pol Pot and others, "that one man had the courage to be evil; and that millions had not the courage to be good", and can be said of the millions of Germans and Austrians up to and during World War II and the Americans during the 250 years of slavery and 150 years of Jim Crow right up to the present mistreatment of immigrants and fellow citizens. Man chooses and enjoys his antisocial behavior designed to make social connections between antagonistic groups almost impossible.

Going further back, religions had their fair share of antisocial behavior. All were equal in the sight of God, but obeyed and interacted only with those with like ideas and those with authority. The social milieu for the group was based on common beliefs and any deviation was punished or ostracized. The 13th century Catholic church in the enforcement of its Inquisition rules against non-Catholics (besides labeling anyone who did not agree with doctrine as a heretic) degreed that Jews and other non-Christians wear yellow badges so that "good Christians would not fraternize or socialize with them" as was a similar occurrence in Nazi Germany. Religious beliefs are capable of bringing people together and driving them apart. Sacred places and rituals as the core of human spirituality, brought people together, developed language and social behavior and gave order to the world. The segregation and separation that followed was not conducive to the health of the society.

Santa Rita di Cascia, Augustinian nun, guardian of lost and impossible causes, sickness, abuse, marital problems, the saint protector against loneliness, died in 1457.

There is no scientific justification for rejection and ostracism of others. Hatred and rejection promotes violence in rich and poor communities. For the poor, the bonds of family and friends mitigate some depressing effects of poverty. (Good Times TV program) For the rich, lack of trusted relationships could be just as damaging as physical poverty. (Dallas TV program) A *stable society that socializes freely and frequently has no need of guns for protection (neither for offense nor defense). Anonymous*

In a society that discourages free and open interaction, decrees that only money can buy comfort and that poverty is the fault of the poor, one can feel lonely in a crowd or any place that people gather. For this kind of loneliness, one has only those who devised and promoted the caste system, the skin color system and the exclusion of snobbery to thank. Closed societies with approved interaction only with people exactly like yourself results in a higher incidence of loneliness compared to open societies with global ideas and diverse interactions.

Physically we live in bigger houses with more space in and around, that offers less contact with others. Loss of community cohesion, as years pass without neighbor knowing neighbor, not connected in any meaningful way, absence of bonding. Collapse of local tribes and putting blame on "others". Replaced by Anti-tribes with no bonds between "different" people, lack of interactions lead to poor health, both mental and physical and widespread use of hatred as a tool.

> *"Without friends, no one would choose to live,*
> *even if he had all other goods." Aristotle*

In the 21st century America, one half of the population hates the other half and not only deliberately avoid interacting, they demonize each other, raising resentment and blame to unprecedented levels. It is almost impossible to communicate effectively with someone ideologically opposite to yourself. The result is a chronic stress on the emotional and physical health of the society. When the focus is on beating "them", there is little engagement, less interaction and no connection. Separation, segregation, discrimination, and persistent hatred is now the standard behavior cheered on by a large segment and revealed in our statistics of poor health.

Disrespect for the dignity of "them" was seen in responses to disasters in New Orleans and Puerto Rico. They, not us, do not deserve any form of help. People died because of neglect, abandonment and resulting hopelessness, and nobody seemed to care. They died because there was insufficient social network in place to save "them". We escaped together.

Social democratic countries with adequate social networks and safety nets in which all citizens bond, are accounted for and accountable, lead healthier, better and safer lives.

Effects of Loneliness On Health

*"Loneliness kills. It's as powerful as smoking
and alcoholism."* Robert Waldinger

*"For modern Indians, loneliness is a natural cause
of death."* Sherman Alexie: Memoirs

The lack of adequate social connections has the same value and influence on health as inadequate diet and lack of exercise. Loneliness creates social cripples with poor communication skills who misread facial expressions, or tone of voice, perceptions of threat, and whose curiosity is often mistaken for hostility. Being involuntarily disconnected from others and feeling isolated can lead to stress induced inflammation, heart disease, cancers, diabetes and dementia. Feeling heartsick, homesick and grief-struck results in that deep sinking feeling of a hormonal rush, followed by the disruption of hormonal balance and the chronic drip of a combination of bad-feeling hormones, that destroys cells, tissues, muscle, nerve and body organs. In the lonely immune system, white blood cells remain on high alert for acute bacterial infection, and maintain a state of chronic inflammation that does long- term damage to normal cells (confirmed by the work of Professor Steve Cole, UCLA School of Medicine in 2007).

Social isolation and lack of connection with others adversely affects the Cardiovascular system, with hypertension, strokes, and myocarditis associated with physical inactivity, poor sleep quality, and high stress hormone release; neurological systems with a profound effect on cognitive pathways and the ability to function intellectually, depression, dementia, memory loss and Alzheimer's; digestive system with indigestion and malabsorption of nutrients; the immune system dysfunctions that lead to increased incidence of infections and general reduced longevity.

Loneliness is at epidemic levels. Many studies highlight its association with cognitive decline and premature death from obesity. Nearly one half of Americans report "feeling lonely" at some time (46%). Feeling lonely is equated to smoking 15 cigarettes a day and one lonely day is the equivalent of one pack of cigarettes. They estimated the effects of loneliness to reduce the chances of reaching a longevity above average life expectancy by as much as 10 to15 years. (Loneliness in Later Life and Reaching Longevity: Findings from the Longitudinal Aging Study Amsterdam. Brandts L, et al. The Journals of Gerontology. Jan 2021)

A Cigna Insurance company survey of 2016, found that antisocial behavior was number one in young people born between 1990 to 2000. Some 47 to 54% reported limited in-person social interactions, feelings of loneliness and that no one knows them well or cares.

The 18 to 27 age group was lonelier that any other demographic group and were deficient in social skills, had a high use of electronic media yet felt "unconnected", had decreased time spent with others and felt that society practiced exclusion and separation that reduced the number of interaction encounters. Some 40% admitted to lacking companionship, that their relationships lacked meaning and that they felt increasingly isolated from others. 43% of all demographic age groups reported loneliness There was a high incidence of alcoholism, drug abuse, dysfunctional immune systems (easy sickness), stress-related disease susceptibility, premature ageing, avoidance of social encounters, inability to make and maintain connections, increased distrust of others, high sleep deprivation, high attachment to cars, guns and electronic devices, negative thoughts, fluctuations in weight, and depression, full of anger, fear and misunderstanding. Rates of loneliness have doubled since the 1980's, partly due to use of electronic connections instead of face-to-face interactions.

Study: "Loneliness kills" as validated by outgoing US Surgeon General, Vivek H. Murthy, MD, in 2017 and was directly connected to opioid crisis, drug addiction, suicide, ill health, violence and the status of chronic stress. The CDC reported that 116 individuals died of overdose daily in USA in 2016, which was more than died from heart disease, diabetes, arthritis, cancer or flu. The lack of social connection, loneliness (15 cigarettes a day) associated with a 50% risk for premature death.

Study: "Loneliness, social support networks, mood and well-being in community-dwelling elderly", J Golden, et al. Mar 9, 2009, International Journal of Geriatrics linked both loneliness and lack of social networks to poor mood and well-being examination of quality of life in a Dublin community. Some 35% of participants over the age of 65, reported feeling "lonely", 9% had "painful loneliness", and

6% had "intrusive loneliness". Symptoms were higher in women, the widowed, and those with physical disabilities. The incidence of loneliness increased with age.

Study: "Older adults reporting social isolation or loneliness show poorer cognitive function four years later", Cacioppo JT and S, Evidence-based Nursing. 2014. They tested 8000 individuals, age 50 and over for social isolation and loneliness as potentially modifiable risk factors for poor cognitive functioning.

Study: "Increased risk of mortality associated with social isolation in older men: only when feeling lonely? Results from the Amsterdam Study of the Elderly (AMSTEL). Holwerda TJ, et al. published online, 06 September 2011. A ten year follow up of men, aged 65 to 85, showed that loneliness has a significant influence on both physical and mental health and was associated with increased rates of premature mortality. There were higher rates in men than in women, for mortality associated with feelings of loneliness and not for social isolation. Mental depression from loneliness was linked more with death than just physical isolation.

Study: The impact of social activities, social networks, social support and social relationships on the cognitive functioning of healthy older adults: a systematic review. Kelly ME, et al. Systematic Reviews. 2017. 6:259, concludes that there is an association between social relationships and cognitive function. Further research is needed to define or identify the nature of this association.

Cognitive function determines functional abilities, quality of life, degree of independence processing speed, and extent and quality of memory. Severe cognitive decline does not appear to be a part of normal ageing, and is affected by modifiable factors like, smoking, poor diet, levels of physical activity, mental stimulation and "social interactions and relationships".

Study: "Greater social connection is associated with 50% lower odds of premature death." The results of an investigation by Julianne Holt-Lunstad, PhD, psychologist at Brigham Young University in 2017, showed that roughly 75 million millennials (age 23-27) and Gen Z (age 18-22) are lonelier now than at any other time, than any other demographic and in worse health than the older generations. Lonely/isolated people are 25% more likely to die prematurely than well connected people.

Study: Death from heartbreak is real. The Takotsubo cardiomyopathy and flash pulmonary edema in a trauma patient, reveal that emotional pain (heartbreak syndrome) elicits a severe increase in stress hormone release that mimics a heart attack. Elderly couples often die within months of each other, even without evidence of serious pre-existing pathology. Menopausal women and individuals under severe physical or emotional stress can die from a "broken heart". Loneliness affecting brains and hearts is measurable and is increasing in frequency. Magnetic resonance imaging (MRI) shows that a reaction to emotional rejection occupies the same brain area as physical stress, both show similar responses to high stress cortisol. High stress hormones reduce immune function in lonely anxious individuals who get sick more often and more intensely. J Emerg Med. 2013 Oct;4594):530-2, Ritchie D et al.

Statistics from National Institutes of Health, (NIH), Bethesda, Md.in 2016 data, reveal that 63,632 died of overdose drugs in one year (more than Vietnam War), and 45,000 suicides (drugs and guns) in deaths from despair and associated with a severe lack of community, friendships, and meaningful relationships. Findings included evidence that the wealthy, even being better informed and supposedly "more connected" are not truly so. Most of the connections are shallow and artificial. The rich are more isolated, less happy, more paranoid, and less fulfilled than are the poor, and their range of interaction is considerably less.

In an IPSOS online Polling Survey in 2018, 47% of the individuals polled felt that loneliness coupled with work demands caused anxiety and was associated with inadequate social skills. Of the 46 million individuals aged over 45, almost half reported chronic loneliness and 55% of those reported suffering from poor health.

In the AARP -Loneliness Study, feeling disconnected was associated with early Alzheimer's. Loneliness was defined as a lack of social connections, feeling isolated, misunderstood, and depressed and associated with a high incidence of dysfunctional immunity, hypertension, early cognitive decline, poor heart health, low energy, obesity, depression, sleep disorders, and gastric problems. *Christakis, NA and Fowler JH, The Spread of Obesity in a large Social Network over 32 years. Jul 2007 NEJM Vol 357:370-379*

There is also a study in which a substantial increase in cases in which like attracted like, person to person spread noted as a contribution to the epidemic, irrelevant to biologic and behavioral trait of obesity spread through social ties with food preferences directly linked to social behavior. It amplified loneliness during a holiday season such as Thanksgiving with the tradition of feeding the poor, invite one or two vagrants to dinner, then ignore them for the rest of the year. The loner withdraws from social circles and loses some of his/her social skills. With time, there is a marked decrease in health, with depression, cardiovascular disease and cognitive decline being the most common conditions. Suicidal thoughts are common.

Management of Loneliness

When we starve bacteria in the laboratory, they direct their own mutation to another state, for survival. When in a lonely and negative, we too can change to a mode of positivity and create a new state. Loneliness, a state of feeling disconnected due in part to a lack of human contact, is a "sickness" can lead to more complications. Humans need interactions, relationships, and connections to function in a complete state. We are not here alone, we have access to each other, we have animals, plants and nature to change feelings of loneliness.

One problem is that we may have evolved past the age when togetherness and social connections were required for survival. Our kind DNA gradually changed to cruel DNA and we do not depend on each other anymore. We use those we can and destroy those "we don't need" and designate empathy and altruism as a bane, a drawback, and a hindrance to the principal goal, which has also changed from survival to "getting ahead".

Initial solutions involve the recognition and confrontation of the problem. One must become aware of what you are doing to promote distance and isolation, then stop doing it. Second, build your self-esteem and gain the confidence to carry encounters to the next level. Improve your basic health with adequate exercise and diet and ensure that you are in good enough physical and mental condition to engage and pursue social connections. Third, fix your social skills. Install and sharpen your basic manners. Seek encounters from a wide range of exposures. Avoidance of certain types and groups of people severely limits your range. Focus on the individual's gifts and talents and not on his/her ethnicity or class status. Fourth should be the easiest. Connect and maintain the relationship. It requires a bit of awareness and perseverance.

Socializing reduces fear and its associated stress hormones. It brings immediate results. The human activity of contact, support and intimacy boosts endorphins and provides a state of well-being fulfills a significant part of purpose-seeking. Natural repair and regulation of the social being in a traditional sense, can then rely on the rest of the basic strategies of lifestyle, exercise, nutrition, mental stimulation, stress control and avoidance of toxins.

Preparation of the immune system to maintain function despite the stress of loneliness and antisocial behavior are effective regulation and repair mechanisms. To counter oxidative stress and related cell breakdown, a diet of antioxidants, fresh fruit, whole grains and vegetables can preserve DNA and cell integrity. Foods with magnesium can reduce the adverse stress response and the omega 3 fatty oils in borage and cold-water fish can reduce abnormal norepinephrine release. Adequate physical activity releases endorphins to burn off excess adrenalin/norepinephrine and coping strategies of avoidance of toxic situations, hardiness development and comprehension of emotional and physiological mechanisms of stress can help with control and successful sense of well-being.

If you feel the need for outside help, do not hesitate to ask for it. Concurrent talk therapy is the most effective treatment for depression. Cognitive Behavioral Therapy (CBT) is effective and safe, but not readily available or particularly attractive. Getting help with understanding yourself and connecting with others, developing the skills necessary to communicate effectively, building on core values and establishing purpose and meaning in life, learning the importance and mechanisms of collective well-being as opposed to pure individualism is a natural repair system for depression.

Unfortunately, modern society demands the immediate fix, complete repair at any cost, Including the acceptance of serious side effects of conventional treatments. Social anxiety and concomitant depression is treated most often with sedatives, tranquilizers, inhibitors, and blockage of impulses, and less often with control and implementation of natural mechanisms.

The USA, for one, consumes 66% of worlds antidepressants. (Harvard blog March 6, 2020) Prozac, Celexa, Effexor, Paxil, Zoloft, and anti- anxiety and anti- insomnia medications, Adderall, Halcyon, Xanax, Transxene and the ever- present savior, Valium are riding at full strength throughout our society. Two out of every three people rely on drugs for their daily function. (And the use has increased in response to the Covid-19 pandemic. Prescriptions increased by 21 % to deal with the emotional effects of physical disconnection.). Opioid crises have displaced car accidents as the leading cause of death for Americans under the age of 50. Loneliness and drugs now go hand in hand. Yet we continue to treat the effects and ignore the causes.

Antidepressants work to ease anxiety and stress by balancing brain chemicals (neurotransmitters) that affect mood and emotions. Many are selective serotonin reuptake inhibitors (SSRI) that increase the levels of serotonin available to generate good thoughts, emotions and actuate sleep. The "happy pill", a precursor to serotonin, is 5-Hydroxytryptophan (5-HTP), which boosts emotional well-being by preventing the resorption of natural serotonin, so that it stays around and keeps working. (Alcohol and some illegal drugs do not last this long and have worse side effects.) Antidepressants may cause nausea, increased appetite, weight gain, reduced libido, fatigue and drowsiness, dry mouth, blurred vision, diarrhea and/or constipation, the same anxiety you are trying to avoid, and severe agitation. Although these medications are promoted as "non-addictive", routine overuse and abuse may lead to physical dependence. Withdrawal symptoms do occur and are more prevalent than previously reported. Suicidal thoughts and behavior is present, especially in younger subjects. According to the latest data (NCHS Data Brief, August 2017), nearly 12% of youngsters 12 and older in the USA have taken an antidepressant medication in the past month.

The choice is not attractive. Get sick and die from excess rejection or loss, enter depression from a state of chronic loneliness associated with isolation or turn to drugs to dull the pain and provide happiness and well-being and risk the adverse effects. It is neither good nor logical if you need drugs to interact with someone, relate and pursue a social bonding to fulfill a basic need. Often the desire is not there in the first place.

Since there is no single cause of loneliness, there are multiple solutions. Encounter, interact, and connect. Venture out and join stuff. Volunteer to match your skills with others' needs. Look at yourself, you matter, you have value, share your worth with someone else. Consider meeting people in local organizations, join a dog walking club, and finding others with positive outlooks and plans. Join a book club, a local community center, a journaling organization and/ or a travel club. Keep in mind that all humans are more similar that we are different and capable of interacting and connecting anywhere and anytime. Observe and sort out your own thoughts and feelings and get rid of guilt, fear, and anxiety. Build your confidence in your own ability to interact and connect. Appreciate others and expand your range to include strangers and foreigners. The more opportunities, the better the chances of connections. Do something "different", approach someone "different", leave your comfort zone and seek new experiences. Develop new interaction skills, a new language is fresh access. Visiting outside the limits of your circle does wonders for the body and the mind.

Still, one of the best time-tested solutions to loneliness is getting a pet. An animal companion can help reduce much of the lonely feelings. The reciprocal care of pets provides stress and anxiety reduction, a plethora of feel-good hormones, and elevation of self-esteem. The act of caring for pets provides stability, responsibility and valuable companionship. Social connections with other pet owners are an added benefit.

There are no moral or realistic justifications for restriction of social interaction between all human beings. However, in the present self-interest mindset and economic framework, many view socializing as a losing position. That sharing space and time with "others" that are of no use to your agenda is wasteful and detrimental to getting and staying ahead, gives way to antisocial behavior with its aura of toughness and strength. All social and psychological studies show that pro-social behavior promotes good health and well-being of the individual and success of the society, and that antisocial behavior is stifling and destructive to both.

Social Media and Electronic Devices

Study: FCD Educational Services (Hazelden Betty Ford Foundation) found that those who used a lot of technology to address and complete their daily functions was at a higher risk of developing similar brain chemistry as that of a substance abuser. The constant and repeated release of hormones (the dopamine effect) of instant gratification was the equivalent of overeating, excessive exercise, and social media use. The study included 1500 kids using electronic devices for more than 3 hours a day and was associated with a 30% incidence of depression.

Electronic device use makes possible the receipt of information from friends rapidly and far-reaching and maintaining lines of contact that might be more difficult otherwise. Positive contact with distant previously lost social contacts, easy information availability, easy "connection" with others, Easy and continuous contact with family and friends. The amount of knowledge available is astounding. Making the proper use of it is imperative.

Electronic device use enhances alone time unless it is overdone. Availability of social technology is the main thing saving the mental states of many during pandemic times. Enables increased frequency of communication, with daily visual and audio interaction while physically distant. Even for telephone date calling and online dating, you need to use sufficient social skills, proper timing, and be able to convey sincerity of intent in order to be effective. If the contact is good, but the content is lacking, either exaggerated or falsified, success might be lacking. The subtle cues of interaction, spontaneous gestures, body position, aura, and "chemistry" are still missing. We all agree that even the best electronic connections are not the same as in person interactions. Too many variables are missing. There is a total absence of touch, smell and taste. The virtual world cannot replace the real world, as all the senses are not engaged.

We connect with those at a distance while shutting out those nearby. While in a crowd, we move forward boldly, with headphones in place, eyes glued to the screen, embracing loneliness and sending the message that person-to-person interaction is off limits. Intense focus on the device while walking, while driving, while waiting, not only is dangerous but hampers the ability to communicate verbally and nonverbally, use gestures and body language, basic human skills. Wearing headphones in public indicates that "I prefer not to interact with you". Either unable or unwilling to socialize, to share space, to acknowledge the existence of another. On my last airplane travel before the pandemic, a 15- year-old boy in the window seat for the 4- hour ride, did not once look up from his tablet to acknowledge presence of anyone. He watched the same one hour program for the entire flight.

Reliance on electronic device use reduces the quantity and quality of real-life Interactions and with the surrounding environment. There is no comparison between the value of a live 3-day conference and a 3 hour zoom meeting.

Negative social effects are evident at any gathering where dining is the main event. The presence of a cell phone at the table means "you are not important" and "any call is more important than you". The device substitutes for and destroys "interactions", sends a negative message, reduces eye contact to zero and verbal communication to grunts. Losing the opportunity to use face-to-face social skills with the person next to you has profound repercussions. Not only for diminished connections—but with the wrong hormones in play, the effects on your cardiovascular, immune, digestive and central nervous system may also be significant. Lack of human interaction in real time promotes the inability to engage, practice and relate. Widespread promotion and availability of electronic devices without a thought of what might go wrong, has exposed people to the best and the worst.

"Facebook gives people power to share and unite a world more open and connected". Mark Zuckerberg...

FBK suggested the need to belong and to "connect", but does not actually fulfill all the requirements. Because of the lack of touch, give and take, and other natural responses, the quality of the interaction can be seriously reduced. The prominence of poor diction, grammar, and spelling contributes to the inadequacy of interactions. FBK further enabled people to lie, abuse, misuse, and spread misinformation with impunity. And they are very good at doing it. People cannot be trusted to do the right thing especially when cruel DNA clashes with the kind DNA. Whichever provides the most satisfaction, wins.

With antisocial behavior across the board, in talk show radio, false news media, and across community borders providing a constant stream of promotions that enable hatred, division, and disconnect. Exclusion is good, and connection is bad. Addiction to bad and sensational news is the normal.

Use and abuse of social media has enabled the free expression of meanness, nastiness, hatred, fear and misinformation hiding behind anonymity. Bullying designed to hurt, and diminish is widespread and extremely damaging. It enables retreat from rather than interaction with people and reduces interaction time, even when engaged. Ever popular slogans and mantras keep the reptilian brain occupied and satisfied with feel-good hormones.

Though we recognize the physical impact of use of social media and electronic devices, we continue to overuse them. Computer vision syndrome, or digital eyestrain, is a group of vision-related problems resulting from prolonged computer, tablet, and cell-phone use. Blue light released by digital devices can damage the light-sensitive cells of the inner lining of the retina, resulting in early macular degeneration. Dry eyes from reduced blinking, blurred vision, nearsightedness and eye fatigue can may also occur. Electromagnetic Frequency exposure (EMF) may result in sleep disturbances, headaches, depression, fatigue, poor concentration and reduced memory. EM waves emitted by some devices have been implicated in reduced levels of melatonin, a hormone essential in regulating the sleep-wake cycle.

High screen time (> 6 hours/day) leads to chronic stress from cortisol, and a reduction in feel-good hormones, serotonin and dopamine, resulting in irritability and heightened risk of depression. The choice to play phone games inside or play basketball outside is becoming more and more skewed to the former. The mind goes into overdrive and the body suffers from neglect. Without face-to-face socializing involving signals, we lose the warmth and relationship to the environment and to each other. Gone also is the end-stage connection. High screen time is especially detrimental to child development and can lead to sleep and mental health issues. Dependency on the device for all social and entertainment activity, foregoing all physical activity may cause a stunted personality and physical growth. Over stimulation from high screen time has been linked to depression, ADHD, and mood disorders. Electronic device use for gathering and managing information is useful but should not be a substitute for face-to-face social interaction.

The inequality gap is growing between levels of society and the internet and electronics have done nothing to reduce the divide and enable interactions. The out of sight, out of mind has probably contributed to widening it. The larger the class gaps, the higher the social anxiety, the lower the self-esteem, more confidence loss, higher rates of depression and poorer health.

As many social connections in the 21st century and in the time of the pandemic rely on electronic devices through a variety of media, all provide insufficient input to ascertain true human character involved in the interaction. The following suggestions may be of some help.

Real life friendships are much better than social media ones. Set aside social media time and include some real-life people time. Use your electronic access wisely, do not let it use you. Instead of spending all your time on Facebook and Twitter, read a book, get informed and then pass it on to your peers, electronically, if you must.

Electronics takes away quality time with others and has a dual effect, social media replacing face-to-face interactions and enabling meeting for face time. Most social connections in the 21st century pandemic time involve electronic socializing through a medium, with insufficient input to discover and examine the true human character involved in the interaction. Try to disengage from media and with masking and social distancing you may still meet and interact with actual people in real time.

To protect vision and mental well-being, limit screen time to two hours a day, go out, and try to meet people. Take advantage of the good that electronic social media provides, "connecting" billions of people in a virtual world, but do not pass up any opportunity to re-visit the world of reality.

Social Distancing

*In a world of Social Distancing, can healthy
social interactions still take place?*

America was built with social distancing in mind. Space—and lots of it —was the basis for wide spread out cities with neighborhoods, many fenced off, and miles of road intra and inter connected. The development and preference for suburbia,1945 to 1960s, over urban life already indicated a notion of "social distancing". Living apart, not knowing your neighbors, dependence on automobile for essentials and TV for everything else, was the ideal world, apart from the group, safe and sound. The environment was already conducive and inviting to antisocial behavior.

*"You never realize how antisocial you are until there is a pandemic
and your (social) life doesn't really change that much."*

*"Social Distancing: Day 47. I struck up a conversation with a spider
today. Seems nice. Turns out he's a web designer." Internet Quotes*

Social distancing is physical distancing that becomes social distancing in practice and effect. Along with mask-wearing, both are essential to survival in a pandemic of high contagion. Standing or passing at a physical separation of at least 6 feet apart was suggested in the USA in March of 2020, long after the pandemic had spread to every state. Limiting face-to-face contact, not talking directly into each other's faces, singing, yelling, and standing too close are all suggestions but not enforced in the USA. Physical isolation in home and hotel quarantine, keeping the sick and those who might have been exposed and infected away from others, was proposed as limiting movement outside the home, banning unessential travel, lockdowns of places where people congregate, restaurants, bars, cafes, churches, schools, no gathering of arbitrary numbers of individuals, discouragement of singing, shouting, and long conversations which carry the airborne virus and enable contagion. Though highly effective, these methods affect both short-and long- term health and well-being of the individual and of the community. At least in the USA, along with lapses in and total rejection of mask-wearing, social distancing was never fully practiced. The six foot rule became three feet. Then it was totally ignored in department stores, licensure lines, rallies, fast food outlets, beaches —you name it. Because of the defiance at the "loss of freedom" and simply not caring about others or themselves, our assessment of the long-term side effects may not be accurate. The spread of viral particles between people is still evident despite efforts at quarantine and social isolation. For those who did practice social distancing, we may look at what has transpired and speculate on what to expect as the pandemic continues.

"I still have a hard time accepting that my chances of survival depend on the common sense of others." Internet quote

A primary effect of social distancing is social rejection and loneliness, and the wider sense of loss of personal and community well-being. Though the absence of contact at cafés, lunchrooms, dinner parties and backyard barbeques have been replaced by virtual contact through electronic media, something essential is missing. These feelings of inadequacy inhibit the social experience, reduce learning and growth and invite tinges of depression.

Already I spend more time with my Samsung galaxy phone than with my friends. It solves problems, provides entertainment, sends and receives my emails, sets up and conducts teleconference meetings. It can order a meal, which I eat alone. Its GPS finds any designated address. It calls an Uber ride if I need to go somewhere, and it issues alerts on which areas are attractive and which to avoid. All is well and good with my handheld device, but it lacks the warmth, creativity, unpredictability and intimacy of a friend. It lacks touch.

Social isolation leading to loneliness, generates feelings similar to post-disaster loss, post traumatic stress disorder (PTSD), and depression. From close quarters may come reactive domestic violence and child abuse, with concomitant increases in substance abuse and feedback into the cycle. One of the first articles to corroborate these events is from the Boston University School of Public Health, Journal of the American Medical Association (JAMA), April 2020, by S. Galea and R.M. Merchant: "The Mental Health Consequences of Covid-19 and Physical Distancing; the Need for Prevention and Early Intervention".

In the physiology of isolation, with a reduction in social support and stimulation of the senses, we adopt the physiology of alone instead of together. The production of social hormones, oxytocin, serotonin, and dopamine decrease and the stress hormones, cortisol, norepinephrine and epinephrine increase. Children attached to parents and family are deprived of learning from other sources. Adolescents may be affected the most in their "formative" years when it is imperative to get out and meet people, create, and form friendships. Isolation narrows the field and the opportunities tremendously besides the natural feelings of separation and ostracism. Learning and growth through socializing, being hypersensitive, affects them more than other groups. Brain development may be impaired and the reactive increase in drug use, legal and illegal, all but guarantee added detrimental effects. (Orbitofrontal cortex thickness and substance use disorders in emerging adulthood: causal inferences from co-twin control/discordant twin study. Harper J. et al. Addiction (Abingdon, England, 2021 Feb23.))

In response to isolation, there is a steady drip of cortisol, the stress hormone, activating inflammatory cytokines, impairing the immune system and keeping it on constant alert, open to sicknesses of corrosive damage to the Cardiovascular system, linking it to diabetes, stroke and heart disease. The increased release of stress hormones may lead to Central Nervous System disorders, prominent of which is depression, in which mental and physical pain use the same receptors. They manifest the science of a broken heart in real time. In Japan, there were more deaths from suicides in October 2020 than from Covid-19 complications, 2153 to 2087.

With our digital technology (I for one have been using telemedicine for patient care) the biggest deprivation is the absence of touch. Without a mother's or nurse's touch, the infant is more likely to become sick. Touch stimulates oxytocin pathways, the natural antidepressant, serotonin, and the pleasure chemical, dopamine, and several other comfort hormones in combination. Touch promotes relationships, trust, dependency, and sustenance. It blocks abnormal cortisol release, reduces heart rate and blood pressure (the calming caress in an anxiety attack) and stimulates touch receptors signals to the vagus nerve (X) to slow the pace of the nervous system activity. Even the touch of a stranger can assuage feelings of social exclusion, and loneliness, such as with a downcast child on the playground being left out from games. Deprivation of touch can lead to depression, anxiety, low relationship satisfaction, sleep disorders, and avoidance of secure relationships.

In the long term, we can associate the avoidance of touch with the avoidance of trust, as seen in studies of feral children in the varying levels of human attachment.

In most Latino communities, "un abrazo fuerte", a hug for at least 20 seconds, the point at which it releases oxytocin is similar to the endorphin release of a long-distance runner. There has been much concern and consternation on how social isolation will play out without this cultural traditional greeting. With touch deprivation, a breakdown of the entire system of encounter and interaction, as relegated to speech, sound and sight, may occur. Without touch, even the basic hug, handshake, and kiss, (especially the French 'bise'), the physiological systems of nerve (weak vagal response), hormones (low oxytocin production and excess cortisol) and pain control (mental and physical) will have to adapt and adjust. Socializing is a fundamental human need. With social distancing, we shall soon see if touch is an essential requirement for human development and survival. On the **positive** side, social distancing may bring some couples and families closer together, enable the realization of the essential need for each other and use of innovative ways of coping and enjoying each other's company. Isolation may encourage the prevention of excessive lifestyle habits linked to diabetes, hypertension, cardiovascular diseases and chronic obstructive lung diseases, and realization that good health matters. My book, Natural Health and Disease Prevention with the six basic strategies for good health, along with many others, enjoyed increased scrutiny and use during the initial months of the pandemic. Isolation led many to start and increase regimens of exercise for the health of the brain and body. Nutritional changes amounted to eating less quantity, eating local, fresh, non-processed healthy food. People understood that stress control is a major factor in immune system function, and that toxin avoidance, such as smoking, excess alcohol consumption, and reduced exposure to airborne pollutants and certain household products could have a positive impact on one's health. Mental stimulation with a reconnection to reading and writing, brain games, and electronic learning, could create, expand and clarify ones thought processes and that physical isolation did not prevent reaching out to old friends and making new ones. Social connection with others came to the forefront because of the realization of its importance. Ask yourself how many new friends have I made and kept during the Covid-19 Pandemic? If zero, then you have some catching up to do.

Substitute the isolation from people with connections to nature. Long walks and new observations accomplish much. In quarantined homes, the increase in empathy, patience, gratitude and appreciation are all positive attributes to the pandemic. The creation and generation of **humor** has been a welcome healthy occurrence. Here are some of my internet favorites:

"Bad ponies make good riders"
"If you keep a glass of wine in each hand,
then you can't touch your face"
"When this quarantine is over, let's not tell some people".
"Pretty wild how we used to eat cake after someone had blown on it."
"So you're really staying inside, practicing social distancing
and cleaning yourself? You've become your house cat."
"I miss being late to everything." Make some up on your own.

New skills developed, like cooking, art, building a new patio, tiling a bathroom, and ways of doing laundry. My teenaged grandchildren mastered these. Novel ways of connecting with neighbors, who may have been previously ignored, organizing communal spaces and innovations in getting together were all in order. The increase in financial acumen and budgeting of time took on new meaning and even fresher importance. Survival.

On the **negative** side, our natural DNA is imprinted and hard-wired for participation, cooperation, collaboration, competition, and engagement with others, using all the senses. Any deviation from the whole will have repercussions. Humans are not fully formed at birth. It takes between 15 to 20 years for development to maturity, with input from the environment and from other humans as essential factors. On the journey from childhood to adulthood, all the senses need to be stimulated to achieve complete brain and body development.

Short term isolation appears to be difficult for bar hoppers, café goers, and office cooler chatters who use this milieu for socializing. There should hardly be and serious loss of social skills but merely delayed acquisition of perceived goals. Even without imposed isolation, many youth prefer to use their electronic devices to communicate and forego face-to-face socializing, especially with adults. Adverse effects would affect those without access to readily available personal digital technology.

The long-term effects of lack of interactions, withholding of the senses, and resultant antisocial and asocial behavior has yet to be tabulated. Though the detailed reactions may differ between children, adolescents, adults and the elderly, the basic damages are quite similar. The effect of isolation on mental health simulates that of disasters, mass shootings, natural disasters, and terror massacres. Like with PTSD, substance abuse disorder, domestic violence, and child abuse (with schools closed), damages may persist long after the event is over. Adverse childhood experiences (ACE) related to trauma, verbal abuse, neglect, dysfunctional home, inadequate schooling, malnutrition, community violence, rejection from peers, and bullying, have increased. (ACE can also be ascribed to At home Covid Effects.)

Social distancing and sheltering at home affect adolescents who depend on socializing as an integral part of their development. Those with privileges, ample electronics, outlets, social groupings, and the knowledge and will to use them, do well. Those lacking adequate access, are affected disproportionately. Loss of contact creates anxiety, impaired social skills, and the lack of opportunity to learn, practice and grow. For most there is a loss of a sense of community, where impersonal and individual feelings replace group activity. The negative effect is again on learning and growth, as one does just enough to get by as the uncertainty of the future is pervasive. The prevention of human interaction raises fears of others, as carriers of viruses, as threat of taking something that cannot be replaced, of permanent damage to body and mind, which may lead to paranoia and panic.

Even more than in "normal" society, the socially isolated turn to drugs for pain relief and as substitutes to ease fears and uncertainties. There has been an increase in prescriptions for stimulants, sedatives, and tranquilizers in addition to the use of illegal drugs. Losing physical interactions dull the senses and the drug culture itself adds to the dependence.

Those with access increase their use of electronic devices for entertainment and daily routines, and a whole new set has added eyestrain and noise pollution to their exposure to toxins. There was a noticeable reactive increase in food intake (comfort food) and the results will be forthcoming. Obesity.

The outcomes after loss or disruption of the natural encounter-interaction-connection mechanism depend on access, individual temperament and ability to handle stressors. Those with access and ability, do well and those without, do poorly. The prevailing emotion elicited is one of **anxiety**. Simple encounters and interactions generate anxiety, as vulnerability to perceptions of threat and distrust, prevail. There is loss of trust between maskers and non-maskers, distancers and non-distancers, vaxxers and non-vaxxers, are deliberately trying to hurt me. There was a flood of anxiety when dt called the pandemic, the "Chinese disease" and "Kung Flu", which created more stress, promoted more exclusion (them vs us), and fixated on the disconnect rather than cultivate connectivity like "we're all in this together" and let us help each other out. Instead, this antisocial behavior cut "us" off from "them". This destructive mentality added to the loss/ detriment/ with most impact on health, loss of interactions, deprivations, loneliness, depression and resultant concomitant diseases.

Loneliness is the most common and feared effect of social isolation. Already lonely people have higher stress cortisol levels, lower immune system function, higher incidence of depression, substance abuse and suicide rates than the socially connected. Quarantine negatives include possible seclusion with quarrelsome, stressed adults, dread of scarcity of essentials, rationing, lack of caring, and fear of contracting the disease. Loss of established social connections, reduced interactions, loss of communicative and emotional reactive skills, loss of academic confidence and purpose. The pandemic and its subsequently imposed isolation have disrupted lives, impaired cognition and deprived us of the use of the arts and music for healing in community gatherings. The absence of live concerts and events has also reduced our interactions with friends and strangers over appreciation of music. Alone, exposure to the arts may help assuage emotional and spiritual isolation, but does not replace the physical presence. Without the interaction of others, we lose a large part of our humanity.

Further isolation of the elderly exacerbates the loneliness, anxiety, depression and other mental problems similar in impact as "not eating" or "homesickness". The broken bonds of social connections lead to feeling lonely, which induces acute and chronic release of stress hormones that affect sleep patterns, cause emotional exhaustion, and may lead to substance abuse, especially alcohol, and all their sequelae. The likelihood of premature death from the side effects of isolation about equals that of demise from the disease. With seniors isolated, out of sight and out of mind, plus recession and unemployment, both physical and mental deprivation hasten the poor outcome.

Suggested Solutions

The UK manual on Mental Health, 2020, suggests Three Steps in the approach to social isolation imposed by the Covid-19 pandemic. First is to outline specific plans to offset loneliness. Use digital technology to connect socially while remaining physically distant. Schedule and conduct meetings online, set up a virtual workplace, attend churches, and structure schooling to focus on learning and include socializing. Do gymnastics and take nature walks to promote feelings of togetherness. Reach out to a group of friends with video and voice calls, use social media and all forms of information gathering and sharing. Second, change destructive behavior. Control and reduce domestic violence and child abuse. Seek and get help by all means available. Balance social distancing and safe place. Follow the rules. Third, make and take the treatment available. Physical and mental care have become "psychological first aid" and are essential in this atmosphere of feelings of isolation. Use telemedicine for care and support.

In practical terms, here are a few additional suggestions. For those who are absolutely physically alone, use touch substitutes. Long hot baths, blanket wrapping, pillow hugging and cuddling with a pet may help to stimulate the touch receptors. Interaction with a pet gives more comfort and satisfaction than you may think.

Solutions for Seniors and Adults

Make ample use of phone, digital messaging, email, and zoom to stay in touch with family and visit with your established friends. Take a special interest in others. Reach out across cultures and expand your range. Be creative, share information, and maintain the importance of acknowledging each. Be aware that loneliness and depression are not acceptable states in which to live one's life, and do not have to happen. When this is all over, ask yourself again, how many new friends did you make during the pandemic? The answer should not be zero.

Vignette #24: When the Internet became available, I set out to reconnect with my High School teachers and classmates who had left an impression and enabled my development as a person. Those who were sincere and genuinely glad to hear from me warranted further connection. I reinforced that their instruction and friendships were worth the effort and asked to keep in touch, share information and play at staying young. When the pandemic came, my network was already in place. We tried to stay in touch regularly, discussing everything from sports, politics, international geography and history, and all sorts of gossip. It was a virtual "tertulia" over coffee, tea or a glass of wine, a panoramic of the past, present and future. The primary item of discussion, however, remains to have a plan and pursue it. "What are you doing now and what are your plans for the year" was the core of many a conversation. My daily contact with at least one person at a great distance reaffirms our inherent values and keeps my world intact.

Use technology to offset isolation, stay connected with the world through virtual travel to old and new places, then share thoughts and experiences. Get outside, walk, set a goal of A to B and back, then do it. With inclement weather, do the mall walk. It is flat and has bathroom facilities. Visit the local gym and follow the rules. Visit the local coffee shop outdoors in a park, or under a tree, visit with locals at 6 feet apart and chat. Make sure that everyone knows what six feet is and if someone refuses to adhere, then leave. Visit restaurants that provide outdoor seating and heating, dining alfresco, take advantage of drive-in social events like celebrations, weddings, religious holidays, and movies from the safety of your car. Use large scale meeting facilities with good ventilation, hand hygiene, and good spacing for small gatherings. Watch and be aware of the rate of infection of your community and the community with which you come into contact. For family use the bubble strategy to keep members and friends confined to those who shelter in place or forego contact outside the bubble, to keep those inside, safe. Note that it does not work if one person belongs to multiple bubbles.

In winter, make use of sports like skiing, sledding and skating that call for coverings, face masks, goggles and gloves, customary isolation already in place.

Doctor visits could be online when possible, provide diagnostics and monitoring by telemedicine, set up as web visits, with registration, diagnosis and treatment. Patients will need to know the technology required and gain the communicative skills to convey your symptoms and signs effectively. For in-person visits, interaction with the staff, waiting room attendees and the doctor should be as before, except for the reduction in touch and greater attention paid to hygiene and disinfection.

"Please Be Responsible for your own Health" was a sign in my waiting room for 30 years. Though most ignored it at the time, perhaps some may pay attention now. The best cure has and will always be prevention, and that is your responsibility. Staying healthy and not getting sick in the first place is the best pathway to a strong immune system that functions well.

The advent of the 21st century and the pandemic have significantly reduced access to professional health care. Home visits by the family doctor disappeared a long time ago. Doctor-patient relationships have changed and will change even more. The emphasis on cost per time spent with the patient, the push to use diagnostics over touch and physical contact with the patient and the reduction in repeat visits, all contribute to less time and attention spent with individuals on a personal basis. The interest of reliability and effectivity of diagnosis, treatment and outcomes, by AI interventions, may be fine, but we have reduced the connectivity of human to human, which cannot be replaced. Insurance companies dictate the quantity, reliability, and quality of encounters, with those with access receiving levels above those without. Limitations on time spent, which diseases are assigned to which physicians, numbers examined per hour and cost, were all in place before the pandemic. Currently the limits have been magnified. In the absence of universal health care where everyone receives near equal treatment, money and access will continue to dictate healthcare. Either you have it and you get it or you don't. Since the mid-1990s, with the widespread use of digital records, during a visit, some doctors sit with a computer, make no eye contact, no touch, and make no meaningful connections. The efficiency of information in is high and the quality of visit is low. The patient often leaves feeling unsatisfied and unfulfilled.

With the pandemic, patients were being told to stay home, gets diagnosis and treatment from Internet apps and visit only for urgent care. Add the fear of contracting Covid-19, fret over diagnosis and treatment plus the stress of obligatory payment and you get a further reduction in immune system function. Visits by telemedicine (send pictures by phone) and call-in prescriptions are now the standard of care.

Reliance on the Internet for necessities to stay healthy: exercise, nutrition (order out or hone your cooking skills), mental stimulation (virtual travel and read more), stress control (relaxation techniques), toxin avoidance (in house and outdoor air pollutants) and social connections are suggested solutions to reduce angst and worry about health.

Social Distancing during a pandemic just may enhance socializing skills and outcomes. Use social connections to offset the stress heart syndrome. Find comfort in the company of those nearby and reach out to those at a distance. Use social interactions to offset the fears and threats of others. Avoid non-mask-wearers and seek like-minded acquaintances. Use the pandemic to educate yourself about the human condition. Read. We are not as indestructible as we think and certainly not immortal. Reach out and ask for help when you need it. Being afraid is okay. Accept help when offered or available. And reach out to help someone else in need. Practice altruism, appreciate each other.

Use the pandemic to enable social change. Stop the separation based on differences and talk to each other. Get together, even if virtually. If you live in the same place, be friends. Invite and include Provide for the less fortunate. Drop the hoarding and share. We are all in this together.

Seniors and adults should lead the way in embracing technology without fear of threat. We have less to lose. Though remote working is not a viable substitute for human contact, make use of technology to communicate, reach out, interact and connect. with family, friends and others as often as possible. Express concern, offer help, share ideas and implement innovations.

My friend, Dr. Stan Gryskiewicz, Founder and Chairman Emeritus of the Association for Managers of Innovation, has the right idea in organizing regular meetings of a group of knowledgeable people to share ideas and help solve problems related to the implementing of innovation. Gathering for over 40 years, this association is quite impressive and owes its success to the group itself. (podcasts at www.positiveturbulence.com) Membership is global and AMI's management is spread over North America. (aminnovation.org)

The opportunity presents itself to bring together those who were previously excluded, victims of social injustice, and those having the wrong zip code. A universal crisis gives us the chance to show compassion and charity, to offset the self- interest and greed of the pre-pandemic society. (*Ironically, a large section of the Congress just voted to withhold needed assistance to the populace*)

Seniors need to interact socially as an essential ingredient to good health and stay connected to the outside world to avoid depression, anxiety and resultant stress diseases. Mentally, the pandemic should have broadened our thought processes and made us more aware of the interconnectivity that we share. We are all the same and need each other for survival. The "Us and Them" does not matter in the face of a common foe, the virus. "We "matter and we need to go forward together. We make and share solutions. We confront and solve problems. Isolation and fewer opportunities may just teach us to reach out more often and be more friendly. We need to contact and interact positively with those who did not get the memo.

Physically, we can implement and make use of outdoor cafes and restaurants, biking and walking paths, car-free zones (to allow for small safe public gatherings, reduced number of city inhabitants (as many fled to avoid the panic and proximity). People are naturally attracted to each other, especially if different (*antisocial avoidance because of differences is not natural*). Try to see the world through fresh eyes. We must learn to embrace and manage diversity, not to shun it.

Before the pandemic there was some degree of social distancing already in place as many preferred texting over speaking, even while sitting on the same bench. HD TV sports game viewing was chosen over stadium attendance. Videogaming was preferred over shooting hoops in the driveway, climbing a tree or hitting balls (golf and baseball). Some continue to prefer zoom or face time to the complexities of a face-to-face visit. This disconnect is a major concern now and will have lasting effects on our sociability. The social kindness DNA is being overcome by antisocial cruel DNA. (Anti-protesters, self-declared Nazis, and white supremacists insisting that police brutality. Targeted drone murder and the January 6, 2021 Capitol riot are okay.)

Faced with a respiratory virus that kills, the initial motivation in some humans was to stockpile toilet paper and refuse to wear a mask.

Some 550,000 deaths later, many still refuse to wear a mask. What message does this convey about our social nature?

Youth

In isolation, the young will not learn to socialize, nor is there any indication that they care. Digital and virtual encounters are no substitute for face-to-face interactions. You cannot read and react appropriately to intentions on a screen. A lot of social distance already exists between us, as separated into "groups" by class and ethnicity. Social distancing just makes indifferent behavior legitimate and encourages more separation by adding new fears. Socializing is essential for brain and social skills development. Homeschooled children are not as socially adapted as group schooled children, no matter what the statistics imply. Instagram and social media are not viable substitutes for face-to-face interactions. How to behave in a society and the use of basic manners take practice and cannot be taught or learned in isolation. Active social modes (posting) are okay for some personal relationships, vs passive scrolling (news, negative influences, etcetera), but do not take the place of a wider range of social encounters.

The long- term effects of physical distancing on social connections are yet to be determined. You cannot substitute for face-to-face contact with its input output and outcomes, indefinitely without incurring some serious mental and physical effects.

Isolated Children

For children deprived of contact with an assortment of other children and the company of a variety of adults, the outcome is not good. Children learning from each other and exposure to other adults are paramount to childhood development. Losing a fount of learning from the extended family means the loss of the full understanding of morality (right and wrong); and insufficiency of knowing how to behave in a society. *"It takes a village to raise a child."* (and a lot of stable marriages to make a village.)

Homeschooling deprives children of the company of mainstream social interactions that are vital to developing the ability to manage in a diverse society. Certain studies support the premise that educating children at home does not affect their social abilities or lead to antisocial behavior. Socializing with other homeschooled children provides sufficient interaction with friends to meet social needs. (R, Kunzman. The Wiley Handbook of home education. Homeschooler Socialization. 2016.) I beg to differ, along with others. It is not biologically logical nor psychologically practical to deprive a child of diverse social interactions. He/she will have a worldview distorted by the strengths and limitations of the parents, especially with regards to religion and human values. Social isolation does not provide sufficient experience for the development of social skills. Without a wide range of interactions, a global view is next to impossible. (S. Lebela. Homeschooling: Depriving Children of Social Development. Legal Issues 2007.) Note that while the Sandy Hook shooter was homeschooled, some 2-million homeschooled children were safe from his reach.

We know that hand- holding reduces physical and mental pain and that a smile and a hug go a long way. Without physical contact and mental stimulation from others, children will suffer from serious effects. Without open avenues to socializing, children are vulnerable to a high risk of loneliness, accompanied by depression and failure to develop normally. As they are vulnerable so they are malleable and can adapt and thrive accordingly. We need to be aware of the symptoms of depression and attempt to guide and protect them from total isolation as well as from disease.

Social interactions are the equivalent of food and sleep. In the face of isolation, maintain a feeling of connection, keep the mental humming, even if the physical has been reduced. With Covid-19 social distancing, one needs to expand the range of socializing, not shrink it. Forget the exclusion, racism, discrimination, hatred and fear altogether. Occasional connection with a small group by electronics is not enough. Reach out and socialize with as many as you can by any acceptable means available.

Unsociable: Asocial: Autism

Having or showing a disinclination for social activity is the definition offered by the Merriam-Webster dictionary, with synonyms or solitary and reserved. In practical terms, being unsociable is associated with being detached in the presence of others and not open to friendly relations. Distant, cold, and standoffish are other terms appropriately given to the ultra-antisocial. The roots may lie in a lack of social skills, limited opportunities, or low levels of kind hormones, or in a core meanness with high levels of bad hormones, feeling fearful and seeing a threat in everyone around you, or lack of motivation to engage in social interaction. Being unsociable is often learned from or the product of a family that was unavailable or unresponsive to their needs during the early years of development. Seeing others as a threat then withdrawing from interactions may be a reaction to low self-confidence, a deep need to be alone or a desire not to make the effort, a release of responsibility, or more simply, differing views on human meaning.

The ultra-rich have little or no contact with the poor. Billionaires become insensitive to ordinary people and "disconnect" in fear of exposing their wealth to scrutiny and possible self. Power and wealth provide one with feelings of superiority accompanied by the right to disconnect from the rest of humanity, because you can.

Wolf people, grow up in isolation, are asocial and subnormal. Inadequate social exposure can lead to decreased brain development.

Most "unsociables" do not seek nor enjoy the company of other people, with reasons usually hidden in their psyches. Avoidant personality disorders manifest by being uncomfortable in social situations giving rise to anxiety and inappropriate behavior. I group the extreme introverts, who focus almost entirely on internal thoughts and actions, with the unsociables. Both are one step past the anti-socials, in being voluntary behavior that can be unlearned and made functional.

People who avoid all social interaction because of clinical conditions that affect their ability to socialize, are asocial. Autism, or autism spectrum disorder (ASD), is a broad group of conditions in which social skills are lacking, repetitive behaviors, lack of speech and non-verbal communications. There are several subtypes, but all involve some degree of disconnect from others. Factors that influence the development of autism include sensory nervous system abnormalities, seizure activity, sleep and gastrointestinal disorders resulting in brain development that affects areas of social interaction and communication. We have associated asocial behavior and its lack of neural development with the abnormal synthesis, release and/or utilization of oxytocin and dopamine. Males are higher in autism and ADD, while females are higher in depression and anxiety disorders. In addition, autistic subjects have shown alterations in the mesocorticolimbic dopamine signaling pathway associated with reduced neural responses in the nucleus accumbens area of the brain. Magnetic resonance imaging (MRI) can make the diagnosis, by revealing a reduction in connectivity and mirror neurons in multiple neural systems associated with an abnormal migration of embryonic cells during fetal development.

Autistic children avoid eye contact, are uncooperative, exhibit little or no trust in anyone else and are totally devoid of social skills. They cannot relate to themselves or to other people and situations. Communications mechanisms shut down or never develop. They usually have an exceptional intellect.

Asperger syndrome as described by the Austrian pediatrician, Hans Asperger, in 1944, is a developmental disorder in which there is an inability to socialize effectively and communicate non-verbally with other people normally. Those afflicted exhibit repetitive patterns of behavior and interests. It is characterized by intellectual or artistic interest, poor social skills, delayed motor development and speech problems. These children were initially treated with communication training, cognitive behavioral treatment and physical therapy. The breakout signs were limited understanding of language, light awareness of others and a slight reduction in physical clumsiness. In 2013, we estimated the existence of 31-million cases globally.

In 1998, a Lancet article linking autism with measles vaccine that made headlines was proven to be false and ill conceived. The association was a coincidence. There is no virologic or epidemiologic evidence to support this claim. The article was retracted 6 years later after enormous damages were done in scaring parents into denying vaccinations to their children, hence endangering the entire group.

The cause is related to a genetic defect at the synapse of neurons required for sensory perception (input), movement (output), coordination, learning, memory and social interactions. Environmental toxins may or may not be involved.

The classic exposé on autism was presented in the 1988 academy award movie, Rain Man, on the interactions of a hustler and his autistic savant brother, an unforgettable emotional and learning experience.

Hyper-Social

The excessively social person cannot exist alone and must be in contact with others at all times or they become nonfunctional. One subtype is the Williams Syndrome, another neurodevelopmental genetic disorder with sociological features. Elfin in appearance, these people are outgoing, friendly and often charming beyond social norms. Often exhibiting special talents for music, they are super happy, trust everyone and exceptionally sociable. Biochemically they have high levels of calcium in the blood and urine.

"Someone with autism has taught me that love needs no words."

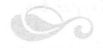

CHAPTER FOUR

SOCIAL EXPERIENCES

Fortunate to have been exposed to "civilized life" in Europe during my teens, I found that meeting and befriending a diverse group of people was not only educational and exciting but has lasted to this day, 60 years later. (*Do the math*). The social distancing imposed by the pandemic has not affected me as it would someone whose circle of friends is less extended, confined to homogeneity and more segregated. Well-equipped with a working set of social skills, keeping in touch with friends close by and in distant places continued as before and even grew.

Social connections depend on genetics and the expression of types of behavior that support pro-social or antisocial, which are directed by the cultural environment in which the interactions occur. Only humans live in cultures bound by tradition and language. Culture dominates genes and human social practices supersede genetics. Although all cultures contain a mixture of positive and negative behaviors, cooperation and altruism are better expressed in some and aggression and self-interest in others.

Of the seventy-two countries I have visited (and the hundreds of others I have read about), I choose to showcase Greece as having a population that is most empathic, sympathetic, compassionate, and friendly to strangers. On my many visits, I have tried to identify the reasons even asking the Greeks themselves why they are so friendly, as compared to the people of other countries. The answers they offered together with deductive reasoning, will be presented in this chapter.

Hospitality in Greece has ancient origins. Xenia is the Greek concept of guest-friendship/ hospitality, generosity, gift exchange and courtesy shown to strangers, those who are far from home. Historically, friendliness toward strangers and guests was a moral obligation. Zeus and Athena were both honored as patrons of foreigners. In a painting by the Flemish master, Peter Paul Rubens, "Jupiter and Mercurius in the house of Philemon and Baucis" (1630-33), Zeus and Hermes, both in disguise, test the hospitality of the Greek village. Having been warmly received by Baucis and Philemon, and not by their neighbors, the gods reward the former, while the latter were punished. This myth serves as one of the templates for Greek behavior toward strangers.

In a modern example, the island of Lesbos, in the northern Aegean Sea, is a destination for migrants. The bodies of two drowned children washed up on shore. The locals took them to Christos, the gravedigger, who assumed they were Muslim and took a guess at their ages As there was no designated cemetery, he buried them in an enclave in the "Christian" cemetery. Locals left plastic flowers and stuffed toys on their graves, and said prayers for their souls. (*story The Next Great Migration, by Sonia Shah)

In Greece, I found that empathy, sympathy, and compassion were all around. Unlike other European countries, with similar claims of economic problems, Greece did not disparage and shut out the Middle East migrants. They faced the problem and offered solutions. They moved them to camps on Lesbos, and other camps and tried to help. I did not hear or see the vehement hatred and fear from the Greeks as from other countries that have much more resources, but they refused to share. These were the very ones whose population migrated to the USA when they were in trouble.

Vignette #25: Personal experience: As my wife and I were moving into our borrowed apartment in Athens, we encountered a neighbor entering the same building. She had just come from the bakery. Greeting us with a smile that could warm an oven, she reached into her shopping bag and gave us each a freshly baked pastry, accompanied with a big "enjoy" written all over her face. Granted, we did not look like refugees, but we do not look Greek either. To her, we were strangers visiting and worthy of a small gift, a "sharing is caring" smile and a decent welcome.

The word for "compassion" (having empathy for the suffering of other beings) in Greek is "eleos", sometimes personified as a goddess, Elea, personification of pity, mercy, and clemency. Charis is the Greek goddess of kindness and life, one of the Charities or Graces. Philotes was the goddess of friendship and affection, and perhaps also the spirit of sexual intercourse. Of the three forms of Greek love, Eros is the romantic, Philia, the friendly one and Agape, the unconditional love without expectations. The highest form, it is the love of a god. Silipitiria, gratitude within condolences in times of mourning may be expressed as,

"I feel sorry with you" or "I feel happy for and with you" in times of success.

Basic Greetings

Greetings are intentional communications used by humans and other animals to announce one's presence. An expression of good wishes, it may also draw attention to another person or suggest what type of relationship, formal or informal, that exists or that is to be expected. Greetings are the basis of politeness and successful interactions. A dog that approaches a group with his tail between his legs, head down and a submissive whimper is more likely to be accepted than one with teeth bared, a menacing growl and demanding to face the alpha. Animals signal status, place in the group, and intentions more explicitly than do humans. Dogs bark with different timbres, pitch, and frequency, plus specific behaviors, tail wagging teeth-baring and sounds that accompany the greeting. Brief bursts of 5 to 10 seconds may show play, move on, fight or look for sex, depending on the accompanying body action. They sniff each other, make an assessment and, if unreciprocated, react according to breed and disposition. When a dog meets his human, the sniff, lick, tail-wag, and happy dance is unmistakable. Human means good. Dogs greet and lick everybody. Wolves lick each other, but not dogs or humans. Animals greet each other, communicate, establish status (dominance), defend territory, coordinate group behavior, care for the young, and seek a mate. Greetings take a major role in the initiation of the interaction.

In 5000 BCE, if a stranger shows up to your cave, offers greetings, then asks for shelter or trade, you would invite him in to share a meal, exchange information (mostly gossip) and stay the night by a warm campfire. If another stranger barges in, ignores the greeting, demands your herd, your women and your cultivated field, the reception would be different. The type and manner of the introduction is all important.

Gestures are basic expressions made upon meeting, which may consist of formal expressions, like handshakes, kisses, and hugs, as determined by social etiquette of the culture or other more informal body language forms. Greetings may be signals like open arms showing that hugs are expected or that crossed arms mean hostility. The accompanying facial expression, body language and eye contact indicate emotions and interest level. When men wore hats, touching the tip with the hand or removing the hat was a gesture of respect. In the Middle East, men offer "salaam", meaning peace, and accent it by placing the right hand over the heart before and after the handshake.

The opposite sexes greet only with a soft handshake. Acceptable greetings are made only with the right hand as the left is considered unclean. Chinese greetings are made with the right fist placed inside the palm of the palm of the left hand and shaken back and forth a few times, both on meeting and on parting. In India, everyone offers the namaste greeting of palms pressed together, held near the heart with the head slightly bowed.

"Adab", a hand gesture and word of respect and politeness in Southeast Asia, involves raising the right hand with palm inward to the forehead while bending the upper torso forward. It may be answered with the word "Tasleem" or a facial expression of acceptance. "Wai" is a gesture in Thailand of placing the hands palm to palm at nose level, while bowing. The elbow and fist bumps are the standard greetings in the current pandemic world.

Basic greetings possibly originated in the Old Stone Age (Paleolithic) when humans climbed down from the trees, stood on the ground for prolonged periods, and walked around in groups from point A to point B, with a purpose in mind. Along the way, they needed some form of signal to summon and identify each member of the group as friend or foe. A reliable and repeatable greeting indicative of good or bad intentions could save a life. They registered the handshake was on papyri and relief slabs in ancient Egypt and Assyria. Homer refers to handshaking in both the Iliad and the Odyssey. The ancient Greek handshake upon meeting in the agora of each one grasping the open right hand (dominant) was a symbol of peace, mutual respect, and agreement on the terms of the encounter. It also showed if one was carrying a weapon and shaking it vigorously could dislodge any hidden weapons (noted also with the medieval knights). A salute was with the right hand to show respect and the absence of a weapon in the dominant hand.

With languages, "hello" or "hi" are greetings in English, which derive from the Old High German for "hala", the emphatic for the word, "holon", to fetch, as in hailing a ferryman. The French used "ho-la", or whoa there. Variants range from "hola" (Spanish) to hallo, hullo, hollo and hillo. "Good morning, good afternoon and good evening" are preferred in many regions. We use some words in both the greeting and the farewell: Good day in English, Shalom in Hebrew, As-Salamualaikum in Arabic, Namaste in Hindi, Aloha in Hawaiian, Ayubowan in Sri Lanka, Kia ora in Maori and Ciao in Italian. Some form of greetings exists in all known human cultures.

In the Latin Romance languages, we make the introductory greeting with respect, Signore, Madame, Senora, Senhor, in acknowledgement of their presence and status. Making the greeting confers likeability upon the greeter, as well. The greeting releases feel-good hormones and suggests more to come. A greeting that is made incorrectly or not returned, may produce an immediate rush of feel-bad hormones, that little sick feeling in the stomach and tinge of disgust.

Every encounter with the intention of interaction in French should start with "Bonjour" in order to get the effect of opening the conversation. Once "engaged", the French are just as friendly, helpful and eager to engage as anyone else is... perhaps more so, as discussion is a full- time occupation in Francophone regions.

Vignette #26: I first met Ms. Joanna Bema, a nurse anesthetist from Ghana, at the St Croix Hospital where I was fortunate to land a student summer job. At my insistence and her delight she taught me a few greetings in the Twi language. "Maa-kyé" (good morning) and "wo ho te sen" followed by "me ho ye" (I am well). I remember as they were audible sounds repeated daily between us. (I do not know how to write them.) Later when introduced to a group of Ghanian physicians at a conference, I used these greetings with the perfect accent, tone and delivery I had learned by imitating Ms Bema. The instant wonder and love that followed has endeared and connected me to that group to this day. Like in the commercial, the event was "priceless".

Good and Bad Manners

Cultures that consistently exhibit interactions with good manners will elicit trust and those with a history and label of bad manners, mistrust. We treat other people with courtesy and politeness because it is correct public behavior. Canada, Norway, Denmark, France, Portugal, Greece, Morocco, Cameroon and Puerto Rico, all stand out as having populations that exhibit basic good manners. In most countries it is polite to offer your seat on crowded transportation to the elderly or the infirm. In some countries this is consistently ignored. In Russia, Poland, Czech Republic, England, USA, you are lucky to make a brief eye contact.

Good manners begin with the proper greeting and parting words and gestures. Treating others with respect that you would appreciate being given to yourself. Behaving with self-control and discipline is indicative of decent training and background. Using "please, may I and thank you" in gratitude for what others do for you, involvement in a conversation without interrupting, and showing responsibility for your actions and words is just decent social behavior.

Covering your mouth and nose when sneezing or coughing, asking for things instead of reaching, knocking before entering a room, and not picking your nose (or certain body parts) in public are acceptable behavior that make life more pleasant for those around you. Good manners are important in all social situations and are about respecting yourself as well as those with whom you are interacting. Being well-mannered makes others feel good and more comfortable in your company, and enables them to admire you, which in turn builds your self-esteem and self- confidence. Respectful behavior makes it easier to start and keep relationships that have more chances of developing into lasting connections.

Bad manners are rooted in the selfish disrespect and disinterest in anyone around you. The antisocial personality manifests as rude, excessive and inappropriate behavior, being unkind, abrupt, and impolite to those around you and is more pronounced if the recipients are the elderly or the less fortunate. Intruding on a small group of people to talk to a few, while ignoring the others are bad manners. Talking with your mouth full of food, loud cell phone conversations in public, yelling and shouting, crowding the person in front of you (and now refusing to observe the 3- to- 6- foot distancing rule), are not acceptable social behavior. This unacceptable behavior implies lack of training, poor education and abject ignorance. A simple unpleasant habit like showing poor table manners can and will seriously limit your social opportunities.

Trust and Distrust

Eye contact, steady and maintained, is essential in initiating an effective greeting and starting and maintaining a conversation. It is the best greeting and interaction skill, followed by body language, head movements and smile that is open and inviting. Good eye contact shows openness to conversation, respect and trust, while "shifty" eyes, looking away then rechecking, or looking past the person, indicate unease when hiding something or telling a lie. Intermittent eye contact may be a sign of shyness or short attention span and is often accompanied by a stammer and/or blushing, A stare or glare may be a display of anger or hostility. Avoiding eye contact completely was common in colonial times, and slaves were severely punished for even looking toward their self-appointed superiors.

Good eye contact reflects sincerity and integrity, enhances a quality conversation, builds and sustains trust, shows confidence, and maintains the interaction. Good eye contact, when listening is a sign of involvement, interest, and respect. Most times, it speaks more than words, rates high in the compilation of social skills and reflects self and intentions. Eye contact says "You are important and I am listening to what you have to say."

The slight head nod supports the greeting, indicates acknowledgement, acceptance and agreement to your presence. (This is not to be confused with the head bobble in India, which is a sign of agreement or disagreement, without saying no directly, or getting a point across, a tradition.)

The smile is a pleased or amused expression, a social greeting, intended to put the recipient at ease. It releases endorphins of both participants, promotes positive, happy feelings, and improves mood and disposition. (*endorphins are feel-good hormones that act as pain-killers, reduce blood pressure, increase heart rate, relax muscles, then relax heart rate and further lowers the blood pressure, boosts the activity of immune cells, increases antibody production, and relieve stress by lowering cortisol*). The opposite occurs when a greeting is ignored, rebuffed or answered with a snarl. A sincere smile labels a person as "likeable" as opposed to those who wear a blank or hostile look. A person with a smile has a good chance of interacting and connecting. A person who never smiles has a hard time maintaining a relationship. One who smiles too much may not be trustworthy.

Words for "friend" in different cultures and languages that bring a smile and good feeling, range from "fren" in Bislama, Vanatau , to "freund" in Munich, Germany, "vriend" in Amsterdam, "ami" in Marseille, "amici" in Pisa, "ven"in Denmark, "van" in Sweden, "vinier" in Iceland, "cara" in gaelic Ireland and "amigos" in Lisbon. "Zanmi" in Haiti, "sadiq" in Morocco, "rafiki" in East Africa, "umugenzi" in Central Africa, "arkadas" in Turkey and "filos" in Greece, add to a long list of greetings that make you feel good.

Blue Zones on Longevity & Quality of Life

The concept of the Blue Zone grew out of the demographic research of Gianni Pes and Michael Poulain, presented in the Journal of Experimental Gerontology. They drew blue circles around the villages they identified in Sardinia as having the highest concentration of male centenarians. In 1999, Dan Buettner. National Geographic Fellow, listed five such Blue Zones where people live the longest and healthiest lives: Japan (Okinawa), Sardinia, Greece (Ikaria Island), (Nicoya Peninsula), Costa Rica and California (Loma Linda). Shortly after, several "blue zone diets" emerged, featuring fruit and vegetables and the Mediterranean diet. An assembly of a Power 9 list of lifestyle habits shared by the longest- lived peoples: move naturally, have a purpose, control stress, reduce the amount of food taken in (80% rule of fullness), plant- slant, moderate alcohol intake favoring red wine, belonging to a community, families first, and maintaining social circles, were promoted. (*In my 2016 book, Natural Health and Disease Prevention, I narrowed these down to: exercise, proper diet, stress control, mental stimulation, social connections and avoidance of toxins.*) The diet of olive oil, fish, fruit and vegetables that hit the bookshelves and the airwaves, took on an almost magical value and healthy living (based on diet and exercise) appeared as a global epiphany.

After visiting Ikaria and other areas with high longevity statistics, I am convinced that the strongest factor that distinguishes the blue zones and other high- quality life expectancy zones is not only the healthy diet, but the stress control, which probably supports the other health factors as well. Low levels of stress promote low inflammation, high immune system function, high cognition into old age which led to good quantity and high- quality life. The trust and respect held by these blue zone people for each other, coupled with their lack of fear of and friendliness toward strangers, fuels an inner peace, free of destructive resentment, self- interest, harmful competition, and worship of materials. I experienced this in Ikaria, where money was not a subject, time passing was of minimal importance and time spent together carried the highest value. People in Blue Zones owe their longevity and high quality of life primarily to the extraordinary low levels of stress in their daily lives.

An Ikaria Report

Ikaria is an island in the northeastern part of the Aegean Sea, near the western coast of Turkey. With Chios to the north, Samos to the east and Náxos to the southwest, it is a quick plane ride due east from Athens. Surrounded by rough seas, it is fairly difficult to approach by boat, and so historically it remained quite isolated. The island supports a year-round population of about 8500, of which a relatively high percentage achieve and live past the age of one hundred years. The lifestyle developed into self-sufficiency out of necessity and all the basic strategies contribute to extending life expectancy and high quality of living. It gained notoriety recently as a Blue Zone where its citizens not only defy the averages but are also in very good physical and mental condition.

Looking past the now commonly accepted Mediterranean diet as the best on the planet, the health benefits of regular exercise highlighted by daily walking, the relative absence of toxins in the food supply and in the air, and the mental stimulation displayed by and on the population, my focus was drawn to the almost complete absence of stress in the daily routines and the positive social atmosphere that permeated life on the island. (*This phenomenon carried over well on visits we made with Icarians to other more stressful localities. And most of my observations were later supported by references from the books, Ikaria, Lessons on food, life and longevity from the Greek island where people forget to die by Diane Kochilas; The Blue Zones: The Secrets of a Long*

Life, National Geographic magazine article, November 2005 and The Greek Blue Zone, Lessons for living longer, by Dan Buettner.

In 2009, the University of Athens School of Medicine released a study on diet and lifestyle of the Greek people over the age of 80 on the island of Ikaria. Reports by the team of D.B. Panagiotakos, C. Chrysohoou and C. Stefanadis found that the features of longevity rested in common behavioral practices consisting of daily physical activity, healthy eating habits, avoidance of smoking, midday naps, and frequent socializing. It involved a combination of pro-social behavior and modification of environmental factors in the extension of life expectancy.

The diet of olive oil, local herbs (rosemary, thyme, sage, marjoram), lemons, dandelion and parsley cleanse, mints, and fliskoumi tea, accompanied by wine with reason (meal) and emphasis on how we eat, slower and with distinctive enjoyment for better and more complete digestion. The bioactive properties of good food provide fuel for function and quality medicines for good health, flavonoids for heart health and blood vessel circulation, low cancer, osteoporosis, and dementia. I do not recall having seen a Greek eating alone. In addition to the stimulation from social dining, the production and release of good hormones (oxytocin and serotonin) from goat's milk, with its high tryptophan- boosting serotonins is a life gift. The preparation and sharing of Icarian herb teas is a delightful social event. Besides containing high levels of antioxidants and mild diuretics, imbibing herbal teas together lends to conversation (usually gossip) that aids both digestion and immune system. The socially driven Kafeneion or coffee meeting is a social event that denies all levels of anxiety, invites full participation and most of all, appreciation for one another.

The cafes and restaurants are full between 8 and 11 pm, with chatting, games, dining and plain healthy socializing as the primary purpose. One cannot sit next to a group and not be included in a Greek fest, no matter the size and most often without occasion. What troubles? Income is not an issue and is not even discussed. It is not important. What matters is you, me and us.

A summary of the results showed that both males and females between the ages of 80 and 90 lived longer when together than when alone. The male to female ratio over the age of 80 in the West is 1:2, while it is 1:1 in Ikaria. One in four people (25%) is over the age of 65 and one in eight (13%) is over the age of 80. These ratios are the best in the world. (Only 3% of the populations of North America and Europe attain this longevity.) Two percent of the Icarians (1/50, are over the age of 90. Ikaria has 3 times more people over the age of 90 than does the rest of Greece. There were three major lifestyle differences, planned daily napping to relieve stress, rejuvenate the cardiovascular system and recharge the brain, afternoon visits to gardens and beehives for physical activity and gathering of nutritious local harvest, and evenings of socializing as group therapy, reassurance of life's pleasures, dancing, singing, volunteering, offering help when needed, where no one is excluded, and the purpose of life in interacting as a major part of a 24- hour period is shared and reinforced. (On the opposite side are the sleep- deprived, stress-stricken western societies that seem to take great pleasure in excluding others and random killing has become a way of life.)

Ikaria revealed to me the possibility of life without haste, threat, or hatred, where spending time with friends and relatives intertwined with rest and quality sleep, provides you with the ability to appreciate and achieve the sense of well-being. Stress control highlighted by open social interactions are the most prevalent feature of all longevity societies. As always, I commend and thank Dr. Andrew Weil of the University of Arizona for his wisdom and skill in explaining the concept of well-being, the details of which may be found in his many lectures and volumes on optimal physical and emotional health through lifestyle measures. Good health is not only the absence of significant disease, but involves mental, physical and spiritual health, mind, body and soul in optimal functional condition.

In 2015, with the help and encouragement of our new Greek family and friends, we organized a site visit to Ikaria to see how these lifestyle features actually worked and to prove that my son's decision to move to Greece because it was "comfortable" and offered opportunities that were not present in his previous residence was a good one.

On the flight from Athens to Ikaria, somewhere over Andros Island, I wondered which of the six basic strategies of health would dominate. Upon arrival, the friendliness of the people and ease of getting our rental car, summoned thoughts of never leaving. Along the way, the rough scrubby, dry landscape was not very convincing. Deriving its name from Icarus, son of Daedalus, whose fashioned wings sealed with wax melted when he flew too close to the sun, plunging him into the sea close to the island. The views of peaceful isolation he must have seen for those few glorious moments in the sky may not have differed much from those of today.

Descending a steep winding road, we arrived at the lovely town of Agios Kirykos and parked just outside our hotel entrance. Inside, we encountered a beautiful interior draped in absolute silence. Perched neatly at the registration desk, was a welcome note attached to a set of keys with our room assignments, breakfast instructions and best wishes for a comfortable and relaxing stay. Absent was any mention of fees or taxes or payment. We were later told payment was on the honor system and would be appreciated whenever it was convenient.

Throughout the hotel there were no clocks, no orders, no indications of anxiety or stress. The wi-fi wiring instructions were plain, and it worked. At the corner grocery store, the answer to the question, "what time is it", was "arga misi" or late-thirty... anytime. We proceeded to walk around the town with ease, returning greetings from the townsfolk in our rudimentary but rapidly improving

Greek. We offered smiles and received the same with a warmth that was immediately felt as genuine and sincere. Though some Icarians move about until the wee hours of the morning, then sleep until 10 a.m., we got to bed early in preparation for our breakfast meeting at an outdoor harbor restaurant with our local hosts. True to form, at 9:00 a.m. the town was still "asleep". Our hosts were right on time and the connection that was made formed quality bonds that hold strong today. A concern for our condition, origins, interests, purpose and impression of their island and town highlighted the first inter-action. From there we organized further meetings and outings with enough "wiggle room" to guarantee comfort and absence of pressure. Nobody wore a watch.

As the town slowly came to life, I could feel that the spirit of "philitimo" was all around. The reactions of people seeing and greet-ing each other, where 80 years old is "young", 90 is average, 100 is respected, and common, and still "working" was extraordinary. "Look at Mr. Popopoulos over there. He is 110 years old and still walks briskly up the hill to pull weeds in his vegetable garden every day. He enjoys the respect and appreciation of the community for his long, successful life.

Thanking my medical training for providing me with the skills and knowledge to ascertain and appreciate the remarkable mental and physical health of these citizens, I wanted to find out why and how they achieved such milestones.

The media response to Blue Zones seemed to focus on diet and exercise as major forces in the shaping the health of Icarians, but my experiences with and instructions from the people seemed to indicate that the low levels of stress and high levels of social interaction played a more dominant role.

*"I am convinced that most disease processes of middle
and old age in the world are due to Emotional and
environmental stress, and less because of genetics." Author*

The environment displayed low levels of both poverty and wealth, with people helping each other to live comfortably and long rather than one group feeding off the poverty of others. Everyone appeared to be a part of the community, interested in and looking out for each other, without fears, anxieties or antagonistic behavior. Everyone speaks to each other and to strangers, easily and sincerely. Diet, mental stimulation (through socializing), exercise and a low toxin environment of fresh air and plenty of sunshine are definite factors, the low stress with its reduction in circulating cortisol and feel-bad hormones with high functional immunity, low disease risk and high mind-body-spirit function appears to be the main factor in directing everything else.

Vignette #27: In some countries, when a stranger enters a restaurant, says "good morning" and is ignored and even snarled at... the instant release of fear and anxiety hormones guarantees indigestion and a lasting distaste for the establishment. Interaction with people in other countries may be so comforting and welcoming that you wish that time would stand still and you never have to leave. Such is the power and conse-quence of a simple social greeting.

Not to imply that there are no stressors present on Ikaria, for some, island life is a significant source of stress. The isolation and feelings of being left out of the mainstream, the lack of access to the latest technology are enough to make you wonder, sometimes. We got back into my rented car and set out on a small tour of some of the other towns and sites. The roads were curvy but well-constructed and maintained.

Though the climate varies between hot, dry summers and cool, wet winters, it is generally somewhere above tolerable and almost inviting. (Between Scandinavia and the Caribbean). The rough seas make maritime travel difficult and impart a ferocity to some of the coastal zones. Homes with workable productive gardens are scattered over much of the countryside and people walking along the roads is a typical sight.

In the villages and towns, restaurants and shops, no one seems to experience loneliness. For the time that followed, in every locale, we experienced friendly encounters, smiles and nods of welcome, greetings extended and offers made, not only with us as strangers but to, from and between each other. Visiting appeared to be on a "no call, drop by" basis. They welcome visitors who show up as some offering of food and drink are always on hand. The main focus is on the visitor and his/her physical and social health, where you are from, how life is there, and how you find us here. There is no mention of material wealth or of what can you do for me if I do for you. "Pleased to meet you" is genuine and has lasting value.

We dropped by a small mountainside factory to see how they press olives into oil. Social interactions involving imparting of knowledge and technique are especially welcomed. On site questions on history, customs, sayings, and behavior are appreciated and answers exuberantly provided. Notwithstanding the friendliness to strangers, the connections within the community are of particular note. The young, the old and the "older" move along, approach a task and complete it, together, naturally and with satisfaction at the accomplishment. At an outdoor lunch café and later in an indoor restaurant, eye contact was all around and conversation included everybody as recipients of basic good manners and genuinely interesting conversation. There was no sense of urgency and no sense of moneyed hierarchy where generosity of spirit is reserved for some and withheld from others. We got the feeling that everyone had a sense of belonging, where time and materials were willingly shared and the group was more important than the individual. And to us, the gestures, implications and communications amounted to the feeling that even though you do not know us, we do not know you, we are human, just like you.

In a socially functional state, your identity is who you are and is important in every situation and in every place. It includes your character and this can be seen almost right away. They like each other, no one hates or fears the "other" and everyone has value. This is a state of no or low stress that is a basis for good health. In direct contrast, there are places, where your identity is what you have, your wealth, status, occupation, position, location, and social class determine your encounters and with whom you interact. They do not need good manners and social skills as one rarely ventures outside the little circle of power and safety, or serve only to move up within the confines of that circle. Interactions with anyone on the downside are undesirable so knowledge and communication skills are unnecessary. In Ikaria, the secret to a healthy stress-free life lies in how you live and the company you keep and not in what you own.

Vignette #28. Some countries harbor the incredible attitude of refusal to provide universal healthcare to all citizens. Besides the deprivation, the additional extreme stress of financial burden and access leads to poorer health. A refusal to take care of each other both socially and physically, is a prescription for an unhealthy society, in which the only solution is to get rid of the vulnerable. In some countries, they control stress by living their lives together, with compassion and cooperation.

(1/5000 in USA reach age 90. In Ikaria it is 1/50)

The Mediterranean diet and a proper attitude toward nutrition are not conducive to obesity and disease. As a result, there is 20%

less cancer, 50% less cardiovascular disease, no depression and no dementia. (In some countries, the level of dementia and depression in citizens over the age of 85 approaches 50%, where both urban and rural social life are exclusive and dominated by fear and anxiety from numerous sources and access to healthy nutrition is limited.)

Fresh, local vegetables and fruit, occasional lean meat, olive oil, garlic, and red wine are loaded with micronutrients that inhibit oxidative stress at the cellular level and prevent gross damages at organ levels. With the bioactive properties of herbs in all meals, and honey (local), wild mint, rosemary and artemisia for blood circulation, serotonin-boosting tryptophan in goat milk, legumes, vegetables (local greens free of toxins), grains, fruit, olive oil to reduce low density lipoproteins and boost high- density lipoproteins, (LDL & HDL), fish, red wine with flavonoids for heart health, coffee to reduce levels of type 2 diabetes, Parkinson's, and heart disease, lots of fiber, and the basic balance of proteins, fats and carbohydrates, Greece has the lowest rates of cancer and osteoporosis, and highest longevity rates in Europe. The Icarian mountain herb, *Sideritis syriaca* also known as ironwort or Shepherd's tea, when accented with oregano, sage, mint, chamomile, fennel and rosemary, acts as a diuretic, lowers blood pressure, eliminates toxins and loaded with antioxidants, enhances general health. The chamomile prevents platelet clumping and helps to prevent cardiovascular issues. The Icarian stew we enjoyed one afternoon, had black- eyed peas, tomatoes, fennel tops, garlic, olive oil, and fish, with sides of hummus, potatoes and a fresh feta salad was "to die for".

We ate better here, but it is "how we ate" that really mattered. They prepare food for the purpose of shared enjoyment. The nutritious value is probably secondary. When biochemical processes regulate digestion and absorption without fear and anxiety and the rush of feel-bad hormones, one benefits tremendously from the dining experience. (Or you may eat in a hurry, vacate the table for the next seating and suffer from indigestion and irritable bowel syndrome for the rest of your life.)

We dined and enjoyed all meals and the company of whoever we were with at the time. Meals that are "shared" and unhurried provide for better health. In most of Europe, a meal is enjoyed in combination with conversation and in Greece, strangers are always welcome. Interesting encounters become interactions that may develop into lasting connections.

In the Mediterranean, a meal without friends, neighbors or strangers to share with is not a Mediterranean meal.

The people of Ikaria walk everywhere, anytime and for any reason. (Cars are small and the cost of petrol is exorbitant). Access to farm plots, gardens where plants grow the best, and bee hives are often out of town, while cafes, the seashore, and meetings with family and friends, can all be done by walking. From my hotel balcony I admired three elders as they walked steadily uphill without teetering or tottering, en route from point A to point B, and perhaps beyond and vowed one day to do the same. After sunset, the evening stroll to visit neighbors, share a meal, gossip, and stay up late having taken the requisite afternoon nap. Regular exercise coupled with a wine and plant- based diet loaded with antioxidant flavonoids and catechins, low stress behavior and good sleeping habits, result in half the seniors (over age 90) still having meaningful sex on a regular basis and maintaining optimal health.

Scandinavians would live longer if they had access to more sunshine. Author

The Aegean island environment with its sunshine, climate control, hills, footpaths and multiple roads, is conducive to exercise and aura of good health.

Similar mental capacity and relative lack of age-related diseases accompany the physical agility of the people as they go about their daily lives. While the incidence of dementias in American seniors over the age of 85 is 50%, the rate in Ikaria is less than 10%. Regular brain exercise through conversation, reading, good nutrition and concentrated purpose and meaning in life, contribute to staying sharp and healthy throughout advancing years. For what it's worth, next door neighbor Samos is the birthplace of the influential thinkers, Pythagoras and Epicurus.

Vignette #29. A Greek doctor, who wished to remain anonymous, told me that the reason Greeks live so long is due to the diet, good rest (regular napping), staying up late, getting up late, no watches, no time limits, no money and no matter…which all added up to low stress.

While the people of Ikaria meet the requirements in three of the six basic strategies of good health, diet, exercise, and mental stimulation, and excel in two, stress control and social connections, the one exception is their approach to toxin avoidance. *All of Europe is in a cloud of cigarette smoke, and Greece is up there among the worst offenders.* According to GLOBOCAN, of the Global Cancer Observatory, in Cancer Journal Clinics, lung cancer associated with cigarette smoking is the most common cancer worldwide and Greece ranks fourth in Europe (behind Hungary, Serbia and Turkey) in new cases in men per 100,000, in 2018. Greek women with lung cancer were not in the top 25 countries, though they appear to match the men in tobacco usage. Greece ranks #28 in global cancer rates, US is 5th.

According to the European Environment Agency, 90% of Europe is exposed to concentrations of air pollutants that are higher than normal. Fine particulate matter, especially from human cigarette smoke emissions and cars in the cities, are minimally affective. Factories located mostly in the countryside, fuel burning, catalytic converters, and intensified agriculture contribute to air and water pollution of rivers. Turkey, Poland and Hungary are the most polluted, Greece falls somewhere in the upper half, and Swedish air is the cleanest.

Cigarette smoking appears to be a "status symbol" especially for the young. "Look at me, I can afford to do this and I am cool". Out of the top 20 highest smoking countries, Europe has 15. (The USA has done very well in reduction of cigarette smokers and has a world ranking of 68th). Smoking may be linked to income, as the lower the income the more the smoking. Whereas in the USA smoking is bad for you and the price has been raised, in Europe there is a relative acceptance of the health risks and the high cost seems to stimulate more sales.

With the most prevalent of the strategies being stress control and socializing a close second, the reasons for the longevity and low levels of heart disease, cancer, dementia and age-related ailments involve a mix of factors. The high life expectancy (#19) despite stressors can certainly be attributed in part to good coping mechanisms. Taking the time and effort to know and love the elderly, treating everyone with respect imparts a particular value to life. Living close to nature, eating fresh foods; aware of both the village gossip and world news; enjoying dancing and traditional lore; staying in love and maintaining relationships, keeping goats, gardens, bees, olive and fruit trees, impart a sense of responsibility and belonging that brings contentment and satisfaction, which prolongs life.

My opinions flow toward lowering the percentage on genetics and raising it for the environment as factors in quality and quantity of life influence this shift. How you live your life is a major factor in how long it will last. To maintain long telomeres, proper nutrition, regular exercise, having a purpose in life that gives it meaning, low stress, avoidance of excessive toxicity, and frequent social interactions with lasting connections should do the job.

We departed Ikaria with a sense of belonging, with the distinct feeling that we would be welcome to return at any time and that we had added some lifelong friendships.

Reasons for Exceptional Hospitality

The Oxford English dictionary defines hospitality as friendly and generous reception and entertainment of guests, visitors and strangers. The synonyms given include gentile, amiable, helpful, cordial, and genial. An acceptable interpretation is the friendly and courteous treatment of others. Associated with the tourism industries of Switzerland, Japan and Latino countries, hospitality implies a sense of community, camaraderie, generosity, and sharing with pride. It can also refer to meeting of and with friends, planned or on the spur of the moment, as expected with the Greeks.

With pride in food provision and preparation, and at the expense of one's own labor and knowledge, most households are self-sufficient: garden vegetables, fruit trees, goat cheese, olive oil from the tree in the yard, and eggs from the chicken coop, "mezedes" and wine from the hillside vineyard, on the menu and often the leading topics of conversation.

My question of "*Why is the hospitality of the Greeks exceptional?*", elicited a variety of responses.

Dr. Illias Leriadis, Vice Mayor and Icarian physician acquaintance, provided several reasons that focused on diet, rest and relaxation. "People stay up late here and get up late and always take naps. No one wears a watch (time) and no clock is works correctly. They don't care about money, so there are no worries. They pool whatever they have to buy food, medicine and wine and what remains is given to the poor. If you need to go somewhere, get a ride or walk. It is not a 'me' place. It is an 'us' place."

An astute observation on Europeans made by **Miles Galin, MD**, traveling companion and mentor, "*They may not be happy all the time, but they are not angry at or with each other.*" (as compared to in the USA where people are unhappy and angry, especially with each other, enough that the blaming of "others" (immigrants) led to the election of an incompetent non-politician as leader of a major country and maintaining him in office for 4 years.)

With particular attention to a low toxicity environment, low stress living, no threats, fears, or anxiety, why are the Greeks friendlier than Russians? Or Hungarians? Or Chinese? Is it the weather? Is it their DNA? Their history? In trying to find out more about why they were so engaging, inclusive, and friendly, I asked some Greeks for their opinions and was directed to the traditional concepts that survive in community life. Philotimo, the pride in sharing food, time, and attention; agape, giving without expecting anything in return—and philoxenia. Hospitality to strangers were the standard replies. From Mr.**John Alfaros**, the General Secretary of Cities and Towns of Greece: since 2007, by direct exchange on Quora. JA: "Geographically, Greeks meet a lot of different people from other countries. From Europa, Asia and Northern countries. Also, the weather and great diplomacy we have, make us friendlier."

Me: "I could accept this…the pleasant weather certainly makes for a more agreeable people." But then shouldn't the Italians, Spaniards, Turks and Egyptians be just as friendly? I find they are not.

Additional reasons for Greek friendliness were offered by Mr. **Moscholidis Giogis** of Piraeus. "Greeks are friendly because of the weather, the sea and islands, like Hawaii, and traditions. The Father of the Gods is Xenios (Philoxenos), Zeus, a friend to the stranger.

The Greek Philoxenia, or Philotimo (love and hospitality to others) is a basic human behavior and we kept all of this."

All this and more contribute to the Greek embrace of the traveling stranger. The unregimented life that allows one to visit or host, often unannounced, and find him/her ready with food and wine and time to spend with a friend. The maintenance of small gardens and bee hives with honey being used in healing teas, topical wound healing, and occasional hangovers. Yamas! (Cheers) for drinking the excellent local wine, hanging out with gossip, laughter, and able to socialize without exclusion or separation of humans for any reason. Easy friendships, spawned by the "power routine of social creatures" with the DNA capacity to cooperate and forge feelings of closeness/intimacy in the production of a together bond have value.

Ikaria has three times the number of people over the age of 90 years as the rest of Greece, so there should be a positive factor in its small size. The island has five times less stress, less pollution, and ten times more trust between residents that in Athens, so its positive statistics are as expected. But why are Greeks in Athens friendlier than in other cities? While sitting in JFK airport, New York, with a group of strangers all waiting for an international flight that was delayed, the first one to strike up a conversation with everybody, was the Greek.

Here is my humble opinion on why. The **Environment** of the country with its abundant sunshine, clear water, pleasant scenery, and fresh air is agreeable deserves at least 15% of the credit for its positive hospitality. The weather alone lifts one's spirits, brightens the personality, and promotes pleasantry. Ample fresh, healthy food, drink and community participation opens a person to more positive thoughts that they are then willing and able to extend to others. When they look and feel cheerful, they can impart good-feelings to others.

It may not seem important, but Vitamin D promotes positive brain activity. It activates enzymes in the brain and cerebrospinal fluid that help make neurotransmitters and promote nerve growth. Normal levels are required for adequate cognitive function, especially with ageing. (Note that 1000 to 2000 IU are required or the amount that your body will synthesize from 15 to 20 minutes exposure daily.) We need functional cognition for effective social behavior to occur. Are people in sunny countries friendlier than those in cloudy ones?

In a country like Greece, they built the ecosystem around the people, not vice versa. This makes it more amenable to an easy life-style. Transportation is available and at low cost, and when in doubt, you can walk to and from most places. In contrast, cold, cloudy gray days in Scandinavia, Russia, and the UK contribute to low vitamin D intake and negative feelings of threat and fear, that suggest that exclusion of others is normal. Yet, Ireland has a long and current tradition of friendliness. But some of the biggest, most vocal nationally syndicated racists in the USA are descendants of the same Irish who experienced similar ostracism and cruelty upon arrival and throughout their assimilation. Irony?

They focused the culture on "belonging", which is the glue that binds everyone together, provides support and makes life worthwhile. There is not any one thing, but the "entire" thing that makes it work.

Location, positioned between three continents, Greece has been at a crossroads of migratory and trading travel since *Homo sapiens* left Mother Africa. Having seen everybody before, they are accustomed to strangers passing through, stopping and staying or moving on. This they associated with greater benefits than losses. Exposure brings little or no fear of "others". In this case, familiarity breeds friendliness. There is no reason to fear that which you know. (*Fear of hordes of Mexicans crossing the southern US border is either based on hate, ignorance or refusal to face the causal history of the situa-*

tion that forces the migration has totally disrupted any meaningful social connectivity.)

Athenians, thinking themselves as more sophisticated and wiser than all the other tribes put together, welcomed immigrants, especially if they had a craft or a talent. Able to encounter and engage with different peoples, and as a diverse group themselves, they could identify with strangers, had ample knowledge of their customs and very little fear. Their own self-esteem gave them the confidence to interact freely and successfully.

The Greeks named some foreigners, "barbarians", since their language sounded like "bar-bar-bar" but did not particularly ostracize or reject them. For the migrants, it was not what their hosts possessed, or what they gave or took from them, it was how they made them feel. Therefore, they stayed.

(*Some modern countries have the resources, and will share, but the welcome is weak. Others are afraid of migrant women and children armed with Spanish and tortillas or Arabic and falafel.*)

Pericles in a speech to the Athenians, suggested that they be "open to the world, though be aware of enemies seeking profit from state secrets." All Greeks not from Athens, were "foreigners". Resident foreigners were "metics", somewhere between foreigner and citizen, who did the jobs that Athenians would not do. They could become citizens. Egyptians, Thracians, and Phoenicians were economically motivated and passed in and out and among the Greeks, without restraint or limitation as long as business thrived. Location facilitated the exposure to different cultures and encouraged interaction and lasting connections.

In terms of percentages influencing Greek hospitality, I give 15% each to environment and location. Perhaps **Genetics** has a role. Because of natural selection in the region, inherited traits of compassionate temperament, selected traits of kindness over meanness, social DNA over antisocial DNA may be in the process of expression.

If there were specific genes for temperament, friendliness and niceness, the Greeks would have a large share. Genetic expression rises and falls with the influence of many factors. For this reason, I give it a mere 5%.

To **Tradition**, I ascribe 50% from the start. Way of life established patterns of thought, action and behavior; based on the way it had always been. Zeus, the god of friendliness, remains an integral part of the Greek psyche that maintains the tribal custom of welcoming a visitor as a guest to become a friend and opposed to an enemy, an invader, though they certainly had their share. Upon the initial encounter, assessment, and designation as friend, the hosts proceeded to enjoy the company and connection with the others. Perhaps the tradition of open acceptance as above pettiness of rejection, connected to the celebration of the greatness of Greece linked closely to the understanding of the plight of strangers, still stands

Sophocles (Oedipus) and Aeschylus (Eumonides) wrote that integrating foreigners added to the safety and protection of the city-state (Athens) and that rejecting them only created new enemies. Citing tradition is well and good, but it alone cannot produce genuine friendliness. We base Greek tradition on the ideas of equality, discussion among equals (agora), and that the best discussions came from within the group and not from one sovereign. They debated and decided together what was best for the group. A contribution from each one required social interaction to achieve. They invited "others" to take part and see the value of new ideas. They showed that civilizations flourished when mingling and mixing occurred and that isolation hampered and delayed development and led to stagnation. In modern times, certain anti-immigrant groups invoke cultural "purity" and are terrified by the arrival of and possible "tainting" by people different from themselves. If they are so "pure" and pure is so good, then by their strength alone outside influence should not be a threat but a benefit. Looking inward and celebrating your own limits is not functional. Looking outward, opening, enlarging, taking in and adapting diversity is a mark of intelligence and ultimate success. Everybody emulated the ancient Greeks, and their open sociability was a factor in their success.

Unspoken Greek rule: The guest always gets the best of whatever there is in the house.

I reiterate the concepts of love and friendship in mythology, philia, agape and eros, which today still play a significant role in Greek life. Philotimo is the love of honor, a complex set of values, entailing filos equals friend, and timi equals honor. It represents a love of and for friends, family and social living; pride in self, and respect for elders, we saw in Ikaria, and community that we see throughout Greece. This concept is practiced, passed on, reinforced and tested daily in the society. There is a heartfelt awareness in doing the right thing and doing for others without expecting something in return. Agape, a Greek virtue, is the highest form of love, charity, and interaction. It is love from the heart, the core of one's being, human and among humans. It is the expression of trust and sincerity that extends beyond family.

"We are like family but better, without all the mess".

I posed the question of Greek friendliness to **Mr. Edward Rowe**, international literature professor, resident Irish playwright and traveler to Greece in the 1960's. "They are like the Irish. They have the same concept of hospitality but with a better climate. (To them) a guest is someone special. Also, they are descendants of a civilization that few, if any, can equal. When I was there, I didn't feel like a tourist. I felt like I had come home."

What distinguishes Greek friendliness from many others? "We developed a friendship based on trust, because 'I didn't want anything from him'", agape in The Magus, by John Fowles, on unconditional love. Your dog loves you but expects to be rewarded, food, treats, caresses, and kindness. If he is a Greek dog, he loves you no matter what.

For the sake of completion, Eros represents physical love, selfishness. Philophrosyne is the Greek female spirit of welcome, friendliness and kindness. She is the daughter of Hephaestus (God of the forge and of Hades, the underworld) and Aglaia (goddess of beauty and splendor, a member of the Charities or Graces).

Religion may contribute another 5%. Greek Orthodox Christianity appears to be more closely aligned and adherent to the New Testament teachings of Jesus of Nazareth, than are other Christian sects. The culture practices hospitality and concern for strangers, especially in the home, and not just pay it lip service. Both the epistles of St Paul and St John's Book of Revelations were written in Greece.

In South America, 2018, Catholic Ecuador shut its borders to Venezuelans, desperate for food and medicines. Catholic Argentina's citizen genocide, mistreatment of the Native Amerinds and African descendants responsible for most of the hard agricultural labor. Not much there in religion to support social connections.

To the remaining **Unknown**, I assign the remaining 10%, which consists in part of positive feedback from feel-good hormones raised from having done the right thing. Please note that all percentages are non-scientific opinions based on personal observations.

Social Interactions are important; the host sees faces at the table and declares, "you matter to me". The guest feels good, I am worth the effort". Everyone has value and the Greeks do this better or at least as well as anybody.

World Friendliness

Subjective surveys taken by travelers either during or after their experiences in the city or country being promoted, are abundant and widely variable. They are in no way scientific or evidence-based, but comprise opinions of the individuals, which are then interpreted to form a comparative ranking.

Looking at surveys for "Friendliness", they questioned travelers on parameters like the ease of settling, feeling at home, finding friends, extent of conversation, and approachability of the locals. InterNations 2019 survey, listed Singapore at #35, USA 33, Panama 32, and Greece at #2. They list the United Arab Emirates at # 20. Being Islamic, half of its population, women, are off limits to interaction with male foreigners. It is my opinion that technically we should not include Islamic countries in any survey that involves "social interactions" and if so, the best score should begin at 50%. Morocco, #13 in this survey, has an excellent rating for friendliness, and rightfully so, but only the men interacted freely. Spain at #11, Costa Rica #9, and Colombia at #6 would be higher in ranking if the interacting foreigner speaks Spanish. Vietnam at #5 and numbers 4 through 1 ranked high on the friendliness scale in every survey I examined (Taiwan, Portugal, Mexico and Oman) despite the language. Interesting.

Likewise, one should exclude racist countries as the skin color of the traveler is a significant factor in initiating an interaction.

Of the friendliest cities, #15 is Sao Paolo with 12-million people and a mass of chaos. Number 10 is Dublin, 8 is Lisbon, 6, Mexico City, then #5 is Kampala (Uganda), 4, Muscat (Oman) and #1, Taipei.

Another friendliest city tourist survey ranked Budapest at 100, Beijing at 75, Reykjavik at 72, Athens at 64, Milan at 60, Lima at 34,

Geneva at 17, Copenhagen at 12, Tokyo at 7, San Francisco at 4, and Helsinki, Stockholm and Singapore in the top positions.

A most- welcoming- to- families survey listed Sweden at number 1, Portugal at 5, France and Spain at 12 and 13, Greece at 30 and Switzerland at 31. It made no mention of the ethnicities or language capabilities of those families or the travelers who interacted with them.

Another most- welcoming- to- foreigners survey from World News, a bit more appropriate to the theme of "social interactions", listed Portugal, Greece, Ireland, Canada, Mexico, Oman and Morocco in the top positions. An InterNations survey listed Portugal, Taiwan, Mexico, Costa Rica and Vietnam and a Friendliest in 2019 survey listed Taiwan, Portugal, Mexico, Cambodia, Bahrain, Oman and Colombia as the leading contenders. The criteria used was "Not afraid of strangers, Curiosity in others, and Ability to interact".

In the opposite vein, countries with the coldest reception to strangers, in this case groups of Mexican travelers were Switzerland, Russia, Austria and Kuwait. All agreed that they were "uninterested in making new friends".

These surveys were on "friendliness" not on "happiness". The happiest countries are not particularly the friendliest to visitors. You may access those results at the UN World Happiness. report. When visiting a foreign country, the evaluation of the reception and interaction with the local population should depend on how they made you feel, your happiness, not on theirs.

Results of a Local Social Survey

With a focus on Greek social connections and their influence on the health (and longevity) of the population, we toured Ikaria and participated in family events with Stelios, Eleni, Giannis and Vikki.

We visited a park, a lake, a mountain cave monastic home, had lunch in a small plaza in Christos with an amazing view and interacted freely with the diners, proprietors and staff. Smiles and greeting were abundant, food enjoyed and conversation stimulating, followed by observation of centenarians walking, chatting, and receiving respect shown by the youth and seniors. Throughout the island the lack of poverty and presence of comfortable, well-constructed homes of medium size was obvious. There were no ostentatious mansions with gates and fencing, and no walls to keep people out. Dinner at the restaurant of Stelios 'son and daughter in law produced more bonding over a meal. We have remained in close contact for the past 5 years.

Why are the Greeks (and others in the world) so friendly and accommodating... aside from the assets of environment, location, tradition, genetics, and religion? (see Reasons for Exceptional Hospitality in the previous chapter).

Ten paper copies of a survey seeking clues to the friendliness of the people in the region were provided and collected on the following day. The participants were confident in their ability to compete, interact, defend if need be and offer thoughts and ideas to contribute to the concept of and reasons for Friendliness in a Social Setting and between Countries. Despite economic woes and world sentiments, the Greeks are confident in future success. Their social skills, verbal and nonverbal language, are natural, direct, warm, and conducive to "connecting". In most cases there was some knowledge of and interest in how and why "others" live the way they do.

The stranger-visitor leaves with the feeling that "I am welcome here, (why?) whether I stay or not, and whether or not I maintain contact."

We said our goodbyes and departed, each one full of feel-good hormones.

Results

Social Connections & your Health Survey: See Appendix 7

Individual Questionnaires (14): age range 40 to 73, males = females nationality: Greece, Puerto Rico and USA

1. Prefer to be with family (1) friends (2)… or both (11)

2. Preference of the company of parents & grandparents: Natural (6), Traditional (3), by choice(5)

3. Respect for parents (2), grandparents (1)…or both (12) all 14 paid more attention to relatives when sick or healthy, and when older.

4. Religion, Spirituality and Health: Church attendance: sometimes (5), never (9) follow teachings of Jesus on kindness to strangers: Yes (10), No (4)

5. Loneliness: Loners prefer to be alone: Yes (10, No (4) Loners are losers: Yes (5) , No (9)

6. Peer group behavior: Internet (11), fashion (3) , global news (9), electronic devices (14)

7. Exercise: planned walk (8), sport (4), gymnasium (5), dance (7)

8. Female social support is stronger & more reliable than male: all (14)

9. Man's best friend is a woman: Yes (5), No (9); natural (5), traditional (5),abstain (4)

10. Acceptance of strangers (filoxenia): Yes (13), No (1); natural(12), traditional (1), or curiosity (1) Acceptance of visitors: all (14) migrants: Yes (6), No (6)

11. Strength of friendships: Natural (13), traditional (1)

12. One friend to share one's heart with: Yes (12), No (2)

13. Stress control via: Accept (pray & forgive): (1) Alter (change of response) (6), Adaptation (cope) (7) and Avoid: 0

14. Relocation: Yes (8), No (6) ; suggested localities: Italy, USA, Canada, France, Spain

15. Level of feel-good hormones highest (3), Stress feel-bad hormones (4), equal levels of both (7)

Interpretation: The mixture of responses makes any deductions difficult and definitely not statistical. *Note those in favor of accepting migrants were Greek, and those not in favor were Puerto Rican and USA. Of those choosing to remain on location, 3 were Greek, 3 were Puerto Rican.* A better survey is required.

With whom do we interact and seek to form friendships and against whom do we hurl our venom? Or as human beings do we naturally need to do both?

Results of ECNS Testing

Method: Upon encountering a person at any venue, I made or attempted to make eye contact, accompanied by a slight nod and a warm smile. When possible, I gave a basic verbal greeting in their language, while continuing to move and not impede or approach them in any way.

In Greece 9 out of 10 people give or return a basic greeting upon an initial encounter.

Of the 65 countries included in the survey, Greece and a handful of others scored higher in positive responses to the greetings of a visitor, than other major developed countries. (Only Puerto Rico, where greetings are a national sport, was better, but due to sample bias, and being on home turf, I moved it to #2 position.) In some countries, friendliness and socializing appear to be natural and sincere. In others, the spontaneous expression of basic manners appears to be such a chore that they ignore you altogether. (Shout out to Russia, Czech Republic, Poland, and China.)

Note that these results are based on the reaction(s) of cultural groups to the greetings offered by a senior, gray- haired, average-sized, well-dressed man with a medium-brown skin complexion and a pleasant manner. Obviously, as a visitor or at home, I made encounters in an open, non-threatening manner and in their own language. All other variables being the same, I made generalizations based on an immediate reaction or lack of any at all. Some of these observations were made in my own "backyard", in offering greetings to tourists along the beaches, streets, shops and restaurants. It is astounding that one would visit my country, and totally ignore a greeting.

% of positive responses to ECNS *

#1 Greece 90	#12 Mexico 80	#32 UK 50	#85 China 30
#2 Puerto Rico 90	#15 Peru 80	#69 USA 40	#90 Czech Rep 30
#3 Nevis 90	#18 Panama 70	#70 South Africa 40	#100 Russia 20
#4 Portugal 90	#20 Spain 60	#74 Hungary 40	
#5 Ireland 90	#25 France 60	#75 Poland 40	
#6 Canada 90	#29 Italy 60	#80 Japan 30	

annotated chart

In Greece, Puerto Rico, Ireland, Portugal, and Canada, nine out of every ten local people offer or respond to a basic greeting. The United States is ranked way down at 69th, only because of friendly and diverse people in NYC and San Francisco. Some Asians (Chinese, Koreans, Indonesians and Japanese), locally and especially when traveling, are a bit lacking when it comes to showing basic manners. They may have social skills and elaborate traditional manners at home, but very few make eye contact and only 2 out of 10 offer or respond to a greeting when traveling.

You don't have to know the language to be "polite".

Russia and Eastern Europe are last on the list as less than 10% respond even when being greeted in their own language from a stranger...totally lacking in basic manners and interaction with strangers. On a scale of Global Friendliness based on the ease of conversation, degree of curiosity and interest in the origin of the participants in the interaction, the following were in the top ten. *

1. Greece
2. Portugal
3. Ireland

4. Canada
5. Peru
6. Cuba
7. Mexico
8. France (Provence)
9. Switzerland
10. Morocco

*Author's personal experience

The ECNS study revealed that cultural impressions and communication skills are major determinants in whether or not an interaction occurs. On the beach walk encounters (San Juan, Puerto Rico), the responses to the eye contact, nod and smile corresponded to the ethnicity of the participants. Nine of ten Caribbean and Puerto Ricans responded positively, 6 of 10 Europeans and only 4 of 10 Americans. Xenophobia is the fear of someone else and lack of basic manners is simply being impolite. When you are a visitor in someone's country, there is absolutely no logical reason to refuse a common greeting upon passing another person in a shared public space. If your life is so horrible and your worries so intense that you cannot acknowledge the presence of a person who gives you a greeting, then you should crawl into a hole and stay there until your antisocial hormones wear off.

The people of Portugal, Greece, Puerto Rico, Mexico, Ireland and Taiwan, countries with histories of traditional manners and friendliness to strangers, are not intimidated by contact with someone who does not look exactly like them. They express their natural sociality and offer or respond to a greeting like normal human beings.

We should note again that happiness is not the same as friendliness. Happy countries, like Sweden and Denmark, are satisfied with their internal and external situations, which do contribute to well-being. But "friendly", is another matter. Genuine friendliness comes from another space, and has a distinct character. Portugal is a lot friendlier than Denmark, but most surveys list the latter as having the happier population.

Positive social interactions within communities provide health benefits. "They like each other", they are comfortable and enjoy one another's company, interactions with ease and freely given, European café scenes and family get-togethers. When they are equally comfortable in the company of foreigners, strangers, visitors, this is friendly.

Global Samples

A subjective assessment of social behavior in some parts of the world, strictly from observations and some participation. In many Latin America countries, like Cuba, Mexico and the Dominican Republic, when someone enters a room of people, they say hello, and when they leave, they say goodbye. In Puerto Rico, when you enter a room or an elevator, you greet everyone. When you leave, you wish everyone a nice day. When you enter an elevator in Cincinnati, Ohio, there is silence, and when you leave, more silence. Eye contact and greetings are considered invasions of privacy, or worse, as threats?

Island life in St Thomas, Virgin Islands in the 1950's and 60's was so upscale, vibrant, and inviting, that many "out-siders" came to work or visit and stayed to settle. The "friendliness of the people" was a huge attraction. Everyone was welcome. The social interactions and connections that occurred (especially evident at Carnival time) made cultural lines disappear and life was good… until so many came, brought their prejudices, and separated into distinct ethnic groups. This dismantled a uniquely cohesive social structure and turned it into the fractured society we see today in which one group hardly ever interacts with another.

Certain people have low stress levels (Greeks and other people in blue zones), low fear response, high acceptance thresholds and frequent or steady release of feel-good hormones that are shared with friends and strangers alike. Their outlook on life is different than that of the uptight big city commuter or the possession- obsessed suburbanite. They are genuinely interested in others and are adept at enjoying the art of socializing. They are more accepting of diversity, genuinely interested in others and more adept at the art of socializing. They are "nicer".

The following array of statements and quips are not intended to disparage or insult any country or group of people and are in no particular order. This section is based entirely on the observations and results of discussions of myself and my traveling companions.

In Blue Zone areas of longevity, all residents have in common secure reliable social connections, basic manners, and a sense of decency toward fellow human beings. In Ikaria, where, social connections are strong, the people are secure enough to extend their hospitality and friendliness to others, whether they are on the island or abroad. It is a delightful place to visit, but a bit too isolated for habitation by high stress individuals. **Greece:** The people sit together everywhere, talk, laugh, dine, invite strangers to join and share, and offer gifts of food and drink. This happens every day in La Plaka, the popular tourist section of Athens. People appear to be genuinely interested in your humanity. To Athenian Greeks, "Kali orexi"(good appetite) is a genuine invitation to open our appetites, share our lives and lighten our burdens. Familiarity with a dozen words in Greek could cement friendships and extend our cultural connections. The importance of saying kalimera (good morning), kalispera (good evening), parakalo and efkharisto , (please and thank you), cannot be overemphasized. The basic expression of courtesy indicates that you are open to conversation and interaction and deserving of kindness and fellowship.

Vaulting over the Southern Aegean, I have read that the Greek Cypriots greet you with "Kopiaste", sit down with you, share a meal, plus news and stories of your lives. It is an invitation to share quality time and special fare in a unique part of the world. In next door Crete, the hospitality often goes overboard, the use of dialects abound, and you cannot help getting caught up in the "volta", (like the Spanish "paseo"), the evening walk of family and friends which may lead to the nearest party or fiesta. While in some western cultures, eye contact is avoided, Cretans will stare, engage and comment on the activities of everyone around them, including yourself. My advice is just to greet, nod, smile and enjoy.

Throughout the Greek islands, I could not help but recall that Hippocrates, born in Kos (Chios) (460-377 BCE.) practiced and taught clinical medicine, that rational medicine consisted of the healing power of nature, that prevention was better than cure, and that the prognosis of illness (outcome) depended as much on factors within the human patient as from outside. Asclepius of Bithynia, my particular favorite ancient instructor in molecular medicine and practitioner of Greek medicine in Rome, has a milkweed plant containing booth healing properties and life-ending cardenolides, named after him. Epicurus, the philosopher born on Samos, right next to Ikaria, noted diseases as acute and chronic and wrote treatises on friendship and pleasure. The intellectual contributions of people in this region supported friendship as part of mental health based on sensible human behavior and social efforts, and that expansion and inclusion of other cultures, languages and peoples were good for human health.

Of course, not to be mentioned is the history of invasions, massacres and human destruction of other humans that took place over the same centuries of productive thinking. Alexander's entire campaign of invasion and annexation, the takeover of Constantinople and expulsion of the Greeks by the Ottoman Turks in 1453, the

Great Fire of Smyrna in which hundreds of thousands of Greeks and Armenians perished or fled (1922); the Nazi annihilation of 1-million Greeks in 1944; Ataturk's expulsion of the Greeks from Istanbul in 1956; the Armenian genocide by Ottoman Turks in 1915; and the Golden Dawn's racist threats and insurrections in the 21st century reveals that the region is far from being "socially perfect".

SARDINIA produces Cannovan wine, which claims the highest levels of polyphenols, arterial cleansers, of all examined wines, so far. The local bars, grape harvests and village festivals occupy important rungs in Sardinian social life. A Harvard study by Dr. Lisa Berkman and associates on "Social connectedness and Longevity", used such parameters as marital status, family, friends, club membership and volunteerism over a 10- year period, to support the premise that high social connectedness was linked directly to longevity. The type of socializing did not matter. Whatever and whenever stress and anxiety were reduced and replaced with purpose and belonging, security and well-being and longevity were increased. In Sardinian cafes and restaurants everyone greets everyone else, with "Buon giorno, como sta" (Good day, how are you) and are genuinely interested in your response. The friendliness extends from the bank and the grocery store to the "passegiata", the customary evening stroll of the family out together with others, walking, congregating, talking and greeting. They exclude no one.

PUERTO RICO, with its culture of "Buen Provecho", is a friendly, comfortable place in which to live and age. The people are amiable, welcoming and well-equiped with basic manners. An "hola, buenos días, buenas tardes, por favor and gracias", go a long way. When you start a conversation with "con permiso", (I ask your permission to speak), a "buenos días" and a smile the whole world opens for you. When I am greeted with a "buenos dias, mi amor, en que puedes ayudarle. mi cielo?" said by a young woman in a store to an older man (myself), my heart melts, every time. "Encontraste todo lo que necesita, Papi?", said by the young man to the same older man, makes my chest swell with satisfaction. Titles of respect said with warmth and sincerity, here are unequaled. Eye contact, smiles, and acknowledgements are the rules of engagement. Even with " no lo podemos, mi cielo" (we can't do it, my heaven), and a smile that would melt a stone, who cares! How can you get mad when your feel-good hormones are leaping with joy.

When you add to this, the "buen provecho" greeting at the start or in the middle or at the end of your meal, your digestion is helped a hundred times. Puerto Ricans entering a restaurant or in the home will offer the Buen Provecho, even if not sharing the food, that serves to wish you well, acknowledge your combined presence and humanity and alert you to their presence. It is a bit more than the "bon apetit" you may get as the waiter sprints away and ducks into the kitchen. It is a greeting from passersby, from the neighboring table, from the chef, from the staff that invites you to enjoy your meal and your time with them. The tradition is friendly, respectful and prevails despite outside influences.

Even on the beaches, the markets, grocery stores, and the post office, people will greet you and invite you to have a conversation. Often curious as to your origins, especially if your accent is not exactly like theirs, they will congratulate themselves upon figuring it out. At Puerto Rican family gatherings, it appears that everyone is welcome. Despite the infrastructural and identity problems, Puerto Rico ranks relatively high on the longevity scale (#38) owing in part to their excellent social connectivity and its positive effects on their collective health. (Nutrition is so-so, exercise and mental stimulation are lacking (cars), stress is everywhere and toxic pollutants abound, though the rate of cigarette smoking is low). There is plenty of sunshine.

IRELAND is very much like Puerto Rico. Having previously benefitted from the expert instruction provided by Irish teachers, eager to test the legendary Irish hospitality, on a visit to Dublin

(1990), my wife and I were stopped by a young man in the street, welcomed and questioned with genuine curiosity, as to our origins and if we were liking our visit. After participating in and enjoying a pub visit, the sights, and a river dance or two, I looked and learned that the hospitality that was mandated by law in old Ireland, and had since become the cultural norm in the new. The hospitality to strangers regardless of nationality that included the greeting at the door, "a hundred thousand welcomes" and "does someone need a drink" is alive and well. I sincerely wish that the warmth, wit, and welcome of the Irish is never lost.

FRANCE: Too often, the French people are mislabeled as being unfriendly and rude. But custom maintains that you must engage and open the conversation with "Bon Jour", and then ask your question or make your statement. France receives an ECNS response rating of 50%, in issuing a greeting and 80% after receiving the same. It offers courtesy and politeness at a high level, but first you have to show an interest and express courtesy on your own. France is a verbal country, speak in French and you get a positive response. Converse and interact and you get much more. Connect and give news and information and receive warm embraces and friendships for life. When you receive "la bise", (the French cheek kisses), you know you have arrived. Just attempting to learn the language, at least trying is a plus in the art of social interaction. Many people speak English and will engage with you, especially if you try French first. Greet before you speak! In France it is imperative. A simple hello, good morning, good evening, or please, opens the conversation, and a thank you, have a nice day, closes it. Warmth and your friendliness go a long way. (*France is the origin of the Art of Conversation, to be examined in Chapter Five*) Friendly with a hard exterior and soft interior, once you make an opening, the French are humorous, knowledgeable, a bit reserved, conservative, and worldly. Though it is difficult to establish a friendship right away, once done, it carries high value and is for life. France is one of the original melting pots of *Homo sapiens*, Neanderthal, Phoenician, Greek, Roman, Carthaginian and others, where at least by now they speak the same language, (notwithstanding Occitan and Parisian dialects), dance to the same music, laugh at the same jokes, and socialize in large and small groups, together.

JAPAN: The Land of the Rising Sun scores well all health strategies except in connecting socially with strangers. It remains a homogenous society in which strangers are not particularly welcome and anyone who does not look exactly like them is suspect. (The tennis champion, Naomi Osaka had a hard time being accepted and celebrated because of her mixed heritage.) When traveling, they do not make eye contact or smile nor do they seem to be aware of or tolerant of the presence of anyone else, besides their own and that of their immediate group. Sorry, but until someone can show me otherwise, my opinion on Japanese global social skills is that they are non-existent. The highest life expectancy of both genders ranks Japan as second to Hong Kong in 2020. The Chinese are much friendlier. Okinawa is a blue zone, featuring stress control with yoga to counteract high financial demands. The system of "Ikigai", the sense of purpose that promotes health and moai "groups of 5 or 6 persons for life" contribute to high degrees of social bonding. The rest of the country suffers high cognitive decline associated with loneliness, from lack of social contacts. As with many Asian cultures, the Japanese celebrate old age with respect and dignity, friendships and purpose, with little connection to the global community. (Japan is high in toxic exposure with smoking (men), alcohol abuse, drugs and "strange" food habits, that often preclude a balanced diet.)

HAWAIANS practice the group healing process of "ho'opono-pono", which focuses on letting go of negative feelings and promoting creativity from that point onward. The hospitality and sociality of the Pacific Islanders is re-known, but suffered seriously from dilution and influence of foreign social misbehavior and impositions of religion.

PERU had an 80% ECNS positive response conducted in the marketplace, streets, train, and countryside. Four out of five Peruvians responded with a smile and a return greeting. On one of my treks in the Andes, along the road I encountered a traveler on foot. Greeting him in Quechua, "allianchu" (hello, how are you) and he responded, "Hal li Kusunchis" (let us chew coca together) leading to a customary exchange of leaves as a social gesture and a conversation (in Spanish). The interaction was laced with curiosity and questions regarding my origin and the purpose in the region. Being somewhat unfamiliar with my appearance, he was pleased with the open and friendly exchange. Before we parted company, he expressed his appreciation for my visit and my respect for his customs.

ENGLAND had a 70% ECNS response with most of the population being rather engaging, expressive, reactive, comfortable with strangers, confident but stiff and a bit reserved even though many are descendants of migrants from somewhere else. The weather is horrible, initial greetings are a trifle standoffish and "How do you do?" is not heard very often. An embrace is rare and reserved for family, if at all. Eye contact makes them feel uncomfortable, and there is a proper order of introduction, with the young to the older, lower status to higher status, and if the same age and same status, introduction of the one you know better to the one you know less is in order. To my ears as everyone in a given region speaks the same regardless of origin, I suspect that they speak to and socialize with each other.

CHINA had a response rate of less than 10%. The people appear aloof and "detached" when greeted by strangers. Only one of ten return eye contact. A higher percentage show some curiosity but then pursue it no further. The Belt and Road Initiative will have to do some serious social training if they wish to engage and connect with the rest of the world, particularly the Third. In the Caribbean, for example, you have to engage and interact in a positive social manner in order to get things done. Aloofness will bring a "schtupps" (the noise made from sucking of air through the teeth) response and all progress will stop.

GERMANY and AUSTRIA cultivate "Die gemutlichkeit", a cozy sense of well-being in a comfortable environment of relaxation, usually alone or with a few friends. Those who do not belong, are excluded. (As a young student, I was welcomed in both countries, treated very well and made long lasting friends. I may have been an exotic exception.)

RUSSIA, HUNGARY, POLAND and the SLAVS are just plainly very unfriendly towards people who do not look like them. The lack of basic manners and extension of courtesies to others is blatant and obvious. My rudimentary language skills often incurred more wrath than acceptance.

SPAIN, including Balearics and all its former colonies, has a history of extreme racism and savage abuse of Jews, Moors, Africans, and Native Amerinds, mass murder and ethnic massacres in name of religion and resource acquisition. A more recent response to strangers, features the fear of "darkening" of the population. The expulsion of entire populations of ethnically different people by the tens of thousands left a legacy of high fear and anxiety and low tolerance that continues to plague the country and its citizens. In major cities, we saw offensive graffitti targeting specific groups they do not like. "Fuera Moros" sprayed on a wall in Avila spoke loudly to my 15% North African DNA. The Spaniards are not friendly to people from its former colonies even though they share the language and religion. They show little concern and offer less assistance when these countries suffer disasters or fall on hard financial times. Instead, Spain prefers to welcome strangers, if they are Nordic, English, Dutch, or Germans. This hesitancy to socialize with "others" limits its scope of social connections to a population within its borders. It is difficult to dismiss its history of exclusion and ostracism and I am not too sure that she wishes to do so. For 400 years, Spaniards dealt out so much pain and suffering, that perhaps they may be afraid of being on the receiving end. So far, they are saved by a strong religion that provides a "forgiveness" doctrine.

The Jack Spaniard wasp in the Caribbean has a vicious sting and shows no mercy. If you let him live after he bites you, he will bite you again.

In Spanish streets and public places there is a low index of eye contact. I am not sure if it is arrogance or insecurity. They appear to have serious issues with being European or Iberian, and always have issues with "purity" of blood. Their apparent refusal to acknowledge their history of horrific behavior towards "others", non-Christians and "Christians" alike, after destroying whole groups of people, now manifests itself in the cultural response of "se cayo", it fell, not my fault, I wasn't there, and proceed as if nothing happened. There is a low index of friendliness, low acceptance of strangers unless you are obviously just passing through and leaving funds. Despite a sense of collective paranoia, modern Spaniards respond 80% to ECNS and their own language. Madrid is friendly, Barcelona less so. When one's main goal is to separate and isolate, the fear and anxiety generated impairs the ability to interact socially with the world.

COSTA RICA, the peninsula of Nicoya) the people use every excuse to socialize: over sports (passion for football), family, and work. With a cadre of reliable friends (trust), and over 7 hours of sleep a night, they are content and relaxed. They exercise (walk), have good nutrition with fresh fruit and local vegetables), low stress in a community of equals setting and pursue the pleasure of daily living. Sharing with their neighbors maximizes joy. With food, family, music, dance, and laughter, it is a Blue Zone and #1 on the Happy Planet Index. Regarding longevity, the life expectancy of men over the age of ninety is highest in the world. It is a mid-income country whose nice welcoming healthy citizens have spare time and a tradition of interpersonal relationships that overshadow materialism and status.

DENMARK has the tradition of "hygge", a condition of coziness, security, contentment, and comfort felt mainly by the self and perhaps a few close family and friends. They describe it as the art of creating intimacy, the absence of annoyance, taking pleasure from the presence of soothing things, like a blanket, a cup of coffee, a candle or a partner. Despite a spirit of cooperation within the community based on trust in their own, there is still a Viking mentality of wariness of the threat of others, which in modern times has drifted into "indifference". There is a mania for candles, a home-cooked meal and cuddling with people you know, but little interest in getting to know strangers. Danes put high trust in neighbors and value personal activities, well-being and social life ahead of material wealth. Paying taxes for most is a sense of duty for the good of the community and that access and opportunity should be available for all to have an equal chance at life. With excellent communication skills, Danes appear to be aloof at times, but are comfortable living and working with "strangers" and do pursue quality social relationships. They treat each other well, with generosity and respect for each other's happiness and successes. The rest of Scandinavia, the Baltic States and Switzerland, appear to be happy and healthy, but not quite "friendly" or completely open to interacting with "others". Some blame the cold, dreary weather for interfering with the true expression of good-intentioned DNA.

EGYPT is one of the 50% ECNS Mediterranean responders in which only half the population qualifies to interact with strangers. The concept of hospitality to guests is a fundamental characteristic in its culture. They ensure you feel welcome and have the skills to do it. Interpersonal relationships carry a lot of weight, reliability and durability. "Nawartouma" (welcome, you bring light to us), and "shukran" (thank you), Dr. Adel Nagdi, of Luxor, for being my friend.

SINGAPORE is driven by economic success. Enterprise and entrepreneurship are rewarded and money and material possessions carry high value. Its population is consistently on both the happiest and healthiest lists. I have yet to visit.

UNITED STATES OF AMERICA is a big place and generalizations should not be made, but it contains the most unhappy people on the planet. In a winner-take-all society, where you increase your chances by creating more losers, the trust and cooperation required for group success that carries over to social success, is lacking. Success is economic, highly celebrated when individual, measured in material possessions, and often obtained at the expense of others. Achievement that involves being above others, generates a resentment and hatred that narrows the field of "with whom to interact". A country cannot always win and still be moral. Obsession with the acquisition of material wealth, attainment of status, privilege and acts of hoarding, generate fear and anxiety and a society of "us and them". Safeguarding wealth promotes distrust of institutions, fellow citizens and much of the global citizenry. Social networks and lasting bonds are few and tenuous and social skills are sparse. In every state, it is not uncommon for someone to sit right next to you and not make eye contact or utter a word. If you greet them, they may look right past you as if you do not exist. If you cannot do anything to their advantage, you have no value.

Generations pass and the basic manners lessen. You have to work hard at forging friendships, and often they remain superficial, fade and frequently disappear. The USA had an ECNS rating of less than 30% overseas, and 20% on the mainland, where only 2 of any 10 casual encounters respond to a greeting. Aloof and adept at looking past or through you, the learned fear is palpable. Members of assigned groups ignore each other in a learned response to fear of threat, of engagement, of the possibility of liking someone and having a genuine relationship. So much fear and anxiety at interacting that avoidance becomes a tradition, passed on from generation to generation, as "the way it ought to be" A country that believes that cooperation, kindness, and sharing are somehow evil and a sign of weakness, will have a difficult time being "social".

To reiterate, the fact that they speak different forms of the same language in the same place is testament to the lack of interaction between assigned groups. The accompanying disrespect and demonization of one group by another severely hampers any attempts of socializing across these artificial cultural lines. (I once endured a 14-day European river cruise with a group of American tourists from the South, that did not once say a word to me or return a basic greeting.) Sorry to bear bad news, but compared to the rest of the world, many Americans are lacking in basic manners and social skills, and the culture that emerges is one of contact avoidance.

From a stress promoting lifestyle on all levels, poor processed diet, unnatural exercise, refusal to socialize freely, intake and exposure to toxins (OTC and Rx drugs, food additives, and recreational) and a fractured society, it is no wonder that the world health ranking is way below its potential. In a separated society, where social connections are confined to small groups, each averse to contact with "others" add to this, the almost complete aversion to interactions and connections with foreigners. US history involves a disgust at having to share space with "others", savages, heretics, slaves, and immigrants that forged a frontier mentality of distrust that carries over to the present fear and hatred of "Mexican caravans coming to take your jobs, rape and steal" and a social response of wall-building mania.

USA has a poor health rating (#34 world ranking in life expectancy at birth: Source: America's Health Rankings, 2019), shorter lives, more heart disease (depression), more injuries and homicides, obesity and diabetes, chronic lung disease, elderly disability, and drug-related deaths than any other developed country. A weak social structure contributes to poor health.

Good health is a human need that requires air, water and nutrients. To maintain the psyche intact, you need energy to establish dignity, that sense of belonging that secures your standing in the world, country, and community. To be dignified, you have to mean something to yourself and have a purposeful life. Achieving a state of dignified health explicitly and implicitly involves other people. Social connections and "socializing" have a lot to do with health.

There are many stories and instances of loners existing quite well, but are they truly "healthy"? The answer is no. Physically, they may appear to be okay, but biochemically they are deficient and physiologically, they suffer frequent malfunctions.

Social connections are necessary for development of the mind and nourishment of the body with ideas and events respectively. External relationships of family and friends provide both mental and physical support, valuable input, suggestions, concern, care when needed, that directly affect health. Internal well-being depends on one's reaction and handling of the range from minor irritations to major crises. "Loners" function or malfunction on a different psychological level.

Stress may be acute and repeated like financial burdens, deadlines, work related, extended commutes, or chronic, long term, perpetual such as racism leveled upon black males in school, streets, home, job or lack of, prison, and women not complying with the expected "norm", academic shortfalls because of inadequate facilities or motivation, etc. and stress from interpersonal relationships and interactions... ranging from simple lack of courtesies on a daily basis to long term repeated lack of concern or attention between one group and another.

Societies that confer and respect the dignity of their own as well as others, are more advanced socially than societies that do not.

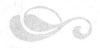

CHAPTER FIVE

BUILDING SOCIAL SKILLS

Why should I be Sociable?

Social interactions and connections are good for your general health.

First: decide whether you want to be sociable. Weigh the pros and cons. Settle on a positive mindset because it is natural, fulfills an inner need, is the right thing to do, and you will enjoy it.

Second: be in good health, so you may function optimally, and maintain good health

Third: develop and use good communication skills as an asset

Fourth: seek encounters and engage in interactions as a natural human activity

Fifth: Take the time and make the effort to manage and maintain your connections

Sociability 101

In preparing to be social, weigh the pros and cons. Am I aware of the health consequences of being antisocial? Do I wish to be healthy or take a chance of suffering from depression and potential cardiac problems? Do I have the self- confidence, self-esteem, and purpose? Do I want to spend the energy required to learn these skills? Do I have what it takes to pursue an active social life (return phone calls, answer texts, show up at meetings) or remain in glorious seclusion? Do I know the consequences of pro-social vs antisocial behavior? Am I ready to express my kind DNA and suppress my cruel DNA? Is socializing with other people worth anything?

Feel-good hormones vs feel-bad hormones

The foremost premise to becoming & being more social is to rid oneself of all inhibitions and restrictions that limit one's access and opportunity based on differences between human beings. The similarities are far and above of greater importance and simply more interesting.

On considerations of "race", it is a societal construct originating within the age of discovery and exploration. As a biological fact, it does not exist. Get rid of it. Think of building a national character based on inclusion and celebration of diversity. Only by including everyone can socializing expand and accomplish its health-promoting goal. Any antisocial behavior will limit one's range of encounters.

Get into the correct frame of mind. "SOCIAL" is not a dirty word. It is not political. Being social, using social skills is an integral part of being healthy. Being social works best when those skills are acquired in the early years (my daughter, Lyn, the "social butterfly" of Mrs. Brown's kindergarten class of 1976 matured into an effective,

303

healthy adult with lifelong friends and deep friendships that have meaning.) Interactions are the openings of a healthy social life.

Functional social skills should have developed by college age, 17-21. Personality development, communications, emotional maturity, acceptance of others, compassion capacity, comprehension of and connection with the world, and reaction to social interactions should all be in place. We see mature interactions in countries like Greece, Japan, Sardinia, Netherlands, and Denmark, where people engage daily as a way of life. In some countries, neighbors do not interact with each other, lack of common courtesies among and between the population, people are distant and aloof, live in separate communities, vote to make policies against each other, competition is fierce and final, and only victory over another is the measure of success. Communities exist side by side for 400 years, but do not speak the same language nor share the same customs and traditions. They vary between indifference and hatred of each other. This venom reflects directly on the health of each community: hypertension, diabetes, obesity all based on stress- induced inflammation derived from challenged immune systems on one side and fear of threat, fear of loss of self-proclaimed privileges, anxiety and depression under the guise of defending a "way of life", on the other, which induces still more stress. The huge inequality gap generates more separation, illness, and deaths that could be eliminated by a willingness to share... simple meals, holidays, commutes, talk to each other, share experiences. "We are more alike than different," stated President Obama. No one listened and instead blamed him for worsening "race relations" when in effect it was fear of change, of integration, of sharing lives that is tearing a country apart, while driving health statistics in reverse.

Natural selection, biochemical and physiological reactions in place, promotes social instincts that favor survival. Poor social behavior reduces chances of success. Selfishness loses to cooperation. Behavior that allows and encourages personal interactions, actions appropriate for group viability, ability to handle familiar and different situations, ability to socialize inside and outside the comfort zone, will develop and progress. Social skills in action, conversation, group dance, engagements, and anticipation of seeing a friend for a sports event that generates genuine interest in "others" not oneself, with highlights on the attitude and time spent with others, nature, and an appreciation for life, are all associated with good health and longevity.

Equipped with social skills to express that we care about each other, there would be no need for the organization and emphasis on "Black Lives Matter". With effective social mechanisms in place that includes everybody, "social" would not be a dirty word and communities would not be designed and constructed to keep out others. Antisocial behavior is unhealthy, stressful, and produces disease that is and will progress to dysfunction.

One day your life will flash before your eyes: Make sure it's worth watching" The Bucket List 2007

"Do or do not. There is no try." Yoda, Star Wars, episode V, The Empire Strikes Back

"An old friend is never an extra guest." Alfred Hitchcock, Notorious

Here are a few basic requirements for developing social skills. First, one must have or develop and display a genuine effort at being interested in others. What they say, who they are, what they are about and how it would feel to engage and interact with them must be considered. One must have the desire and nerve to break away from the selective group and engage others, with the mindset to exchange and try something new. Being selective and aloof will severely hamper the social skills. Have a social purpose. Find a group of people who challenge and inspire you. Spend quality time with them. Focus outward instead of inward. Have a genuine curiosity in others, care about being with others, interacting and gaining knowledge and experience. Open your mind and extend your range. The higher the quality of the interaction the greater the mental stimulation, the more the feel-good hormone release, the better the health.

We know the comfort of similarity. Group A resembles group B, and will naturally interact because of less fear, less threat and more limitations. When group A meets a disparate group C for first time, they may each reject the other or fight and bring damage to both groups. Expand your range early when it is easier to join forces, share resources, accept and adapt to one another's strong points. Realize the benefits of being with others and the damages of confrontation and antagonism. Overcome differences by understanding that all humans are the same. Separate "races" do not exist biologically. Include and engage everyone that you can in conversation, support and activities. Groups that refuse to learn this natural fact and act accordingly will be in constant antisocial mode and at odds with everything that life offers.

Basic Social Skills

Self- confidence is the first of the basic social skills. Trust in your abilities, good qualities and sound judgement. Take comfort in your decisions, without fear of consequences, especially about other people. Viewing yourself in a positive light (self-esteem) enables better interaction with others. Knowing who you are and what you are about reduces anxiety, widens your comfort zone and increases feelings of belonging. When you value yourself, in relation to the world, it is easier to engage with others. With internal validation, any external approval can build more confidence. Self-confidence takes practice. Encounter, engage, interact and make the connection. Believing in yourself enough to present for others to accept, be realistically comfortable in your positive traits and skills. Become good at one skill at a time, make the effort, test it, then move to the next skill. Build on your self-worth. Socialize.

Make a good physical and emotional appearance. If you have a flaw or an oddity, embrace it, make use of it. Know that those who don't accept you are themselves not worth being around. Believe in and practice affirmations. "I can do this, I've done it before, and I can do it again." Be sincere. If you talk the game, make sure you can deliver the same. Express achievement and success without bragging. Use inner and outer skills, such as music, art, languages to augment the interaction where appropriate.

With a desire to be sociable, develop and use the skills to build on experience. Remember the young teenager who wanted to become "un homme du monde" and use his skills to interact with and learn about others. Along the way, he developed a confidence in body language, eye contact, use of language, delivery style, and word content plus an altruism (*selfless concern for the well-being of others*) and a "compersion" (*good feeling in the presence of another's joy*) that found for him a solid place in an international community of those with similar attitudes, interests and training. With basic social skills in place, the better you are the better the quality of the social interaction will be and the greater the chance of a long- lasting connection.

Good health is an integral part of building self-confidence. Appearance and mien are skills. You can socialize better if not coughing, wheezing, or on a respirator, not in a wheelchair, can keep up, and not talking about all the medications you are taking. You are a lot more open to quality encounters if you are not relying on the clinic or a physician's waiting room as your main contact with people. The six basic strategies of good health are well worth repeating. Practice them. A balanced natural plant-based diet with portion-size control; daily physical activity with emphasis on structured exercise at least three times a week; read, (at least 20 books a year), improve your concentration and mental skills, be informed so that you have something intelligent to discuss; get sufficient sleep, reduce stress; avoid toxins and toxic behavior; and be sociable: expand your range, engage with people who do not look like you, smile more often, be polite, avoid rude people, try to interact with at least five new people a week that you don't know, by direct communication or by ECNS non-verbal greetings; avoid high risk behavior, excess alcohol, drugs, unhealthy food, and polluted air.

Keep in mind to appreciate your worth, strive to improve and maintain sincerity. Be positive and enjoy being around people. If you are depressed and negative, you are not nice to be around. Those living in disadvantaged neighborhoods face greater health and mortality risks than those with access to healthy lifestyle. Yet living in an exclusive, isolated mansion may have similar effects. Both may involve high stress living leading to poor health, one with threats and anxiety and the other with fear and loneliness. Money may not lead to social connectivity. But access, opportunity and a good dose of self-confidence will increase the chances. Having solid trustworthy friends, a social network to call on in good times as well as bad, for comfort and support contributes greatly to one's health.

Eye contact is the first and foremost method used to interact and communicate with each other. It is a non-verbal way of expressing basic good manners. Upon initial encounter, eye contact and a smile reach out in a positive manner that says, "You are safe with me; I am a friend; I am open to interact". The eyes focus on personal appearance, the return of appropriate gestures, and body language, that are constructive and approving, not dismissive or neglecting. A basic greeting establishes worth, that this person has value. "You are important and pleasing, you matter". If not, you are not worth enough to look at.

Eye expressions can be emotive, happy, inviting, hopeful, or anxious, frustrating and evasive, and the interpretations just as variable. Eye contact, on greeting and during conversation is a baseline for a friendly conversation. (Note the doctor-patient and iPad interaction…no eye contact, no touch, no connection… made worse now by pandemic induced tele-health.)

Body language accompanies both gestures and verbalization and should be appropriate. "How you say it" comprises significant non-verbal clues that may or may not gather the interest in what you are saying. The person you are addressing should be the most important at the moment, so looking askance, past them or with the mouth curled, snarled, or beaming, shows receptivity or rejection, antagonism or disinterest. If you say nice words with an angry face, it has little value.

Basic Manners should be assertive and not aggressive, open and not closed. Ignoring someone who offers you a simple greeting is offensive and insulting. Refusing to note the presence of "another" in a shared space in a positive manner, is rude.

Vignette #30: My wife and I were standing under a sturdy scaffold in the middle of New Orleans enjoying a Mardi Gras parade. It was drizzly and cool. Two couples were standing on the scaffold directly above us. One of the women was laughing and swinging her arms, unintentionally spilling globs of beer from her cup down on my wife's coat. When we pointed out the infraction and politely requested that she be more careful, she replied "you really oughtta move", and continued to spill the beer.

There is no excuse for this type of behavior of one human to another. This encounter was totally lacking in basic manners. Showing respect to others is a basic sign of regard, class and humanity. In the event of insult and cruelty, be kind to unkind people. Tolerance is healthier than anger and resentment.

Communication is most effective when face-to-face. The posture and gestures should be non-threatening, as with a show of hands, a handshake, and a smile. The verbal action should consist of saying the right things at the right times to produce the right effects. It should be adapted to fit the situation and the audience. Use a softener to introduce the subject, appropriate tone to gather interest and reduce the natural defense mechanisms of the listener. Bring attention to the content and delivery of what you are saying. Attract and maintain contact. Give and receive feedback. Do not wander or get distracted. Sometimes it is better to talk less and listen more.

Conversation control comes from the brain's amygdala, seat of physical and emotional Well-being. Tone of voice, gestures and expressions should mirror what you are saying. A good communicator is genuine, invites comfort and keeps the listener involved in the story. In using both sides of the brain, right for emotion and left for logic, the speaker should be able to get his/her point(s) across. (Remember the Neolithic hunter relating to the group what he had just seen and heard. It makes a big difference if his story is of a sparrow building a nest at the cave entrance or a warning of an approaching leopard.)

The listener's attention and response are important as well. Sometimes a repetition of what the speaker has just said or a "me too" inclusion response can keep the conversation going to its natural conclusion. Any unsolicited interruption, especially in mid-sentence, over-talking or wandering off is a sign that you may not be listening. The listener should choose the appropriate response to signal to the speaker that the communication was understood.

With communicators, as with all social modalities, zip code matters. The environment, both original and immediate, plays a big role in how, what, and why a particular communication is offered and received. It is a fact that poor kids hear a fewer number of words per hour (600) than rich kids (1200). Some spend more time alone or with one parent, compared to others with both parents, a nannie, tutors, visitors, and a complete social family. Some kids have less exposure, less access to knowledge, (books, travel, parents with interest, exposure to conversations), and less opportunities to develop social skills. Early conversation, content and number of words spoken to a child contributes to later social skills. Around the campfire, stories designed to keep children in, safe, (Grimms Fairy tales), the read-me-a-story-before-I-go-to-sleep interaction confer advantages of communication. Kids without this opportunity, have less access to social skills. For this reason, I do not agree with nor recommend homeschooling away from other children and influential adults, nor abbreviated curricula like putting doctors through 6 years of schooling instead of 8, where there is less chance and opportunity to develop bedside manner and social skills. Doctors are teachers and must be able to communicate as part of the skill of medicine. I do not wish to offend but, without sufficient interaction of other students, teachers and campus life, many graduates are seriously deficient in basic social skills, especially in communication. Insufficient time and instruction find one lacking in the skill of having a basic conversation that leads to a connection.

The tone of voice should match the content. The conversation should be comforting and not combative. If the speaker is upset and uncomfortable, the listeners will be too, resulting in an unhealthy feedback. We should attempt to show and tell and use words, body language and emotions that validate what you are saying. Make it clear that you made a sincere effort to carry on a conversation. With foreign listeners, make the effort to learn the language, or at least parts of it, as an indication of respect and expedience.

For an **interaction** to occur, one must have the proper mindset, and be positive, considerate and accepting of each other's appearance, attitude and venue. Here again, zip code matters. Certain communities are structured to encourage gathering and encounters, and certain cultures are more open to socializing than others. Inner city neighborhoods, gated communities, the front porch and steps and the open backyards either encourage or discourage interactions. Eighty percent of Greeks spend time with neighbors, 80% of Americans do not. Some people use public spaces to engage and converse, others do not.

In seeking interactions, you choose the appropriate space, where there is already a high frequency of encounters, preferably with a diverse group of people. Get into the mental zone of engaging, move forward, enjoy the interaction with familiars and venture over to engage with someone who does not look or sound like you. Learn and use the culture. Invite and be invited to participate. Form a network of relationships nearby, then widen it to include the fringe. Expand your comfort zone and follow up on newly formed acquaintances. Get to know the people with whom you are engaging, be authentic and pleasant to be around. Avoid being critical, crabby, and self-pitying. Being open to learning, teaching and showing respect for the opinions of others, is a sign of class and humanity.

Kindness created the tribe and still has some value in all cultures. Social behavior involving one person at a time, improves physical and emotional health, and enhances immunity through better nutrition and lower stress levels. Antisocial behavior is destructive, decreases immunity and contributes to an inner sickness that may become consuming.

Pointers on engaging in social interactions go back to self-confidence, self-esteem (I am worthy), and the investment of interest. Practice the skills of eye contact, communication, body language and basic manners. Understand the same social cues when they are returned to you. Show up, speak, and listen well. Interactions will add quality and quantity to your life.

Perhaps the most difficult skill to master is to **include and accept** people who may not be attractive or responsive. Reaching out and taking the initiative, shows flexibility and range. Ignore the negatives. Do not refuse to interact or choose selectively because of skin color or economic status, accent or different culture. Every encounter may be an opportunity to expand horizons and experience, and no matter the outcome, every adventure in socializing has some value.

Do not be afraid to engage, put down your devices and talk, engage a European, Asian, African, Indian, practice and develop your skills. Be open for all to join. It will surprise you. We are more alike than different. We all discuss the same subjects, in similar ways and appreciate the knowledge that is around us. (Exclusion keeps you dumb.) Dismantle the divide that limits the pool of available encounters, ignore the institutionalized separations, cross the lines, interact and connect.

The English landscape painter, John Constable, alleged that "Nothing is ugly in this world". Likewise, no one in this world is not worth at least a greeting, and perhaps a small interaction for your health and theirs. Everyone has value and one needs to be socially active with functional skills and enough exposure to get a talented group of friends. Abraham Maslow's 1943 paper, A Theory of Human Motivation, discusses a hierarchy of needs in building friendships as based on mutual trust, shared purpose and generosity. When all are present, commitments are a lot easier. Connections require like-minded people willing to risk loving and being loved to rise to the level of friends. A mix of give and take must cater to the needs of both parties. To have a good friend, be a good friend. You are born into your family, but you choose your friends... well. *Social Connections are seriously reduced by and with the pandemic. There are less opportunities for new interactions and existing social connections are curtailed.*

Be human and humane is the Golden Rule of social skills. Whatever you desire to receive, you must give. Show compassion and sympathy to others, especially to those who are suffering and distressed. Be liked as you are, happy, positive, and kind. A "nice guy finishing first" type of guy is always preferable to a brash, self-centered, arrogant, uncompromising snip. Make a good first impression, then maintain it. This image lasts long after the initial event has passed. Accentuate your strengths and minimize your weak traits. Being human (noun and adjective) is taking responsibility for ourselves, each other, and the environment; being humane (adjective) is having human traits of compassion and kindness. Be aware that lack of humanity devalues every other quality. Failure to acknowledge or offer to assist those in misery or suffering is inhumane.

Vignette #31: We are a lot like crayons. Some of us are sharp, some are pretty, some are so-so and some are dull. Some have weird names, and all are different colors, but they all live in the same box...together. Using only a few to dominate the picture is never a s grand as when all are used to their potential.

High quality social interactions depend on the goodness of human nature and is next to impossible as long as humanity continues its obsession with material possessions. *Climate change destruction of the environment is being ignored in favor of resource extraction and the money it generates. The refusal of anyone to cooperate with global society and wear a mask during a pandemic is classic antisocial behavior on the inhumane scale.*

Managing relationships once we form them takes more effort than the initial interaction. When we make the list of all the qualities we want in a relationship, make sure we have the same qualities to offer. In a group of like-minded people, it is easy to give and receive love to and from others. As long as trust exists, you accept, communicate and share experiences, in relative comfort. Keep friends close, show appreciation, express thoughts and feelings. Spend quality time with novel ideas and solutions, laughter or in deep conversation intended to ease any worries or stresses. Friendship reduces the pain sensitivity when dealing with mental or physical duress. It is okay to grow and change in a relationship, when truth is expressed at all times. A small group of trusted friends and a network of supporters contribute to well-being, resilience to PTSD in the environment and the ability to cope. From Diagnosis and Complementary Therapies, "Women with more social connections have better survival". The support of true friends contribute to higher cancer survival rates that loneliness. That empty feeling in the pit of the stomach signaling the biochemical release and presence of feel bad hormones (chronic cortisol) empty feeling also indicates the erosion of nerves and damage to cellular tissues. One may avoid depression by maintaining social bonds to assist with motivation, energy, and purpose. Seclusion associates with poor health. Alone or in negative company, one blames others (often parents) for difficulties and losses. This only reinforces the problem and establishes the victim mentality, which seldom moves forward. Having friends strengthens your immunity, by increasing your white blood and T cells, your cardiovascular and neuroendocrine systems, to help overcome Herpes simplex rises, shingles, and recurrent cold sores and papilloma. Social support helps reduce blood pressure in hypertension. (The Health Benefits of Friendship. Fix.com/ Consumer Health ews; and "Friendship" a new book published by W.W. Norton & Co., January 2021, by Laura Denworth, science journalist.) The perception of loneliness leads to high cortisol release while the perception of social connections associates with reduced cortisol and increased serotonin and dopamine.

Once in place, value your connections and keep them safe.

Ten Basic Social Skills

1. Self-Confidence
2. Eye Contact
3. Body Language
4. Basic Manners
5. Communication
6. Interaction
7. Include/Accept
8. Connections
9. Be Human & Humane
10. Manage Relationships

Social Hurdles

Socializing begins in the mother's womb, with signals from mother to fetus, and the fetal response. If the mother is depressed or anxious during pregnancy, the stress hormone, cortisol, may reach and affect the baby. At birth, the cultural norms of the society, and emotional and physical experiences direct the child's development as pro-social or antisocial. Failures in attachment at the family level causes insecurity, anger, and self-hate. Exposure to physical and mental abuse, absence of caregiver, chronic pain, neglect and depression, and lack of opportunity to start and hone one's social skills are major sources of inability to socialize. Research shows that children lacking close relationships often lack conscience and affectionate emotions, empathy, trust and guilt, and have a high probability of becoming psychopaths.

What may at first appear as external shyness at different levels, fear of rejection, poor social skills, and misconceptions on socializing, may actually be the consequence of deeply ingrained antisocial feelings and erupt as acute anxiety panic attacks. The imbalance of excess stress hormone, cortisol, and depleted neurotransmitter, dopamine, triggers emotional and physical effects that are averse to positive social interactions. To achieve success, one must want to fix and overcome the imbalance, remove the negativity, discard the bad feeling experiences and seek social interactions by consciously developing and using social skills.

Initial step is to identify two types of "others". An in group, the one most in proximity, would be the easiest to approach. Practice social skills until confident and comfortable. Then search for and engage the out group. It is a bit more challenging, but with your new skills, all is possible.

Vignette #32: At a high school graduation ceremony in 2015, were 508, multicultural, well-accomplished young people. The first notice was that they self-segregated into groups. They did not seem to even know each other. In the same class, one ethnic group didn't know members of another "group". Hyphenated students all labelled with "minority "status separating into groups. Though they all had four years of access and opportunity to interact, they didn't, and the society deems it okay to separate into their "natural" groupings. All spoke "American" with different accents and were content to remain locked into their own cultures. As I watched them accepting their diplomas and resuming their seating, there was a lot of discomfort implicit in their indifference to each other. Social skills or not, "They do not like each other".

Social Skills Associated Strategies

1. Invest time and effort in family and friends Socialize with people outside your work or school
2. Join a club

3. Volunteer
4. Act nicely, be generous
5. Be active mentally and physically
6. Keep healthy, experience nature
7. Focus on the happiness and value of others
8. Keep learning
9. Set goals and reach them

The Art of Conversation

Began with the encounter of two Paleolithic hominids some 500,000 years ago with a common purpose to get something done. The control of fire and setting up shelters to ensure optimal conditions for safety, rest, and nourishment, required organization. Cooperating and working together for maximum success required specializing and vocalizing. Grunts and gestures were used to express desires, intent, satisfaction and recommendations. Along the way, thinking man set about making plans for reliable nutrition and better, more efficient quarters at future sites. Both would provide them with more leisure time for campfire chats, storytelling, teaching, learning and enjoying each other's company. Social interaction through conversation has been developing for a very long time.

Fast-forward to Athens, Greece, where the Demos encouraged walking and talking on the *Stoa poikile* (painted platform). The *agora* (marketplace) composed of streets and squares, was where Socrates "socialized", conversed with people, asked questions about their lives, exchanged information that was of value to both participants and held discussions on the art of living well. Athenians mastered social conversation, competitive debates, diatribes and discourses. Dialogue built social connections and became a basic tool in the formation of all aspects of human society.

In the coffee houses of 19th century London and Vienna, the focus was on conversation as a major past time. But it was in the Parisian salons of Madame Pompidou and Madame de Staël and the cafes of Saint Germain that the art of conversation peaked. Verbal interactions were taught in schools and L'Education Nationale still cultivates the oral tradition. Codes and taboos involving mistakes in French grammar or language usage were designed to smooth the rough edges and develop proficiency. From behavior at a bus stop, over lunch, at a picnic in the park, at the pool, or at work, to the eloquence on display at elegant dinners, the oral culture of the Paris salons dominated the in scene. If unable or refuse to take part, no invitation was extended.

Words in Paris mean more than in New York City

Basic conversation required language skills of articulation both ways (listen and speak), be able to command and hold attention (include not exclude), and present interesting content with flawless delivery. Appreciation, positivity, responsiveness, and correct interpretation were expected on the other end.

Tips for achieving proficiency in the art of Good Conversation

1. Listen with interest. Get others to talk about themselves (hobbies, ups & downs, occupation, likes and dislikes, challenges, and struggles, past and future, then offer positive feedback. Show interest like you really want to be there and they are the most important item of the moment. Show that you are listening.

2. Interpret correctly. Be aware and distinguish between heavy conversation and light points so that you may respond appropriately. Avoid overreaction or under reaction. Avoid raising

or lowering your voice inappropriately. Tone of voice conveys the message as much as content.

3. Regarding the center stage, do not interrupt. Give others the spotlight sometimes. Do not cut in or cut off with opposing or competitive information. It is rude, elicits a negative reaction and shuts them down. (*Mooneyism: "Someone I know has already done this, or already has that." This response takes away from the import of the speaker's content.*)

4. Be responsive. Show interest in what is being said. Send signals indicating you understand and appreciate what is being said. Keep eye contact, head up, and hands assisting. Avoid a negative attitude.

5. Let your assertions be self-explanatory and prepare to back up your claims. Take responsibility for your own words and implications and prepare to face the consequences. In case of a disagreement, show tact, yield gracefully to an objectionable statement, and decline further discussion to avoid argument.

6. Do not be combative. Be uplifting, instructive and accommodating.

7. Use your conversation skills as tools to engage, include, build bridges and seek comfort.

8. Be able to say, "yes, I understand, you did well." Be supportive, not critical. Avoid competing, especially in subjects of money, toys you own, intelligence, religion and politics, unless you agree wholeheartedly, then use your skills to reinforce.

9. To keep a pleasant conversation going, focus on them, not on yourself. What is important to them and how you can fit into their lives and bring comfort will enhance connections and secure bonding.

A conversation where both the speaker and the listener are equally involved, shares knowledge, stimulates the mind and is beneficial to the health of both.

In modern France, where the cuisine is superb and dining is a form of art, the real pinnacle is the conversation at the table/ at the cafes/ at the restaurants/ at the home. The French attitude toward food is that in which the meal should not be eaten unless they enjoy it with others. The company, relaxation, information exchange, laughter and act of dining, stimulate the digestion and placate all the other organ systems together.

In 2010, UNESCO, the cultural arm of the United Nations, designated the classic French dinner (*le repas*) for 20 or more participants as "an element in humanity's intangible cultural heritage". To share such a meal with family and friends satisfied hunger and the social practice of celebrating important moments in the lives of individuals and groups" is good for health, both individual and collective. The Spanish tradition of *sobremesa*, sitting around the table long after the meal is over, chatting and laughing (socializing) for up to and over an hour, is good for digestion, releases positive hormones and indicates that the meal was good and that one is among friends. (This is very different than jumping up from the table, eager to leave or being asked to turn the space over for another seating)

In other modes of conversation, letters provided permanence, but the time lapse due to distance may dull some of the impact. The telephone reduced the distance but removed the face, gestures, body language, and pose, and the Internet gave interaction but takes away privacy, in addition to the lack of face-to-face feel.

Conversation allows you to practice and show off your social skills, builds confidence, your liking to be with other people, seeking and allowing friendly and pleasant relations, and instills value on socializing and supports overall good health

Social Cues & Rules

"Focus on how to Be social, not on how to Do social."
Jay Baer, American writer and digital market speaker

Treating people as individuals and not as groups exposes one to a wider range of social interactions and greatly enhances your chances of good health. Expanding the range and scope of your social interactions, increases the chances of functional connections and increases the (magnitude) of your mental and physical health. Hiding behind a computer sending out alias insults and rudeness to get the point across, while avoiding the consequences, has no value.

Social cues are the recognition of and response to the opportunities put in place, by both nature and society to encourage and enable socializing. Ingrained from infancy, the baby's recognition and response to the mother's smile, eye contact, response to cuddling, comforting sounds and touches, these actions are signals that promote development throughout childhood and adolescence. Any vacancy or lapse can signal antisocial behavior. Aberrant cues in the adult can make the difference between kindness and meanness.

Look at the individual, not the group. (*Dr. Martin Luther King, Jr "character not color".*) Avoid focusing on the group behavior. Stop choosing a small narrow range from which to make friends. Broaden your range, make friends outside your narrow group. Forego the mocking antisocial behavior that fuels certain groups, look at character, not appearance. Engage and the experience might surprise you.

Avoid too much alone time in favor of being with others. Loneliness is a state of mind and can be overcome by reaching out, interacting and (hopefully) connecting.

Volunteer whenever the opportunity arises. Helping others will lead to reciprocation and put you in contact with other like-minded volunteers. Giving meals to the elderly and doing community service will lead to interacting. Join a choir or a group that helps others. Meet and greet provides pleasantry and opportunities. Give something to someone daily.

Be passionate about something, dance, sports, stamps, gardening, cooking, cars, art, and music. Take the cue and use your talent to share with someone with similar interests.

Look into spirituality. Share with a close- knit group on the same spiritual level, like Bahai or Buddhism. Belong to a real spiritual community. Church groups serve both social and spiritual needs.

Be a good friend to the ones you have, quality over quantity. Do not criticize or ostracize your friends or may end up with none. Highlight what you like about your current friends and let them know it. Make someone laugh and you laugh yourself.

Family should be a priority over all others. In most cultures, it is an honor to care for parents and grandparents. Take as many meals together as possible. Visit. Arrange and go on shared outings and activities, and repeat trips to favorite destinations. Include, love and care for the elderly as the highest levels of social investment. Through natural selection, kinship prevails. We choose favored relatives to form groups based on trust in sameness to ensure cooperation and yet divergent enough to admit new DNA. In *Homo sapiens* as in nature, we require variety for the forward evolution of the group and its ultimate survival.

For the extended family and close friends, the importance of frequent invitations to share information and offer solutions should increase with age and is a reliable studied positive factor in cancer survival rates. Strong family ties of Italy, Greece, Portugal and Japan, where elders are included and respected, knowing that someone cares, are a boost to health, especially to Central Nervous System and

Immune system function. Regular socializing in a comfortable setting is good. The German, Kaffeeklatsch, (*from Klatschen, meaning to gossip*) and the British, "go sip", blend information with the local watering hole.

With relationships, you will never be alone.

Failure to make eye contact, looking away upon confrontation, high levels of electronic use, looking out the window on a commute, unable to speak coherently, speaking only of oneself, displaying limited knowledge, zero global awareness or concern for others, and unable to engage, maintain or follow up appropriately, are signs and cues of poor social skills.

Make use of cultural knowledge and language skills. English has two billion speakers. Use it to connect. Attempted interaction is more important than language perfection. Use a different idiom to communicate when necessary. The effort is appreciated (except perhaps in Russia and other "cold countries" that traditionally see foreigners as a threat.) Use your ability and make the effort to extend across cultures and adapt to styles and content that work to connect. Foreigners do it with us all the time.

Welcome diversity. Do not reject it. Language is important but "coping and adapting and persevering is more important". Open yourself to socializing with all "groups," even if you possess only a token knowledge. Learn Japanese etiquette of bowing, saving face, avoiding conflict, extreme politeness, punctuality, and respect for silence and each other. Examine the Scandinavians' politeness, cleanliness, bilingualism, Hygge and Lagrom comfort, and interest in world culture.

Differences are okay. It is the "appreciation" of the differences that count. Do not risk trying to be what you are not, but an appreciation and cursory understanding of the culture goes along way in making a connection.

Pick your environment, a place in which to socialize. The UK has pubs, France has cafes, Germany beer halls, and Greece restaurants. Some places have a history of saloons with an "atmosphere of exclusion" that developed into noting that "invites" socializing, except for a select few of the same people. Societies based on separation have difficulties with socializing, resulting in an epidemic of loneliness fostered by the society itself. A society that deals in hatred and threat and does not try to be polite, will invariably have to deal with poor health.

Management of Social Life

"I never had any friends later on like the ones I had when I was twelve." Stand by Me, 1986

Ageing "starts" anytime in adulthood, especially when you think you have "arrived" or feel affected by change. Life-changing events such as losing a loved one, changes in living arrangements, loss of previously reliable social connections, and contemplation of retirement generate feelings of uselessness. Loss of control over one's life and activities of daily living, loss of independence, driving, ambulation, responsibility for financial affairs, loss of Intimacy, long-term relationships, sex, age-related memory loss, onset of dementia, loss of privacy, subject to mistreatment, response to mistreatment, access to health care, attitude towards health care, paying for health care and preoccupation with failing health, all make deep cuts into one's social life.

As a group, most adult men do not do friends very well. (Women are much better). The competition for "toys", position and prestige, depending on the society's values, take up most available time. Friends were plentiful and became more difficult past the age of puberty.

Solution to sudden isolation involves the adoption of the six basic strategies of good health. Maintain healthy habits. Regular exercise, preferably with a group, and balanced healthy nutrition with good weight control is imperative. Buffer stress and keep mentally stimulated with solid social connections of like-minded friends with whom to share worries and concerns, special interest tours, cruises, and spas. (nationalgeographic.com/travel/sustainable) Keeping and maintaining good relations with family and friends stimulates the mind and provides security and freedom from the fear that ageing brings. Stay connected. Be positive. Read, do puzzles, relaxation and hobby workshops and classes. Volunteer and /or join groups. Teach your native language in a foreign country. (voluntourism.org)

Your management of social skills while ageing will determine your levels of social connections. The delivery of and response to "shaming" is one of the most common social experiences of ageing. What drives you to shame another? The answer lies in the insecurity of the shamer in transferring one's negative emotions to another. Self-confidence rids you of the need to bully or insult another. Have compassion. Find the spot that comes from experience in developing relationships, where a connection comes without conditions. Find that "sweet spot" on the basketball court from where every shot goes in with a soft "swish"; or the spot on the bat where every baseball goes over the fence; that spot on the wedge where to golf ball lofts high, lands and rolls into the cup; and the spot on the racquet where the tennis ball hots the corner line. That is the spot where connections and relationships merge into what leads to contentment and well-being, what is important in life.

Forgiveness plays a major role in stress control. Instead of punishing those who have done you wrong, get rid of emotional pain by ending cycles of hatred, fear, and thoughts of retribution. Use skills of mindfulness, empathy, compassion, and above all, compromise to reach a stage of resolution and absence of conflict

Gratitude is rewarding. Well-structured relationships (absence of source of stress) lead to mood improvement and stable health. The effect of giving and the effect of receiving with genuine appreciation are both positive experiences. (as opposed to selfishness, hoarding, resentment and indifference, sources of bad hormones that lead to poor health.)

Compassion has the power to change humans on all levels, physiological, emotional, neurological, and cellular). Sincere concern for the welfare of others can lead to better health within the human being and the society. It can change the way we express genes and lead to less stress, more "happiness", and better health.

Resentment in later years will kill you. Get rid of it! Constant release of stress hormones leads to reduced immune system function and premature death. (Remember that acute stress can and will strengthen the immune system and the sympathetic system, like when friends help in a crisis but only when turned off at the end of the triggering event.) Chronic stress leaves the system turned on, which leads to ruin and destruction.

The basic social skills of seniors are clear when you show up and listen well.

(Pardon the repetition, but some items are well worth repeating)

1. Engage. Use and improve your social skills.
2. Have a purpose, a goal, and pursue it.
3. Do as you say.
4. Make time for someone else.
5. Make no excuses.
6. Take the right path, not the easiest.

7. Ditch regrets, forgive yourself first.
8. Give up bad habits and hastily made choices. Think it out, weigh the input against the consequences.
9. Live your life, not someone else's.
10. Communicate with others and respect their views.
11. Enjoy your own company. Be able to use time for creativity and self-development.
12. Take responsibility. Invest time and effort in something worthwhile. Own it.
13. Give up on the wrong people. Holding on might make us seem strong, but letting go strengthens us.
14. Stop worrying and talking endlessly about money. Learn the concept of "enough".
15. Use up saved money. Reward the sacrifices made to earn it. It is not wise to invest at this time. Use it for peace and quiet or a loud raucous time, but enjoy it yourself. Don't worry about the financial situation of your children or grandchildren. You taught them. Now it's their own responsibility to take care of themselves.
16. Keep a healthy lifestyle. Get tested, stay informed.
17. Do not stress the petty stuff. Live in the present and future. Do not dwell in the past.
18. Keep up with the fashions appropriate to your age. Avoid reckless behavior.
19. Embrace the years, avoid bitterness and bitter people.
20. Respect the opinions of the younger generations; give advice, not criticisms. Help them realize that yesterday's wisdom still applies to today. Do not use worn phrases like "in my time", this time is yours too.
21. If you must live with children or grandchildren, keep your privacy. Visit often but maintain your own space.

22. Keep hobbies or make new ones. Travel, cook, hike, read, dance, have a pet, garden, play cards, dominoes or chess, golf, paint, volunteer, start a collection or spend time liking the one you have.

23. Accept invitations (even if you dislike it); baptisms, graduations, birthdays, weddings, conferences and leave the house. Visit museums, parks, and recreation areas.

24. Conversation: talk less and listen more. Avoid long stories and no complaints or criticisms. Accept situations as they are and find good things to say.

25. Smile, laugh and enjoy this age. Ignore what others say about you or what they think.

26. Pain and discomfort come with the numbers. Do not let it become the entire focus. Accept it as part of the life cycle.

27. Forgive whoever offended you and if you offended someone, apologize, and ask forgiveness. Do not hold on to resentment. *"A grudge is like taking poison and expecting the other person to die."* Forgive, forget, and move on. (*unless it was a huge offense, then enjoy the revenge*)

28. Savor your firm beliefs, but do not force them on others. Likewise, live your faith, not theirs.

29. Write things down, share knowledge, keep your memory sharp. Use the health effects of "journaling".

30. Avoid loneliness. Maintain existing relationships and form new ones.

*Happiness is when what you want, can get
and must do, are all the same thing.*

Social Solutions for the Youth

Already in possession of digital expertise, use these skills to interact and connect with others in positively. Make and keep new friends. Lean toward acquiring information and sharing rather than just "posting". Learn and practice basic manners in on- line greetings, salutations and sign-offs. At six feet apart and masked, may still "interact" and show courtesy. Seek and gain exposure by planning, engaging and interacting with those you know, then with others. Monitoring is in order, but the parent should not coddle, shield over-protect or otherwise obstruct the child from interacting. Facetime with grandparents and friends is important and so is interaction with others outside the family. "*It takes a village to raise a child*" still stands firm.

Social Solutions for Children

Expose them to people and ideas from outside the immediate family. Children learn speech and language skills from each other and from exposure to adults other than their parents. They need a wide range of exposure and frequent interaction. Depriving them of these contacts has a profound effect on their motor, mental and social development. The absence of knowledge and experiences from extensions of the family (aunts, uncles, cousins and grandparents) leads to a less than full understanding of morality and the mechanics of behaving in a functional society.

Manage the worldview with emphasis on the diverse society through mental stimulation as a basic strategy for good health. Instill and maintain feelings of connection with others. Do not allow them to be cut off. Use electronics, family, and neighbors to keep their minds anchored in reality.

Work on the social skills. Teach, drill, practice, re-cap and drill again. Children must be able to communicate and feel comfortable with others. They must learn and use basic manners in order to have a chance at socializing in later years.

Touch: Smiles and kind words accompanied with a hand-squeeze, a reassuring back- slap and a hug, go a long way in supporting still fragile psyches. The touch receptors are still immature and in need of positive stimulation and activity. The handshake is almost gone. Though lacking the physiological sensory input, the social implications of the fist bump and elbow rub remain.

Look for and identify signs of loneliness and failure to thrive from nutrition and exercise. Children are magnificent at adapting and getting back on track to good health. Being aware of the signs of depression, will help to guide and protect them from total isolation and associated disease. Maintain feelings of mental connection, even if the physical one has been reduced.

Social Skills in a Pandemic

When not allowed to gather, visit and touch freely, attend events where new people would be present (cafes, schools, bars, sports events, extended family events), or otherwise be deprived of the opportunities to practice one's social skills (speech, eye contact, body language), a significant part of the human physiognomy is gone. Expression and temperament that make up one's character is impaired, and for younger individuals the damage could be serious.

We rely on electronic devices to socialize for us. (Some people write better than others and some are more comfortable in front of the camera than others.) For basic manners, inclusion and acceptance, making connections, showing humanity, and managing, this medium is lacking.

Electronics may distort or misrepresent the truth and is prone to faulty interactions (not who you say you are) and deceptions. A few such encounters could lead to severe weakening of the social interaction process through a serious loss of trust. Virtual face-to-face loses the art of reading intentions, nuances of emphasis, loss of blush (shame), and expression of baser emotions. The level of satisfaction and gratification cannot compare to a face-to-face interaction in real time.

Interpreting the individual's nature is questionable. The Strange Case of Dr. Jekyll & Mr. Hyde, a Robert Louis Stevenson classic highlighting the duplicity of human nature (good & evil) in the same person and the prosocial vs antisocial, unstable, fearful, impulsive, emotionally swinging self- destructive character, can camouflage and deceive from end to end.

On Internet learning, the material may be there, but the instructor-student and peer interaction, influence, and participation cannot be replicated.

Negatives: Social distancing and quarantine, low frequency of encounters, engagements, and events, interrupts some interactions and connections and prevents others from occurring for the first time. The ongoing result is a loss of adequate mental and physical stimulation, reduced access to companionship, family and friends, intimacy, opportunities for new encounters, and overall independence. Reduced communication and disuse of social skills, though present before the pandemic, leads to a level of disconnection we never experienced before. The interruption leads to reduced learning, impetus to learn, misperceptions of threat and exaggerated hostility, indulgence in substance abuse and multiple medications, failure of self-care, child abuse, and disruption of the sense of community.

Physiologically, fear and anxiety promote the release of stress hormones (cortisol, norepinephrine, epinephrine), reduce the production of feel-good hormone (oxytocin, serotonin, dopamine), which reduce immune and metabolic system function (mainly cardiovascular, digestion, and cognition). Change uses a lot of energy and we become fatigued in trying to cope.

Physical loneliness (social isolation) is already the #1 global disability and cause of mental and physical decline, and the pandemic made it worse. It associates with hormonal changes (↑ cortisol and ↓ serotonin and dopamine) that lead to anxiety and depression, with signs and symptoms of homesickness and heartsickness. Grieving in the wake of the pandemic and the deadly effects of societal unrest have taken center stage. Under no circumstance should someone be made to grieve alone.

Loneliness is as lethal as obesity and smoking.

Depression promotes the release of stress-related inflammatory cytokines associated with immune system dysfunction, heart disease (arrhythmias, myocardial infarction, hypertension, congestive heart failure, COPD, and stroke), diabetes, cancers, dementias (vascular and Alzheimer's), neurodegenerative and autoimmune diseases: Systemic lupus erythematosus (SLE), multiple sclerosis (MS), amyotropic lateral sclerosis (ALS), enteritis, ulcerative colitis, celiac disease, irritable bowel syndrome, thyroiditis, psoriasis, and pernicious anemia.

The science of a broken heart

We compound antisocial behavior when fear and anxiety result in arrogance, greed, Selfishness, and any mistreatment of fellow humans. Stress affects the immune system by reducing the reaction to viruses, weakening the cellular response, disrupting function that results in the breakdown of tissues and organ systems and making the pandemic worse.

Late effects of isolation in a pandemic are breakdown in organ systems resulting in poor health, accelerated ageing, degenerative diseases, cognitive decline and premature death.

Cuddling of children is good, but "coddling" by overprotective parents while failing to instill basic manners and humane principles, can have detrimental effects on their development of useful social skills and ultimate independence.

Loss of contact with grandparents (knowledge, family history, warmth and continuity) through isolation and attrition(time-related), can lead to displacement and premature death.

Positives: The pandemic has the potential to and is bringing couples and families closer together when in the same vicinity with an increase in tolerance and understanding of the natural need of each other. Coping and enjoying each other's company, showing more empathy, compassion, patience, gratitude and appreciation of life and the senses (sight, sounds, smells, tastes and touch).

The tendency toward the development of healthy habits while reducing the bad ones, increasing awareness of the importance of a strong, functional immune system through good diet/nutrition, regular exercise, mental stimulation, social connections and avoidance of toxic exposures may help to prevent stress- related diseases.

Exercise, physical activity, walking, biking, aerobics, weight training, yoga, and tai chi, may give rise to new observations, experiences and acquaintances. The release of endorphins and serotonin provides a concentrated boost in mood. Working out is effective therapy, rage and envy are not. Focus your energy on the positive pole and discard the negativity.

Humor: laughter really is a marvelous medicine. Make up new jokes and recycle old ones. Stay open and positive. Try intergenerational and international humor.

Use the opportunity to develop new skills (or improve on old ones): cooking, art, construction, renovations, inventions, organization, and hobbies. Start and improve on digital technology skills for communication with others. Engage and maintain.

In pandemic limitations, our prosocial DNA moves toward helping each other, respecting distancing, wearing masks, good hygiene trying not to spread the virus, and promoting the common good. Antisocial DNA of not wearing masks, paying no attention to distancing, disrespecting the vulnerable, not staying away from contacts, estrangement from family, and belittling of fellow citizens comes from the fountain of self-interest being promoted in certain segments of the society. Exaggerated destructive behavior has a serious effect on individual and societal health. A reduction or absence of positive daily hormones, endorphins, oxytocin, serotonin, in the collective circulation leads to an increase in stress diseases, heart, hypertension, depression, and dementia in the whole community.

Individually, choosing to interact with others with kindness and caring and maintaining a positive attitude and healthy well-being is more desirable than pursuing the antisocial route and risking poor health with potential breakdown of the external and internal organism.

Social distancing reduces both family and group interactions. Use of electronics for communication, virtual visits, tours, learning, and entertainment are almost mandatory. Trying some of the old ways may not be such a bad idea. Go through old photo albums (online or virtual) and share, play games (emotional connections? love games? connection games?) We did not always have TV and movies. Stage a trivia night with different topics to broaden the world view. Cook together, same meal, different kitchens. Take online classes, join a book club and share. Take on- line dance lessons and workout classes.

The successful management of friendships indicates the strength of the friendship. Be able to list your trusted friends on both hands (should be six or more). Assure yourself they have your back at all times and that they know that you have their backs without expecting anything in return.

On social media devices: move away from devices and toward people, one at a time. Use electronics for information and a "definable" small group of regular friends and family. A thousand social media friends are not as valuable as your #4 real friend. Take uninterrupted time alone to regroup, organize, and reinforce purpose. Put away the device when in the company of others. Talk, express with your eyes and voice and body now more than ever.

Social limitations allow you to spend more time with the right people, quality over quantity, and to work on the development and delivery of your own special "character". Commit to updates. Take and hold others responsible for keeping in touch. Focus on the good times, maintain across geographical distances and be there for your friends.

"Socrates never had a phone". Ben Saase

"Home is the nicest word there is." Laura Ingalls Wilder

For Physicians: Getting to know your patient involves not only origin, family genetics and consumption history but also a thorough social history. How he or she relates and interacts determines his/her connections and has a significant impact on one's health. The degree of stress present has a huge effect on the metabolic status. Emotional needs and desires, presence or absence of trust, history of strong ties or destroyed ones carry the same import as habits, bad or otherwise. Assess the personality in degrees of social or antisocial and determine how it affects health.

In a Post Pandemic World: Some places have significant levels of success. The Singaporeans possess high social cohesion and trust in government (though only 30% downloaded the tracking app, 70%

declined). What worked so well to contain the numbers, was "proper human" response", high cooperation in testing, contact tracing, mask- wearing and social distancing. They trusted each other and their government to do the right thing. When everyone has value and recognizes it in his/her fellow human being, things can work.

Solution to the problem of antisocial behavior: Live up to the promise of social equality. Take every opportunity to reach out across community and cultural lines, widen the range of exposure and inter-action, increase your knowledge and be more "human".

Socializing is good for your health.

EPILOGUE

"The wealth of a civilized nation (is) the strength and resonance of social relations and bonds of social reciprocity that connect all people in common purpose."
Wade Davis, The Unraveling of America,
Rolling Stone , Aug 6, 2020.

Hoarding money and toilet paper and laying blame on "others" during an epidemic is a sure way of destroying mankind. Author

Reasonings

Narcissistic self-promotion or engagement? Attachments to one another or fences and barbed wire? Prosocial or antisocial behavior? Which one will determine the future of humanity?

Both the social and antisocial individuals are products of their biological makeups, experiences and expressions of their environments. Low stress, low toxicity exposure, low negativity, high social connections, balanced diet and ample physical activity can and will promote togetherness and good health.

Every human being is worth at least a simple greeting. And when you take the time and make to effort to listen and interact, it shows that you value that person. Ignoring or otherwise showing indifference to another human indicates devaluation and is never good.

Chapter one is an appeal to one's curiosity, to tap into one's scientific and humanities knowledge and establish the importance of socializing to the essence of being human. Socializing releases feel-good hormones and was the dominant behavior of the pre-settler, nomadic humans. Antisocial behavior releases and is promoted by chronic stress hormones of fear and anger and are the initial innate dominant behavior of later more settled early humans. Feel-good hormones (oxytocin, serotonin, dopamine) give positive feedback from good intentions and positive activity, that give us empathy, compassion, kindness, altruism, leading to cooperation, productivity, sharing, all essential for survival in ancient times.

Feel-bad hormones (cortisol, epinephrine, norepinephrine) in high doses, repeated releases and for prolonged periods have detrimental effects on one's health by compromising the immune system, nerve, muscle and eventually all organ systems. Man can be kind and/or cruel, depending on genetics and their expression. Mental and physical pain use the same neural pathways. Cognition, compassion, empathy, and kindness are essential elements for survival and produce morality, trust, cooperation and collaboration. Meanness, cruelty, hostility, humiliation is prevalent in modern human activities and promote the acquisition of wealth and power as the sole purpose in life. The resulting inequality leads to antisocial behavior from both sides.

Chapter two is an attempt to elicit those feel-good hormones that friendship and welcoming behavior stir up. The health benefits of social connections, kinships, acquaintances, friendships, kindness to strangers, include nutrition (digestion, absorption), exercise (endorphins, circulation), mental stimulation, avoidance of toxins and toxic behavior, and stress control that promote and improve human function, prevent depression and increase the quality of life.

Being connected and healthy increases longevity. Though in-person, face-to-face interactions are best, connecting by technology also works.

Chapter three releases those feel-bad hormones of antisocial behavior. Inflicting rudeness, hostility, and humiliation upon others may give the perpetrator a brief chemical lift, but the feedback and repercussions are detrimental to both mental and physical well-being. When snobbery, the Us vs Them conflict, materialism, selfishness, self-interest and antisocial behavior dominate and are mistakenly assumed to be essential for success of the individual, the effects of chronic stress hormones will eventually lead to a dysfunctional societal life. The behavior of the society is a direct reflection of its soul. We need each other to survive. Others can hurt and damage our chances of success. Antisocial heartlessness, unchecked, spawns and maintains wars and elements of destruction in societies that continue today.

Chapter four, Social Experiences, connects us with storytelling and global examples of human behavior with which we can relate. Nature exists in positive and negative polarity, and so do human beings. People have both good and bad genes that make good and bad hormones. The good hormones are present at birth and are prominent and innate as beneficial to society. Expression of bad hormonal behavior is learned by bad influences associated with material gain and self-interest. Pro-social and anti-social behavior are influenced disproportionately by the environment and specific situations. Human failure to treat each other with respect and kindness is giving rise to antisocial behavior as the new normal. Empathy and Xenophobia can exist in the same person, in the same society and in the same country. Which one emerges depends on the environment, history and circumstances.

In a Pandemic, social DNA is helping each other, respecting distancing, wearing masks, practicing good hygiene and trying not to spread the virus in promoting the common good. Antisocial DNA is not wearing masks, no attention to distancing, disrespecting the vulnerable, promoting self-interest, staying away from contacts, estrangement, and refusing to get vaccinated. Certain societies and countries perform much better than others.

Chapter five provides instructions and protocols on how to initiate and improve social skills, premised by the fact that: One can learn and perfect effective social skills despite a pandemic.

Good health requires a nutritious diet, adequate exercise, stress control, mental stimulation, avoidance of exposure to toxins, and solid social connections. (the 6 basic strategies) In the United Nations Great Assembly Hall (New York City), there is a tapestry, which reads "Human beings are members of a whole, in creation of one essence and soul. If one member is afflicted with pain, other members uneasy will remain." Written by the Persian poet, Saádi Shirazi in 1250 AD and cited by President Barack Obama in his memoir, A Promised Land (2020). A high prevalence of connections is good for global health. Without them, the world may become more disconnected and move further backwards.

All my books have a unified theme: that each of us has value; everyone is worth something. With Social Connections and your Health, everyone deserves at least a greeting or acknowledgement that he/she exists. Every human being is a part of a complex multitude of organisms, the microbiome. Each individual contributes to the health and well-being of the whole. It is difficult to put an exact value on social connections, so this book attempts to present the highs and lows. It is a commodity that is difficult to measure, to quantify, so "quality" more than quantity is emphasized. As expected, more questions arise that there are answers.

How many friends does one need to avoid loneliness? How many and what quality of friends? Are two good friends worth as much as four so-so friends? Are the social connections of a 20- year-old that much different than those of an 80- year- old?

When we refuse to speak with each other, refuse to interact,
refuse to acknowledge each others' value, there is no connection.
One group starts killing the "other", which will retaliate and the
killing will continue until there is no one left. Sound familiar?

I must emphasize the importance of socializing within and across diverse lines. It may take a lot of coaxing and impressing that friendliness is good for physical and mental health and is ultimately essential for the survival of the species. Tapping into the natural urge to meet, greet and accommodate offers far better outcomes than to meet, feel threatened, inflict harm and pursue the elimination of that which is perceived as a threat... (and take possession of whatever they had). Sound familiar, as in colonialization, exploitation, racism, exclusion, and genocide.

This fear of human diversity is a purely antisocial phenomenon. Africans & Muslims coming to Europe, brown Mexicans coming to USA, eliciting deep feelings of animosity and fear. One would think we would have gotten away from this nonsensical behavior by now, but those who know better (educated professionals) still separate and group people by skin color,

("Blacks" and "Whites" mentioned on USA news daily as if they are separate species; medical records start with identification of the patient as black or white, an assessment made by a clerk) and participate and condone separation and negative interaction.

Not a Good Outcome by any standards

If we fail to establish genuine positive connections in an
individual, national and global basis, the negativity will destroy
us all... mentally and physically, from the inside and out.

How long will it be before *Homo sapiens* truly obtains and retains enough wisdom to realize that all humans are the same race, tribe and people and stop with the hatred, indifference and social injury. We have been loving and killing each other for several million years. How much longer do we have to evolve and in what direction for the antisocial behavior to stop. Which way will we choose on the management of social interaction, a smile or a gun? Are we going to define our humanity as based on "every man for himself" into which destruction is hard wired or as a system of social bonding and issue-solving for the common good that boosts the chances of survival and stress-free comfort of the species? The latter is a far better choice. Caring about each other as human beings, irrespective of differences, will be a great contribution to world health.

Of the ideals of societies, Liberty, Equality and Fraternity, only the last embodies the principles of inclusion, trust, cooperation, and community. Socially, it is the noblest and the most difficult to achieve. Humans are social, relying heavily on interactions that lead to bonding to connections in building communities and functioning through effort and reward. When these social ties are not allowed to form (as in USA segregation and discrimination), or are broken, the fabric of the society weakens and eventually breaks. It is pathetic that some people are still marching in protest of not being treated fairly and others can storm and occupy their state and national capitals and receive a slap on the wrist and a pat on the back. I thought the species was better than this. But.

A society needs intelligent cooperation to survive intact, to overcome a pandemic, and to resolve life or death issues on tribal identification or risk collapse. Author

Summary Points:
1. Social behavior and health are closely interconnected.

2. On the progression from hunter-gatherer egalitarianism in which engagement, movement, interaction and cooperation were essential traits, to indigenous societies with tendency to exclude, isolate, wall off for protection (and to keep members in), to selfish agrarian society with me- me mentality, severance of connections with "others", between members within the society and with nature.

3. From cooperation to conflict, from kindness to competitive cruelty, from charity to theft. Market and economic demands reduce the need for compassion, brotherly love and cultural solidarity to the detriment of social relations. The change from social to antisocial behavior is becoming the dominant force.

4. The splitting and disunity of humanity into dominant and submissive parts, the failure to socialize properly that ensures participation of all, for the good of all shifts the advantage to the few that will do anything to keep that domination.

5. Social behavior depends on the expression of biological genes driven by economic needs (survival) and cultural norms. As the latter outperforms the former, as humans are responsible for our own social behavior, we can change it, to something better.

6. Human social behavior depends on the degree of morality and self-interest in human reaction to our economy-based material world. We face a choice once more of using social skills to uphold humanity or continuing in pursuit of the perfect unequal world that favors the strong few against the weaker many and speculate on exactly when the machines will take over.

7. With Whom do we socialize? We have a broad range (quantity) and narrow range (quality). Choose the best in each group. The number of trusted friends needed for good health

(3-4), number of good acquaintances (30-40). Self-worth is a big determining factor.

8. Snobbery, envy, exclusion, initially link more to mental health than to physical, in that negative feelings and displays appear to be on the surface. Eventually they seep into the psyche and are detrimental to general health. Insincerity and condescendence release both feel- good and feel bad hormones. The chronicity does the damage. (The hypocrisy of evangelical Christians releases feel- good hormones only if the hypocrisy is truly believed).

> *"We are all in the gutter, but some of us are looking at the stars." Lady Windermere's Fan.*

Basic Social Skills: Adherence to the Golden Rule would change the face of social interactions tremendously. *"Do unto others as you would have them do unto you"...Luke 6:31,* is the essence of social management. Self- worth is based on give and take, equally, and on being humane as a human being. A society that is balanced would encourage the obliteration of "lines" between people, join the Us and the Them, and remove the fear of "others", and still promote the safety and survival of all. Interact.

Make Your Own Blue Zone

Arrange to live in your own Blue Zone. Adopt and adhere to all six basic strategies of lifestyle for good health, practice social skills and reduce stress levels to close to zero. (Ikaria)

Use the Protocol for the Six Basic Strategies of Good Health in the Appendix

"Everyone you meet has something valuable to teach you." (take a little time to listen for their communication might just increase your ultimate survival Author

The Future of Social Relations

With the New world Order, globalization and entry of 2.5 billion people into the world economy and geopolitics renewal of networks and collaborations, <u>connections</u> are of increasing importance. One of these days, humanity will evolve and be able to see past the class and status erected in the Neolithic Age of agriculture and material possessions, and past the assignments of place by skin color of the 16th and 17th centuries and past the social upheavals of the 20th and 21st centuries. There will come a time when superficial features do not hold as much weight as they do now, and we can appreciate the enormous value of each person. And the importance of one's life will be judged in terms of how and with whom did you connect, help and love. Or, the time will come when Social Engineering takes over and we lose what it means to be truly human. Like in the Brave New World of Aldous Huxley, who without opinions or individuality, and the obsession with achieving happiness, the humans were deprived of any meaningful relationships. We are rapidly approaching these goals and processes with our pill-popping culture and social media zombies... Unlike BNW we are being controlled by fear and emotions. Our happiness is rooted in enjoyment of material possessions in solitary. We are made content with self-medicated happiness that Prozac and Zoloft provide while our urges for the pleasures of bad behavior are stemmed by alcohol, Ritalin and Quizlet. And our out-of- control social media thrives on emotional slogans, worship of celebrity airheads and absence of reason because it takes too much effort to attain. Friendships are too difficult to forge and do not provide the same rewards that forging enemies brings.

To achieve these goals, with social engineering you buy a brain, genetically manipulated to create "good and happy" and digitally maintained to provide happiness by rejecting neighbors and others that might be an inconvenience to one's "feelings". The science of relationships will be replaced by technological idiocy of artificial reward for the lack of relationships.

Human value or artificial happiness, social or
antisocial beings, we have the choice

APPENDIX

FEATURES OF HUMAN BEHAVIOR

SOCIAL	ANTISOCIAL
Compassion	Heartlessness
Kindness	Meanness
Compersion	Envy
Empathy	Snobbery
Altruism	Selfishness
Acceptance	Fear
Forgiveness	Revenge
Diversity acceptance	Racism
Equality/Sharing	Privilege
Community	Social separation

APPENDIX B

RECOMMENDED STRATEGIES FOR GOOD HEALTH THROUGH A BLUE ZONE LIFESTYLE

Based on six strategies for good health,
from Natural Health and Disease Prevention...
Alfred L. Anduze, MD

1. **DIET** is Nutrition... balanced: proteins, carbohydrates and fats; fresh food, organic, HOW we eat, dining (vs US fast food, restaurant's quick turnover) together, sit and converse and digest; high Quality is better than quantity lower the incidence of GI tract issues (associated with stressors)
2. **EXERCISE**: keep moving, walking, purposeful movements, biking, rowing, swimming, hiking up and down hills, hiking, nature walks
3. **STRESS RELIEF**: best = avoidance, low incidence, attitude towards time is healthy, 4. Sleep, relaxation, home coziness, Hygge and Lagrom, don't inconvenience anyone else, seek

contact, communication, Nap, siesta and good sound sleep experience

4. **MENTAL STIMULATION** : increase reading, seek information from multiple sources (books, internet, classes, and from each other: develop and maintain a strong life purpose

5. **SOCIAL** CONNECTIONS : *very strong…* low inequality -> low separation, Inclusive societies, (not exclusive like in USA); Communicate (multilingual !!!), Social skills, smile and make eye contact, Trust and unity Education systems = *strong*

6. **TOXINS AVOIDANCE**: clean environments, aware of and against chemicals and processed and refined just for profits; their medicines are natural >>> pharmaceutical; Health care is clean and equal access as a right;

APPENDIX C

SOCIAL CONNECTIONS PROTOCOL

Goal: To provide confidence on an encounter, upon starting an interaction and following through with making a connection.

1. Self-confidence (reduce internal social anxiety (internal) , reduce external stress, increase sense that you belong there, achieve feeling of satisfaction
2. Social Skills... work on basic manners, approach, body language (non-verbal), be engaging not threatening; inclusive, not shutting anyone out, show openness, comfort, be appropriate to specific situations
3. Communication Skills ... Eye Contact, Nod, Smile, use verbal ability, appropriate mode of expression, share knowledge and experience without boasting
4. Social Interactions ... increase frequency of encounters, increase range of Interactions (cross cultural) -> diversity improves chances of success, openness to friendships
5. Social Connections trusted friendships take time and work -> increase sustained release of feel good hormones, give more than you take -> good health

APPENDIX D

PROTOCOL FOR LONGEVITY

Six Basic Strategies for Good Health
Greece, Ikaria: 33% of population lives to >>90 y/o
Italy, Acciareli 10% of population is >>100 y/o

Featuring social connections

1. Social Connections: the brain produces and releases endorphins & tryptophans, the GI tract produces serotonin, & cortisol inhibitors. Successful social interactions -> reduced cortisol response -> reduced inflammation-> low heart disease, dementia, cancer and diabetes

2. Stress Control: positive mood, attitude, emotions, avoid stressful situations, quality time with family & friends, hobbies, pass the time doing useful purposeful things Icarian Greeks excel at "Stress Control and Social Interactions"....with frequent social activities: dancing, dining, festivities, community, spending quality time together -> regeneration of body, mind & spirit -> slows ageing process...

   Emotional/physiological & psychological rewards of "togetherness"

   No moneyed hierarchy; shared materials & shared time

Value = acknowledgement, interest & investment in other human beings

Sense of Belonging, spiritual community, total involvement

Family = priority, the highest degree of socialization

Sense of connection (everyone knows your business & looks out for you)

Sense of responsibility, reciprocity; Group is "us" not "me". No one is alone.

3. Diet: fresh local in season vegetables, fish, red wine, herbal teas & plant spices -> good digestive enzymes (variety of food types) + Social Dining: Mediterranean diet = olive oil, garlic, onions, fruit, vegetables, fish, hydration, Vitamins B12,& D for brain function, , C for immune system, protein to keep muscle, plus turmeric to prevent inflammation

4. Exercise: walk daily, bone and muscle strength, dancing: keep circulation high -> avoid dementias, db, osteoporosis, heart disease from arteriolarsclerosis, cancer ; work the garden forever

5. Mental Stimulation: -> conversation, puzzles, read, write, discussions, news, art, creativity, travel... Always have plan for the future.

6. Avoid all risky behavior, pollutants, toxins (kitchen alum foil, canned goods, processed food, too many medications, do not smoke or drink alcohol to excess...

APPENDIX E

SOCIETY BUILDING SOLUTIONS

1. Socialize/ ↑ social interactions between ethnic ally diverse groups, between rich and poor, between religions, between educated and uneducated…
2. Limit the separation/segregation
3. Dispel communication problems / learn to communicate
4. Dispel subjective problems / hang ups
5. Dispel belonging problems / who belongs and who doesn't (all are equal human beings)
6. Include/ stop excluding "others"
7. Recognize the similarities / ignore the differences (all humans are more alike than different)
8. Get your self-worth from interacting/ sharing/ participating
9. Realize that your health is closely associated with your social attitudes and connections
10. Stop the Separation of people based on everything or anything

APPENDIX F

SOCIAL SOLUTIONS FOR ISOLATED YOUTH & CHILDREN

1. Digital expertise: learn and use to interact and connect with others in a positive manner; keep and make new friends. Lean toward acquiring information rather than posting.
2. Basic Manners: learn and use. Practice on line and whenever in contact with others; At 6 feet apart, you can still interact" and show politeness.
3. Exposure: plan and do engage and interact with others; Parent should not coddle or shield or obstruct the child from interaction. Facetime with grands and friends is important and so is interaction with others outside the family. "It takes a village to raise a child" still stands firm.
4. Children learn speech and vocabulary from other children and extended family adults. Conversation is important.
5. Morality instruction and demonstration is essential for teaching how to behave in a society.
6. Social Skills instruction and practice: Courtesy and Politeness are essential to social interactions
7. Watch for signs of and avoid Loneliness (Depression) at all costs.

APPENDIX G

SOCIAL SOLUTIONS FOR SENIORS

1. Keep good relations with family and friends, stimulates the mind and provides security and freedom from fear that aging brings. Stay connected. Upgrade and maintain the quality of present companionship. It is mandatory that one not be "alone" in later years.

2. Cope with change, accept life-changing events, retirement, loss of companions, change in living arrangements, loss of control over one's life and activities of daily living,

3. Be kind to others as to your own; Take an interest, smile, include, engage, interact and expand your range.

4. Use social media and digital devices to communicate with family and old friends, and make new ones; Use to gather information and share; keep learning. Interact with the experts, the youth, for updates and new technology.

5. Positive outlook; half-full glass; show gratitude and appreciation; set goals and purpose, keep or make new career(s). Use this as a chance to improve your health.

6. Get rid of Negative thoughts, can't do's, old hatreds, notions of revenge

7. Exercise, walking, biking, stretches, weights, moderate sports; (serotonin and endorphin mood boosting producers and cardiac health); get sunshine 15 to 20 minutes daily. It is healthy and stimulates the senses.

8. Follow Nutrition requirements of a balanced diet (protein, carbohydrates and fats) local and fresh where possible, ensure that your vitamin and mineral intake is sufficient; Be aware of the health benefits of turmeric (anti-inflammatory mood booster, B vitamins for continued growth and normal metabolism, and magnesium for lowering stress response. Reduce salt and sugar intake, metabolism is more important than taste. Balance your gut bacteria to ensure good digestion and elimination.

9. Do not dwell on medical problems, make sure to have access to healthcare; address and take care of yourself; keep appointments, avoid taking excess medications, be aware of indications and side effects, ask and do; Use available treatment hotlines as "psychological first aid" when you feel in need of help. Use telemedicine for explanations and simple but essential prescriptions.

10. Volunteer: Make time to join organizations and interact with others and make a difference no matter the impact.

11. Acknowledgement and acceptance of pandemic losses and grieve for a lost year(s). Loss of contacts, planned vacations, and special events (birthdays, proms, parades, holiday travel, sports) and being grateful for the health of family and friends, developing new skills, gaining knowledge and making new contacts are all good for mental health.

APPENDIX H

SOCIAL CONNECTIONS & YOUR HEALTH SURVEY E

(circle or check your response)

Feel-Good hormones are released when you are happy and relaxed (*dopamine, serotonin, oxytocin, endorphins*) and "bad" hormones released when you are sad, alone, angry, depressed, helpless (*cortisol, epinephrine, adrenalin, H+ ions, reactive oxidative species).* Good hormones promote good health and bad hormones promote sickness, high inflammation, damage organs and shorten life. *Answer : Yes or No Neh or Oxi*

1. Do you prefer to be with family?   friends?   both?

2. Do you prefer to be with Parents?   Grandparents?
    Is this Natural?   by Tradition?   by Choice?

3. **Respect:** Which do you RESPECT more?
    Parents or Grandparents?   or both?
    Do you give attention if they are sick?   More   Less
    Do you give attention if they are healthy?   More   Less
    Do you give attention when they are older?   More   Less
    (is there any stress attached to ageing?)

4. **Religion & Spirituality** play important parts in your health.
   Do you attend church Every week?   Sometimes?   Never?
   Do you follow the teachings of Jesus on brotherhood, kindness
   to strangers & helping others?   Yes   No

5. **Loneliness:** Do you know any people who <u>prefer</u> to be alone?
   Yes   No
   Are loners considered to be losers?   Yes   No
   Are loners unfortunate & have no support?
   Are loners insecure & alone by choice?

6. **Peer group behavior:** Do you follow European & American
   fads?   Yes   No
   a) Internet news   b) Electronic devices
   c) fashions   d) traditional or global news

7. **Exercise:** preference for …(*check as many as you do*)
   a. Sport   active work
   b. Planned   walk gymnasium
   c. Dance   (*how often & how much energy do you expend?*)
                              low / medium/ very high

8. **Female** social support network is better than male & is based on
   "Trust". (*check as many as you believe are true*)
   a. Women express feelings better _____
   b. Women have "inner circle" security (individual reliability)

   _____

   c. Women have outer circle support (+ group friends)

   _____

   d. Women have greater circle support (+ male friends)

   _____

9. **Men** have pals, companions, colleagues, but few 'friends". A man's best friend is most likely to be a woman.   a. Yes or No
   b. Is it Natural or Traditional?

10. Liking "Others" /**Strangers**/ someone of a different nationality. (*Filoxenia*)
    a. Is it Natural for you?   b. Is it Curiosity?
    b. Is it Traditional/ Custom?   c. Visitors okay?
    d. Migrants okay?

11. **Strength of Friendships**/ Your Group *of friends*?
    a. Is it Natural?   b. Is it Traditional?
    c. Do you stick together no matter what?
    d. Would you do anything (within reason) for a friend?
    e. Do you turn against each other (*easily?*)   (*with difficulty?*)

12. *Do you have ONE FRIEND that you can share your heart with, and be perfectly sure that it is safe.?*   Yes   No

13. **How do YOU control Stress?** (*aware of the biochemical reaction?*)
    a. Accept (pray & forgive)   b. Adapt (cope)
    c. Alter (change your response)   d. Avoid

14. **Relocation**: Given the opportunity and access, would you live anywhere else? Where?

15. Objective: Self- Assessment
    Your Level of Feel-Good hormones vs Your Level of Stress hormones:
    High   High
    Medium   Medium
    Low   Low

Ónoma: (*optional*)_____

Ilikía: _____

Katochi: _____

Ithagéneia: _____

APPENDIX I

SOCIAL SKILLS PROTOCOL

1. SELF-CONFIDENCE make sure you are prepared, healthy and willing to engage
2. EYE CONTACT upon greeting and during a conversation
3. BODY LANGUAGE "how" you say it is as important as what you are saying; use non-verbal cues, like a smile or a frown, or accompanied with a sigh or a laugh; be accepting, not rejecting; On the rebound, show interest in what someone else is saying; address the person as the most important item at that moment.
4. BASIC MANNERS. greet, be assertive and respectful, not aggressive. Do not ignore a greeting. Return the greeting in an "open" manner, not closed or offensive, or hostile. It is insulting and neglectful to "ignore" the presence of another person in a small, shared space.
5. COMMUNICATION: face-to-face skills. Issue an idea or an opinion with immediate feedback, emphasize your point by body language, tone, content, see the reaction, the emotion, the feelings… learn the language or at least parts of it, to show respect; acknowledge the presence and value of another.
6. INTERACTION mindset, be positive, inclusive, considerate and accepting; pleasant to be around, not criticize, not defensive or self-pitying, doubtful or sour; be flexible, cooperative, open

to learning, be respectful to and of others, it will be returned, show class and intelligence, admiration and honor, avoid airs of superiority; be humble and mindful; especially to and with elders

7. INCLUDE/ACCEPT reach out for encounters, expand your range, access and opportunities; do not exclude

8. CONNECTIONS seek like-minded but exclude no one because of differences, everyone is an opportunity for a connection, look for surprising benefits; all friendships have value.

9. BE HUMAN & HUMANE be liked as you, flexible and happy, positive and inclusive, welcoming and open; When you list all the qualities you want in a relationship, make sure you have the same qualities to offer. (not aggressive, self-centered, arrogant, unwilling to compromise)

10. MANAGE RELATIONSHIPS establishing and keeping friendships takes quality time and is well worth the effort, maintain contact, interest, and focus on giving

APPENDIX J

FUTURE OF SOCIAL RELATIONSHIPS

1. New World Order entry of additional 2.5 billion people into the economy and geography

2. Egalitarianism or Self-interest materialism

3. Pro-Social or Antisocial behavior

4. Natural or Self-medicated happiness

5. Natural relationships or Socially engineered matching

REFERENCES

Achor, Shawn: The Happiness Advantage: How a Positive Brain Fuels Success in Work and Life. 2010

Alexander, Richard D. The Evolution of Social Behavior. Annual Review of Ecology, Evolution and Systematics. Vol.5:325-363, Nov. 1974. Museum of Zoology and Dept of Zoology, University of Michigan, Ann Arbor,

Andrews, Bill. Social Skills: Build self-confidence, manage shyness, and make friends. 2018

Anduze, Alfred: In Search of a Stress-Free Life, (*biochemistry and physiology of stress hormones*), Yorkshire Publishers, Aug 2017

Appiah, Kwame Anthony: The Lies That Bind: Rethinking Identity; creed, country, color, class, culture: Liveright Publishing Corporation, Aug 20, 2019

Armstrong, Sue: Borrowed Time: the science of how and why we age. Bloomsbury Sigma, Jan 24, 2019

Barlow, Julie & Nadeau, Jean-Benoit; he Bonjour Effect: the secret codes of French conversation revealed. St Martin's Press, NY, 2016

Bernier, Olivier: Pleasure and Privilege: Life in France, Naples and America , 1770-1790. New Word City, 2018

Boehm, Christopher: Moral Origins: The Evolution of Virtue, Altruism, and Shame. Basic Books, Perseus Book Group, 2012

Borland, J.M. etal ...Albers H.B. (2018): Sex-dependent regulation of social reward by oxytocin receptors in the ventral segmental area. Neuropsychopharmacology, 1.

Bregman, Rutger: Humankind: A Hopeful History. Little, Brown & Company, June 2, 2020

Brookes, S.K., etal: The psychological impact of quarantine and how to reduce it: rapid review of the evidence. The Lancet. Vol.395, March 14, 2020, p. 912.

Brown, Brene: Daring Greatly: and The Gifts of Imperfection Buettner, Dan: The Blue Zones, 2nd edition: 9 lessons for living longer from the people who've lived the longest. National Geographic, Nov 6, 2012

Buisman-Pijlman, et al, The role of oxytocin in positive affect and drug-related reward. Pharm Biochem and Behavior, vol 119, pg 1-88, Apr 2014

Buttigieg, Pete. Trust:America's best chance. Liveright Publishing Corporation, 2020

Christakis, NA and Fowler JH, The Spread of Obesity in a large Social Network over 32 years. Jul 2007 *NEJM Vol 357:370-379*

Christakis, NA, Blueprint: The Evolutionary Origin of a Good Society. Little , Brown Spark Mar 26, 2019

Cacioppo, John T & Patrick, William. Human Nature and the Need for Social Connection. Neuroscience, Aug 10, 2009

Cohen, S. etal. Social Ties and Susceptibility to a common cold. 1997. Journal of the American Medical Association, 25, p1940-1944

Conrad, Peter. The Medicalization of Society: On the Transformation of Human Conditions into treatable disorders. Johns Hopkins University Press, 1st edition, June 11, 2007

Cozolino, Louis. The Healthy Aging Brain: Sustaining Attachment, Attaining wisdom (Norton 2008)

Dawkins, Richard. The Selfish Gene: University Press, 40th edition August 1, 2016 deWaal, Frans.The Age of Empathy: Nature's Lessons for a Kinder Society, Broadway Books, Sept 7, 2010

Dfarhud D, et al. Happiness and Health: The Biological Factors: Systemic Review article. Iranian Journal of Public Health. Nov 2014

Doyle, William. Aristocracy: A very short introduction. Oxford University Press, Nov 25, 2010.

Dunbar RI and Schultz S. Evolution in the Social Brain. Sci 317 (2007) British Academy of Centenary Research

Epstein, Joseph: Snobbery: The American Version. Mariner 1/1/2002

Figes, Orlando. The Europeans,: Three Lives and the Making of a Cosmopolitan Culture. Metropolitan Books. Oct 8, 2019

Fuller Torrey, E. (MD) Evolving Brain, Emerging Gods: Early Humans and the Origins of Religion. Columbia University Press, Sept 5, 2017

Giles LC, Glonek GFV, Luszcz MA, Andrews GR. Effect of social networks on 10- year survival in very old Australians: the Australian longitudinal study of aging. *J Epidemiol and Community Health 2005:* 59:574-579; doi: 10.1136.jech.2004.025429

Gladwell, Malcolm. Talking to Strangers. Little, Brown and Company, Sept 2019

Graeber, David. The First 5000 years, Melville House, 2011

Harvard Study of Adult Development: Can Relationships boost longevity and well-being? Harvard Gazette. https://news.harvard. edu June 2017

Harwood, Jake. Communication and Music in Social Interaction. Cognella Academic Publishing. Oct 20,2017

Henderson, L and Zimbardo, P. Shyness, social anxiety and social anxiety disorder. Social Anxiety: Clinical, Developmental and Social Perspectives. 2010;2:65-92.

Hills, Susan. Loneliness no more; a comprehensive guide to break free from loneliness, social isolation and depression forever. May 6, 2015

Keltner I, etal. The Compassionate Instinct: The Science of Human Goodness. W.W.Norton & Co, Inc. (2010)

Kochilas, Diane: Ikaria; Lessons on Food, Life, and Longevity from the Greek Island where people forget to die. Rodale Books, Oct 14, 2014

Kroenke C H, Kubzansky LD, Schernhammer ES, Holmes MD, Kawachi I. Social networks, Social Support, and Survival after Breast Cancer Diagnosis. *J of Clinical Oncology,* Vol 24, No 7 (March 1), 2006: pp. 1105-1111. Doi: 10.1200/ JCO.2005.04.2846

Lieberman, MD. Social: Why Our Brains are wired to Connect. Crown Publishers, New York. 2013.

Loucks, EB, Sullivan LM, D'Agostino RB, Berkman LF, Benjamin EJ, *Science Daily,* May 2, 2005. Social Connections: Could Heartwarming be Heart-Saving?

MacMillan, Margaret. War: How Conflict Shaped Us. Random House, Oct 6, 2020

Marantz, Andrew. AntiSocial. Viking/ Penguin Random House. 2019

Martin LJ, et al. *Curr Biol. 2015.* Reducing social stress elicits emotional contagion of pain in mouse and human strangers.

Martin LJ, Tuttle AH, Mogil JS. The Interaction between pain and social behavior in humans and rodents. –NCBI *Curr Top Behav Neurosci. 2014*

Miller, Madeleine. Song of Achilles: A Novel. Harper Collins, 2012

Mithen, Steven J. The Singing Neanderthals: The Origins of Music, Language, Mind and Body. Harvard University Press. 2006.

Murray J, etal. Risk factors for Antisocial behavior in low and middle income Countries: A Systematic Review of Longitudinal Studies. Crime and Justice(Chicago, Ill) 2018 Mar 26; 47(1):255-364

Orth-Gomer, K, Rosengren A, Wilhelmsen L. Lack of social support and incidence of coronary heart disease in middle-aged Swedish men. *Psychosomatic Medicine, 1993*, Vol 55, Issue I 37-43.

Olds, J & Schwartz RS : The Lonely American: Drifting Apart in the Twenty-first Century. Boston: Beacon Press, 2009

Pappas, Stephanie. The Social Mind: Brain Region bigger in Popular People. Live Science, Jan 31, 2012.

Powell J, et al. Orbital Prefrontal Cortex volume predicts social network size: An Imaging Study of Individual Differences in Humans. Proc Royal Soc B: Biol Sci 279 (2012)

Putnam, Robert D. Bowling Alone. Simon & Schuster, Aug 1, 2001.

Reich, David: Who we are and How we got here: Ancient DNA and the New Science of the Human Past. Pantheon Books, New York. 2018

Reeves, Richard V.: Dream Hoarders: How the American Upper Middle Class is Leaving Everyone Else in the Dust, why That is a Problem, and What to Do About It. (Social Mobility) Brookings Institution Press, 2017

Reich, Robert: The Common Good. Vintage Books, New York. Feb 20, 2018

Ridley, Matt: The Origins of Virtue: Human Instincts and the Evolution of Cooperation. Penguin Books New York, NY, 1996

Rutledge RB, et al. Dopaminergic Modulation of Decision Making and subjective well-being J. Neuroscience. 2015

Sapolsky, Robert M. Behave: The Biology of Humans at our Best and Worst. Penguin Books, New York. 2017.

Saase, Ben: Them: why we hate each other...and how to heal. St Martin's Press, NY. 2019

Schwartz, Barry. The Battle for Human Nature: Morality and Modern Life. August 17, 1987. W.W.Norton & Company

Seyfarth, Robert M. and Cheney, Dorothy L. The Evolutionary Origins of Friendship, Annual Review of Psychology, January 2012. University of Pennsylvania.

Slater, Phillip. The Pursuit of Loneliness. Beacon Press, 3rd edition, July 1, 1990

Small R, et al. The Power of Social Connection and support in improving health: lessons from social support interventions with childbearing women. BMC Public Health 2011

Spitzberg, BH, Cupach, WR (2002). Interpersonal Skills. In Knapp, ML & Daly, JA (2002), *Handbook of interpersonal communication*. Thousand Oaks, CA: Sage publications.

Thackeray, William Makepeace: Book of Snobs (1848), May 17, 2012

Theroux, Paul: The Pillars of Hercules. Ballantine Books, April 13, 2011

Tomasello, Michael: Becoming Human: A Theory of Ontogeny, Harvard University Press, Jan 7, 2019

Turner, Jonathan. A Theory of Social Interaction. Stanford University Press, July 1, 1988

Wansink, Brian: Mindless Eating: Why we eat more than we think. Bantam, New York. 2006

Weil, Andrew MD: Spontaneous Happiness: A New Path to Emotional Well-Being. Little, Brown and Company. 2011x

Weir, Kirsten: The lasting impact of neglect (early deprivation -> reduced ability to connect). , Monitor on Psychology, June 2014,

Wilkerson, Isabel. Caste: The Origins of our Discontents. Random House, 2020

Wilkinson, R and Pickett, K. The Inner Level. How more equal societies reduce stress, restore sanity and improve everyone's well-being. Penguin Press, NY 2019.

Wilson, Edward O.: The Meaning of Human Existence, Liveright Publishing Corporation, NY. 2014

Wohlleben, Peter: The Hidden Life of Trees, Greystone Books, 2016

Wrangham, Richard: The Goodness Paradox. The strange relationship between virtue and violence in human evolution. Pantheon Books, 2019.

Zakaria, Fareed: Ten Lessons for a Post-Pandemic World. W.W. Norton & Company, 2020

Certificate of Registration

This Certificate issued under the seal of the Copyright
Office in accordance with title 17, *United States Code*,
attests that registration has been made for the work
identified below. The information on this certificate has
been made a part of the Copyright Office records.

Shira Perlmutter

United States Register of Copyrights and Director

Registration Number

TXu 2-266-862

Effective Date of Registration:
May 04, 2021
Registration Decision Date:
July 14, 2021

Copyright Registration for a Group of Unpublished Works
Registration issued pursuant to 37 C.F.R. § 202.4(c)

Title
_____

Title of Group:	Social Connections and your Health and 1 Other Unpublished Work
Content Title:	Social Connections and your Health
	Broken Down People

Completion/Publication
_____

Year of Completion:	2021

Author
_____

• **Author:**	Alfred Lee Anduze
Author Created:	Literary Works
Work made for hire:	No
Citizen of:	United States
Domiciled in:	United States
Year Born:	1948

Copyright Claimant
_____

Copyright Claimant:	Alfred Lee Anduze
	PO Box 776, Maricao, PR, 00606

Rights and Permissions
_____

Name:	Sharilyn Anduze
Email:	papaya4615@yahoo.com
Telephone:	(958)658-0368

Certification
_____

Page 1 of 2

ACKNOWLEDGEMENTS

Thank you to the residents of Ikaria Island, a confirmed "Blue Zone"... Stylianos and Eleni Plytas, and Giannis Bilitsis, Viki Baki, and in Athens, the Nomikou family for providing living examples of how social connections enhance your health. Their natural and easy adherence to the basic strategies that promote good health, contribute to a high quality of life and eventual longevity. Our time spent together will always be cherished.

To the people of Athens, with whom we interacted daily and freely, for their smiles, laughter and assistance when and where we didn't have a clue. On the streets, in the stores and restaurants, and in the museums, I always felt accepted and appreciated.

To Dr. Lionel Sewpershad, Professor of Sociology and Anthony Welling, Professor of Geography for your friendship, guidance, advice and motivation to undertake and finish this work.

To Mr. Edward Rowe of Ireland, Professor of International Literature, Mr John Alfaros, General Secretary of Cities and Towns of Greece, and Mr Moscholidis Giorgis of Piraeus, for their insight and comments on what it means to be "social" in words, thoughts and deeds that makes Greeks so much friendlier than most.

To Dr Stanley Gryskiewicz, founder and CEO emeritus of the Association of Managers for Innovation, for the benefits of his 40 years of bringing people together to share ideas and help implement solutions.

With gratitude and appreciation to the people of Puerto Rico for their social graces and inimitable music...who though at the time of this writing are still undergoing tremendous stress and strain from the devastation of two hurricanes and the lack of efficient recovery, are able to express warmth and kindness to others in their daily routine activities.

To the people of southern France, Mediterranean Italy, southern Spain, Portugal and the Republic of Ireland, whose traditions place great importance on family and social interactions which enable their health.

Thank you to Ryan and Samantha Sheehan, of Yorkshire Publishing, for your patience, loyalty and expertise.

And special appreciation and gratitude to my wife, Sariluz, for indulging in my passion for research and writing of controversial facts and opinions...and for trudging through the first and second readings and offering criticism and reassurance.

And a grateful recognition to all my true friends, past, present, and future.

CPSIA information can be obtained
at www.ICGtesting.com
Printed in the USA
BVHW041740171121
621861BV00010B/100